# CONTEMPORARY NEUROPSYCHOLOGY AND THE LEGACY OF LURIA

T0227407

# INSTITUTE
# for RESEARCH
# in BEHAVIORAL NEUROSCIENCE

Jason W. Brown, Series Editor

# CONTEMPORARY NEUROPSYCHOLOGY and THE LEGACY OF LURIA

**Edited by**
**ELKHONON GOLDBERG**
*Medical College of Pennsylvania*

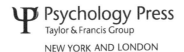

**Ψ** Psychology Press
Taylor & Francis Group

NEW YORK AND LONDON

First published 1990 by
Lawrence Erlbaum Associates, Inc., Publishers

Publishrd 2014 by Psychology Press
711 Third Avenue, New York, NY 10017
27 Church Road, Hove, East Sussex BN3 2FA, UK

First issued in paperback 2014

*Psychology Press is an imprint of the Taylor and Francis Group, an informa business*

Library of Congress Cataloging-in-Publication Data

Contemporary neuropsychology and the legacy of Luria/edited by
   Elkhonon Goldberg.
         p. cm.
      Festschrift for A. R. Luria.
      Includes bibliographical references.
      ISBN 0-8058-0334-3
      1. Neuropsychology. 2. Luriia, A. R. (Aleksandr, Romanovich),
   1902-1977. I. Luriia, A. R. (Aleksandr Romanovich), 1902-1977.
   II. Goldberg, Elkhonon.
   QP360.C663 1989
   612.8'2—dc20

ISBN 13: 978-1-138-87600-2 (pbk)
ISBN 13: 978-0-8058-0334-1 (hbk)

# Contents

# Contents

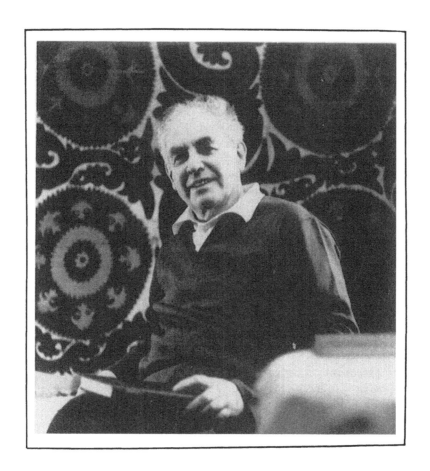

Alexandr Romanovich Luria (1902–1977)

# Contributors

D. Frank Benson, M.D.
Augustus S. Rose Professor of Neurology
University of California Los Angeles School of Medicine
710 Westwood Plaza
Los Angeles, CA 90024

Arthur Benton, Ph.D.
Professor Emeritus
Department of Neurology
University of Iowa Hospital and Clinic
Iowa City, IA 52242

Edoardo Bisiach, M.D.
Professor
Istituto di Clinica Neurologica dell'Universita di Milano
Via Francesco Sforza, 35, 20122 Milano (Italy)

Jason Brown, M.D.
Professor of Clinical Neurology
New York University Medical Center
530 First Avenue
New York, NY 10016

Nelson Butters, Ph.D.
Chief, Psychology Service
San Diego VA Medical Center
Professor of Psychiatry
University of California San Diego
School of Medicine
3350 La Jolla Village Drive
La Jolla, CA 92161

Michael Cole, Ph.D.
Professor of Communications
Laboratory of Comparative Human Cognition
University of California San Diego
Extension Building M, Room 165
Mail Code X003
La Jolla, CA 92093

Elkhonon Goldberg, Ph.D.
Professor of Psychiatry and Neurology
Director, Division of Neuropsychology
Medical College of Pennsylvania/Eastern Pennsylvania
    Psychiatric Institute
3200 Henry Avenue
Philadelphia, PA 19129

William C. Heindel, Ph.D.
Postgraduate Research Scientist
Department of Neurosciences
University of California San Diego
School of Medicine
3350 La Jolla Village Drive
La Jolla, CA 92161

Paul D. MacLean, M.D.
Senior Research Scientist
National Institute of Mental Health
P.O. Box 289
Poolesville, MD 20837

Allan F. Mirsky, Ph.D.
Chief, Laboratory of Psychology and Psychopathology
National Institutes of Health
9000 Rockville Pike
Building 10, Room 4C
Bethesda, MD 20892

Karl H. Pribram, M.D.
Professor of Neuroscience
National Institutes of Health
Department of Psychiatry
Jordan Hall, Room 402
Stanford University
Stanford, CA 94305

H. Enger Rosvold, M.D.
Former Chief, Laboratory of Neuropsychology
National Institute of Mental Health
P.O. Box 289
Poolesville, MD 20837

Oliver Sacks, M.D.
Professor of Neurology
Albert Einstein College of Medicine
119 Horton Street
Bronx, NY 10464

David P. Salmon, Ph.D.
Assistant Research Neuropsychologist
University of California San Diego Medical Center
ADRC (H-204)
225 Dickinson Street
San Diego, CA 92103

Donald T. Stuss, Ph.D.C. Psych.
Professor of Psychology and Medicine
Director of Research
Rotman Research Institute of Baycrest Centre
University of Toronto
3560 Bathurst Street
North York, Ontario Canada M6A 2E1

Herbert Vaughan, M. D.
Professor of Neuroscience, Neurology and Pediatrics
Albert Einstein College of Medicine
Kennedy Center, Room 903
1410 Pelham Parkway South
Bronx, NY 10461

# Introduction
# Tribute To Alexandr Romanovich Luria (1902–1977)

It has been said that a human is alive as long as the memory of him or her is preserved in the minds and hearts of other people. This larger definition of life is especially true for scientists and artists and is the ultimate measure of their creative accomplishments. More than a decade has passed since Alexandr Romanovich Luria's death in 1977, but the process of discovery of his intellectual legacy by the Western scientific community has hardly reached its peak. As I am watching his growing impact on the science of the brain and the mind, it occurs to me that my own, personal relationship with the memory of my professor, mentor, friend, and tyrant is following a similar course. While in daily interactions at close quarters admiration and closeness were interspersed with disagreements and frustrations, with the distance in time and space (I left Luria's lab and Russia to come to this country in 1974) a larger sense of his impact on my life has emerged, and the magnitude of his influence on me, both intellectual and personal, has become increasingly apparent. The way I think and practice my profession, the way I interact with people and get things done, all have the profound impact of my teacher and of my long relationship with him as his student, his associate and his friend. I turned out, after all, to be much more impressionable than it felt at the time!

In the age of increasing scientific specialization, Luria's range of contributions was nothing short of astounding. His intellectual odyssey is summarized in an autobiography, *The Making of Mind* (Luria, 1979). Although Luria is best known as a founding father of neuropsychology, this was a relatively late interest of his.

As a very young man, Luria became intrigued by psychoanalysis and published, at the age of 19, a little book with his review and critique of the Freudian theory. At approximately the same time Luria corresponded with Freud, and many years later, when the very name of Freud was anathema in the Soviet Union, he acknowledged privately the importance of Freud's influence on his subsequent intellectual development.

Though intrigued by the role of the subconscious in the human psyche, Luria was bothered by the lack of objectivity of the psychoanalytical method. He attempted to develop approaches of measuring the subconscious through motor and visceral responses, which resulted in the book *The Nature of Human Conflicts* (1932). The fate of the book was strange. It was published in the United States but never in the Soviet Union, presumably because the very subject of subconsciousness had been declared off limits for Soviet scientists by the crude ideological censorship of the times. Luria's work on the quantitative measures of subconscious responses has a ring of modernity to it in light of the current interest in implicit knowledge and memory. One can only hope that in the ideologically relaxed climate of today, *The Nature of Human Conflicts* will see the light of day at home, in the Soviet Union, almost six decades later.

In the 1920s, Luria began to work closely with Vygotsky. Although they were only 6 years apart, Luria always considered Vygotsky his mentor, and credited him with much of his own subsequent ideas and approaches, sometimes to the point of self-deprecation. He was always loyal to Vygotsky's memory, both intellectually and personally, at the times when Vygotsky's work was being denounced in the Soviet Union from evey pulpit and his name held in disgrace. One can surmise that the effusive way in which Luria talked about Vygotsky, often reducing his own work to a mere implementation of Vygotsky's ideas, was a token of gratitude, the best he could do for a close friend who had died young and in death was brutalized by his compatriots. This was a touching gesture of human decency and civic courage in a man who did not usually strike you as a rebel. As soon as the political climate permitted, in the late 1960s, Luria intitiated and orchestrated—with his characteristic cool efficiency so out of place amidst the chaotic goings-on of the everyday Soviet existence—the publication of the collection of writings by Vygotsky.

Together with Vygotsky, Luria embarked on the development of "historico-cultural" psychology. Its main thesis, summarized by Vygotsky (1934), was that higher cognitive functions are in large measure determined by culture and arise as the end products of the internalization of certain external cultural devices and representational systems. Many years later, this thesis was to color Luria's work as a neuropsychologist, and probably shaped the Lurian brand of neuropsychology more than any other theoretical premise.

This kind of theorizing prompted two lines of research: developmental and cross-cultural. Luria undertook both. Together with Vygotsky, he launched a series of experiments designed to study language acquisition, regulatory influences of language on behavior, and the secondary influence of language on preverbal cognitive structures. Although the main thrust of their developmental program was basic and theoretical, Vygotsky and Luria were aiming also at practical, educational applications. However, in 1936, historico-cultural psychology was declared "idealistic" (not as opposed to "cynical," but as opposed to "materialistic," the ultimate accusation of heresy in the Soviet political vernacular of the times), and its educational applications were banned by a special governmental decree. The theory of historico-cultural psychology developed by Vygotsky and Luria in the late 1920s and early 1930s was exonerated (gradually) only three decades later.

In the area of cross-cultural studies, Luria launched an expedition to remote parts of Central Asia to study the effects of literacy and social change on the types of inference used by the natives. Although an intended implication of this work was to show that the social changes promulgated by the Soviet regime changed the logical structures used by the tribespeople in the direction of cognitive maturity, the sword appeared to be double-edged, and Luria was accused of implying that his subjects, "the builders of socialism," were less than completely civilized. Rather ironically, Luria who was Jewish, was branded as a "Great-Russian chauvinist," which was a dangerous label at the time (but probably not quite as dangerous as that of an "idealist"). The project had to be terminated and Luria never returned to hands-on cross-cultural studies. The findings of his expedition to Central Asia remained buried for years, and Luria was able to publish a book summarizing this early effort only 40 years later (Luria 1976a), with the relative relaxation of ideological taboos.

The late 1930s must be regarded as the turning point in Luria's career. He went to medical school (adding a medical degree to his full professorship in psychology), turned to more biological aspects of psychology, and ultimately to neuropsychology, which was to bring him worldwide recognition.

We will never know to what extent this change of direction was the next logical step in pursuing his intrinsically unchanged intellectual agenda, a natural stage in the unfolding of an internally consistent line of inquiry, and to what extent it was a matter of political expediency necessary to ensure his professional survival.

Arguments can be made to support both hypotheses. Vygotsky and Luria turned to the studies of brain-damaged populations, notably aphasics, to test some of their basic hypotheses concerning the relationship between language and thought. It could be said that they discovered in brain-damaged populations a valuable technique to gain insights into normal cognitive structures, and this is what motivated Luria to turn to neuropsychology. Indeed, cognitive theory was always close to his heart even as a neuropsychologist, and the questions he asked were ultimately about fundamental properties of normal brain-behavior relations for which brain-damaged populations were but a point of departure.

On the other hand, science in the Soviet Union was becoming increasingly oppressed and ideologically charged. Scientific ideas and theories were judged—arbitrarily and capriciously—on the basis of their "ideological sound-ness," and the threat of accusations of being "ideologically alien" or "idealistic" (as opposed to "materialistic") was the Damoclean sword over the head of every scientist, capable of terminating one's career, and even one's life. Social and behavioral sciences were particularly vulnerable to ideological censorship, and

Luria was confronted with the terrifying examples of the two individuals who had made formative impacts on his development, Freud and Vygotsky, being ostracized and branded "bourgeois pseudoscientists." His own cross-cultural studies had ended in disastrous accusations of heresy. It was clear that certain fields of inquiry were more hazardous, and put their practitioners in greater personal danger, than others. Although none was totally secure (genetics and cybernetics turned out not to be), natural sciences were allowed more breathing space than explicitly social sciences and the humanities. It is possible that Luria, always a survivor, retreated into neuropsychology almost by default. With the areas of his primary interest, developmental and cross-cultural, effectively destroyed by ideological taboos, studies of the brain might have offered the hope of a relatively unviolated career.

The turn toward the studies of brain-mind relationships and brain injury was facilitated, or possibly even prompted, by the family tradition. Luria's father, Roman Albertovich Luria, was a prominent physician and professor of medicine, interested in what is now called "psychosomatic medicine." He had a strong intellectual influence on the young Luria and wanted him to become a physician. In his student years Luria was interested in medicine and took some medical courses. Although he chose not to pursue a medical career at the time, these early interests must have affected his later decisions, when he found himself on the career crossroads and under political pressure.

In all likelihood, both intellectual and pragmatic considerations played a role at that turning point in Luria's career. World War II provided another ingredient which sealed Luria's career change. Everyone was called upon to contribute to the war effort, and the development of remedial programs to help head-injured soldiers was Luria's charge.

It is certain that Luria's early cognitive, cultural, and developmental interests shaped the unique way in which he pursued neuropsychology. As I pointed out earlier, he was interested above all in the basic issues of brain-behavior relationships. Specific clinical issues played a subordinate role in his scientific program. It is ironic that in many neuropsychological circles Luria's name is associated primarily with diagnostic techniques. He himself regarded the development of assessment techniques almost incidental to his career. This is not to say that the compendium of the ingenious bedside tasks that he designed or modified do not represent an important aspect of his contribution to neuropsychology. Although Luria's intellectual preferences were toward theoretical issues, temperamentally he was a doer more than an armchair thinker. I think that his fondness for diagnostic work, both for designing procedures and for actually examining patients (which he continued to do one morning a week until the end of his life) reflected the need for tangible, practical, concrete accomplishments, an emotional complement to the highly theoretical work reflected in many of his books.

Luria eludes compartmentalization by bias, as a "biologically," "cognitive-ly," or "clinically" minded neuropsychologist. He eludes also compartmentaliza-tion by topic, such as memory, hemispheric specialization, and so on. Instead, in his long career he evolved as a designer of a general theory of brain-behavior relations in humans, with multiple and profound implications for applied neuropsychology, both diagnostic and remedial. He evolved as such gradually, and the understanding of this process may help to assimilate the concepts and ideas contributed by Luria to the field. This process had an underlying logic, which appears to have persisted throughout his career, and to have determined the progression through various topics toward the completion of his "grand picture."

It was his dual competence, both with respect to cognition (as a psycholo-gist) and the brain (as a neurologist), which accounts for the uniqueness of "Lurian" neuropsychology and the explanatory power of his concepts. Luria was able to go beyond the simplistic brain-behavior dilemma of the first half of the century: narrow localizationism (phrenology style) versus equipotentialism. Luria formulated his concept of functional systems which were neither. He was probably the first to state explicitly and succinctly that (a) behaviors, skills and traits as they appear in the lay, real life nomenclature are not the units appropriate for cerebral localization; (b) the identification of localizable elements of cogni-tion is in itself a nontrivial task; and (c) the relationship between the "lay" and the "localizable" nomenclatures is not a simple one-to-one mapping. In Luria's terms, a behavior or trait is the product of interaction of many cognitive elements, each mediated by a different brain structure or region. Such a con-stellation of interacting brain structures, each mediating a particular cognitive dimension, constitutes a distinct functional system. Conversely, any given cognitive dimension enters a variety of behaviors and competencies as defined in terms of the lay nomenclature. Furthermore, according to Luria, externally similar behaviors can be controlled by differently composed functional systems with different cerebral representations in different individuals, or even in the same individual at different developmental stages.

The latter set of assumptions was a direct application to neuropsychology of the premise formulated earlier by Vygotsky (1934). In its extreme form, the premise implies that individual human cognition can only be understood in the light of cultural anthropology and through development, as the end product of the internalization of codes pre-existing in the culture in an overt, external form. These codes, apart from their obvious function of communication, also provide cognitive strategies and representational systems and are crucial for the develop-ment of self-regulation and volition. The child acquires cultural codes largely in the course of language acquisition. Likewise, the child's capacity for self-regulating behavior developmentally evolves as the internalization of that which initially had been a form of interpersonal verbal interaction. It follows from this viewpoint that the neuropsychological structure of cognitive processes and their dissolution could only be understood in developmental and cultural contexts. This conviction colored all of Luria's subsequent research into brain-behavior relations.

For the scientist who introduced the concept of "functional system," narrow compartmentalization of interests would have been an unlikely outcome. The very notion of "functional systems" dictates that various contributions to behavior must be studied in interaction. However, it is not surprising that in establishing priorities of inquiry, Luria was guided even as a neuropsychologist by his belief in the pre-eminent role of language in the formation of representational and self-regulatory systems. The neuropsychological structure of these systems, the relationship of these systems to language, and the dissolution of language in brain pathology were the subjects of his early contributions to neuropsychology. The results of these efforts were summarized in three major monographs, *Traumatic Aphasia* (1947), *The Role of Speech in the Regulation of Normal and Abnormal Behavior (1955),* and *The Higher Cortical Functions in Man* (1962). The latter book provides the most complete account of Luria's work in neuropsychology and is dedicated to the memory of Vygotsky.

In his rendition of linguistic representations, Luria was more concerned with the structure of the code and its disintegration than with the finer neurological aspects of the underlying diseases. This is evident in his taxonomy of aphasias: It reflects the dysfunctional cognitive processes rather than the presumed neuroanatomical lesions. Although brain pathology is Luria's material, his conceptualizations are formulated with a normal cognitive model in mind.

Luria's interest in these topics never became extinct. With respect to linguistic representations, he attempted to integrate his studies of brain pathology with refined psycholinguistic approaches (Luria, 1976b). His interest in regulatory behavior culminated in a whole program of studies of the frontal lobes, which spanned at least two decades and resulted in a 700-page edited volume which is not available in English (Luria & Homskaya, 1966).

In the course of these studies, the extreme assumption of the preeminence of verbal control in self-regulation gave way to a more eclectic and hierarchical view of executive functions. Both the hierarchic theme and the de-emphasizing of the role of verbal mediation (thus setting the stage for considering other, nonverbal representational systems) reflect another human interaction which left a powerful trace in Luria's work—that with Nicholas Bernstein, a prominent Russian physiologist and mathematician, and a close friend of Luria's.

Already in the 1920s and 1930s Bernstein introduced the concepts of internal representations and plans guiding behavior, and of the hierarchic nature of such representations and of self-regulatory processes. At the same time he introduced the concept of feedback and proposed that the reflectory arc be replaced by the reflectory loop as the building block of neural control. In so doing, he foreshadowed the pivotal concepts of lateryear cybernetics and cognitive psychology. The ideas of hierarchic cognitive controls guided by the images of the future, to-be-achieved products (*Solwehrt* in Bernstein's terminology), are central to the contemporary attempts to conceptualize the functions of prefrontal systems. These concepts undoubtedly had a powerful influence on Luria and contributed to his interest in later life in the frontal lobes.

Predictably and sadly, the third major intellectual influence in Luria's life shared the fate of the first two. Like Freud and Vygotsky, Bernstein was ostracized in Russia for his incompatibility with the Pavlovian doctrine, which by then had become the only sanctioned theoretical framework. For a number of years he could not pursue his research or publish his work, but lived to see the beginnings of his exoneration in the 1960s. The book with the summary of his ideas was published only in 1966 (Bernstein, 1966), three decades after these ideas had been formulated. As in the case of Vygotsky, Luria's loyalty to his friend at the time of adversity was exemplary.

Luria's early cultural-cognitive interests resulted in the progression of themes which, in a sense, ran contrary to the classical neuroscientific progression. Luria started with the cortex, rather than the brainstem; with the singularly human, rather than with that which is invariant across species. In the latter part of his career he began, as it were, to descend the neural axis, thus moving toward the completion of the picture.

The logic behind this strategy of inquiry is outlined in an article in *Scientific American* (1970), where Luria offers a somewhat simplistic but didactically useful conceptualization. According to it, the brain consists of three processing blocks which control, respectively, perceptual integration, programming and executive functions, and arousal-activation. Later in his career, Luria became increasingly interested in the "arousal-activation" block and in the ways in which it interacts with the other two. This interest took the form of the modification of the early representational and executive themes.

The modification of the executive theme led Luria to refine his conceptualization of prefrontal functions, as reflected in the second edition of *Higher Cortical Functions*. In the first edition, the description of prefrontal pathology was largely limited to the convexital, dorsolateral prefrontal syndrome with its predominantly sequential executive deficit. In the second edition, the extensive description of the orbitofrontal syndrome has been added, with its predominantly affective and activational manifestations.

The modification of the representational theme led Luria to embark on a series of studies of memory and orientation impairments following limbic and mesencephalic lesions. These studies are summarized in *Neuropsychology of Memory* (1974).

Given Luria's strong interests in language and in the interface between culture and cognition, it comes as no surprise that his early efforts in neuropsychology were dominated by the explorations of the left hemisphere. In the very last years of his career, Luria embarked on a series of studies of the right hemisphere. It turned out to be the last on his list of themes. With Luria's record of prolific writing, it is probable that, had he lived a few years longer, an extensive volume on the right hemisphere and hemispheric integration would have appeared. As it stands, the chapter added in the second edition of *Higher Cortical Functions* reflects only initial stages of this inquiry. In this chapter, faithful to his concept of functional systems, Luria rejects out of hand the feasibility of linking specific tasks with one or the other hemisphere in an absolute sense. Instead, he proposes that both hemispheres participate in most activities, but provide different contributions to them. Luria's preliminary observations with regard to the limited, but nonnegligible semantic competence of the right hemisphere and the unequal degrees of hemispheric advantages for different aspects of phonemic and orthographic competence are in agreement with the more systematic studies conducted in the West.

No account of Luria's career in neuropsychology can be complete without a word about his clinical contributions to neuropsychological diagnosis and remediation. It was clearly a subordinate, secondary facet of Luria's career. This does not change the fact the many neuropsychologists and behavioral neurologists know Luria mostly or even solely through his diagnostic techniques. They should not seek in Luria's work a neuropsychological battery, since his disregard for methodological considerations such as standardization, quantification, validation, and reliability was quite notorious. What his approach does contribute to applied neuropsychology, is a matrix, a logic of examination which in spite of its methodological looseness, offers an extremely systematic internal organization and dimensionalization of cognition, because it is rooted in a cohesive brain-behavioral model. It also offers insights into how qualitative variants of a "failure" on a task can be utilized in a branching tree of hypotheses testing. His clinical approach in many ways foreshadowed and served as the basis for the currently popular "process approach" to neuropsychological diagnosis.

Such is the story of my teacher's career as I see it. He was a complex man living in complex circumstances, which is reflected in this account. I felt that this complexity had to be conveyed to the reader because sycophantic accounts offend the dignity of those whom they intend to flatter. Alexandr Romanovich Luria died in the summer of 1977 at the age of 75. He did not complete the job of designing a general theory of brain-behavior relations, yet he contributed mightily to the ongoing effort to develop one, and to the emergence of neuropsychology as a mature science.

Contributors to this volume either knew Luria personally or experienced his scientific influence, and their chapters reflect this affinity. Some contributors chose to write explicitly about Luria, and others present their own findings and ideas, which are intellectually connected with various aspects of Luria's work. The spectrum of subjects covered in this volume reflects the range of Luria's interests and contributions. They include cultural and developmental psychology (chapter by Cole), neuropsychology of language (chapter by Stuss & Benson), frontal lobes and executive control (chapters by Mirsky & Rosvold, Pribram, and Stuss & Benson), memory (chapters by Butters, Salmon, & Heindel, and MacLean), hemispheric interaction (chapter by Bisiach), history of neuropsychology (chapter by Benton), "romantic science" (chapter by Sacks), and the theory of brain-behavior relations, both in their spatial and temporal aspects (chapters by Brown, Vaughan, and Goldberg). I hope that this volume will be a fitting tribute to the remarkable man, Alexandr Romanovich Luria.

Appreciation is due to Dr. Edoardo Bisiach for contributing the photograph of Alexandr Romanovich Luria for this book.

This volume was conceived and much of the work on it accomplished (including my chapter in this volume) during my visit at the Institute for Advanced Studies of the Hebrew University of Jerusalem in 1986. The hospitality and generous support offered by the Institute provided a unique environment for creative work and scholarship and deserves my deepest appreciation.

Elkhonon Goldberg

## REFERENCES

Bernstein, N. A. (1966). *Outlines of physiology of movements and the physiology of activity*. Moscow: Meditsina Press (in Russian).

Luria, A. R. (1928). The problem of the cultural behavior of the child. *Journal of Genetic Psychology, 35,* 493–506.

Luria, A. R. (1932). *The nature of human conflicts*. New York: Liveright.

Luria, A. R. (1947). *Traumatic aphasia*. Moscow, English translation, The Hague: Mouton, 1970.

Luria, A. R. (1955). *The role of speech in the regulation of normal and abnormal behavior*. Moscow. English translation, London: Pergamon, 1961.

Luria, A. R. (1962). *The higher cortical functions in man*. Moscow. English translation, New York: Basic Books, 1966, 1980 (2nd ed).

Luria, A. R. (1970). The functional organization of the brain. *Scientific American, 222,* 66–78.

Luria, A. R. *Neuropsychology of memory*. (1974). Moscow, English translation, Washington, DC: Winston, 1976.

Luria, A. R. (1976a) *Cognitive development*. Cambridge, MA: Harvard University Press.

Luria, A. R. (1976b). *Basic problems of neurolinguistics*. The Hague: Mouton.

Luria, A. R. (1979). *The making of mind*. Cambridge, MA: Harvard University Press.

Luria, A. R., & Homskaya, E. D. (Eds.) (1966). *Frontal lobes and regulation of psychological processes*. Moscow University Press (in Russian).

Vygotsky, L. S. (1934). *Intellectual activity and speech*. Moscow: Sotsekgiz (in Russian).

# 1

# Alexandr Romanovich Luria: Cultural Psychologist

*Michael Cole*

*Laboratory of Comparative Human Cognition*
*University of California, San Diego*

For the current generation of psychologists, the title of this article may appear to be an anomaly. True, Alexandr Luria published one small volume recounting research he undertook in Central Asia in the early 1930s (Luria, 1976). However, this work is not the basis for characterizing him as a cultural psychologist. In fact, if this single venture into cross-cultural research were the sole basis for my thesis, it might appear at least an exaggeration of a minor tendency, if not an outright misrepresentation of the man who was known widely in the 1960s and 1970s for his work in neuropsychology and mental retardation.

I have chosen my theme quite deliberately and with full knowledge that during the last 35 years of his life, Alexandr Romanovich devoted most of his research energies to the study of the brain bases of behavior. I know this aspect of his work first hand; I spent the better part of the 1962–1963 academic year commuting daily to the Burdenko Institute of Neurosurgery, where I participated in the neuropsychologial research program that was occupying his attention at that time.

However, partly as a result of unforeseen events in my own career I came to know particularly well not only the research conducted in Central Asia, but the scientific projects that Alexandr Romanovich had undertaken as a young man in the heady decade following the Russian Revolution. Drawing on his writings from this early period (Luria, 1932, 1978) and his retrospective account of his intellectual journey (Luria, 1979), I want to argue that in the period between 1920 and 1930 Alexandr Romanovich formulated (in collaboration with Alexei Leontiev and Lev Vygotsky) a systematic approach to human psychological processes in which the human capacity to create and use culture was *the* central tenet of his psychological thought to the end of his life. I will argue further that all of his later research and theory can not be properly understood if his commitment to the idea of cultural psychology is ignored.

## THE INTELLECTUAL CONTEXT

To begin with, it is important to take seriously the fact that Alexandr Romanovich began his career at a time when modern psychology was just beginning to take shape. European psychology was then embroiled in a series of interlocking debates about what kind of science psychology could be. Should it be an experimental science, modeled on the natural sciences, or a descriptive science, modeled on history and the humane sciences? Were psychological laws restricted to "nomothetic" generalizations applying to populations or "idiographic" laws that could illuminate the causal dynamics of individual human minds? Was it necessary to choose between subjective and objective approaches to research? Was psychology to be restricted to a laboratory science, or could it be expanded to apply to people's everyday lives and serve as a basis for promoting social progress?

His earliest efforts, like those of many of his contemporaries, were to resolve the "crisis in psychology" engendered by the divisions that arose when several of its practitioners (Wundt in Germany, Bekhterev in Russia, and others) began to champion a "new psychology," which sought to be experimental, nomothetic, objective, and very much a laboratory science. He admired this line of work, but he was also attracted by those who argued that the new psychology was sterile and ultimately inhuman. He was especially attracted by Wilhelm Dilthey's arguments for a *reale Psychologie,* which would study human beings as unified, dynamic systems, conditioned by their historical circumstances, who could be studied as they live and behave in the real world. However, he was bothered by what he considered to be the shortcomings of Dilthey's approach, which did not accord with his ideas of what a scientific psychology should be.

## CULTURAL PSYCHOLOGY: WUNDT AND DILTHEY

Although it has not found its way into our textbooks on the history of psychology, the idea of a cultural psychology was very tightly bound up in the argument among turn of the century psychologists about the possible nature of psychology as a science. Somewhat ironically, in view of his canonization as the "father of experimental psychology," Wundt himself forcefully argued that the study of culture must be an integral part of psychology, in fact a full half of the enterprise (Wundt, 1916).

The first half of the new science, which Wundt called psysiological psychology, was assigned the task of analyzing the contents of individual consciousness into its constituent elements in order to come up with universal laws by which the elements combine. To this end, subjects were carefully trained in methods of self-observation (introspection). Experiments conducted with this goal in mind concentrated on the qualities of sensory experience and the decomposition of reactions into their components.

*Volkerpsychologie,* the other half of Wundt's psychology, was conceived of as an historical, descriptive science. To it was assigned the study of "higher psychological functions," including processes of reasoning and the products of human language because they extend beyond individual human consciousness. He argued that

> A language can never be created by an individual. True, individuals have invented Esperanto and other artificial languages. Unless however, language had already existed, these inventions would have been impossible. Moreover, none of these has been able to maintain itself, and most of them owe their existence solely to elements borrowed from natural languages. (Wundt, 1921, p. 3)

Wundt believed that the two enterprises supplement each other; only through a synthesis of their respective insights could a full psychology be achieved. To those who would claim that *volkerpsychologie* could be entirely subsumed under experimental psychology, Wundt replied that while attempts had frequently been made to study complex mental processes using "mere" introspection,

> These attempts have always been unsuccessful. Individual consciousness is wholly incapable of giving us a history of the development of human thought, for it is conditioned by an earlier history concerning which it cannot of itself give us any knowledge. (Wundt, 1921, p. 3)

In this connection, Wundt makes an additional methodological claim which is central to the history and current practice of cultural psychology: "folk psychology is, in an important sense of the word, *genetic psychology.*" Significantly, Wundt's approach to the study of development goes beyond the study of ontogeny (individual development) to investigate "the various stages of mental development still exhibited by mankind." He adds: "*Volkerpsychologie* reveals well-defined primitive conditions, with transitions leading through an almost continuous series of intermediate steps to the more developed and higher civilizations." (p. 4). A finer articulation of a close affinity between developmental and cultural psychology, and the need for cross-cultural research as one basic tool of cultural psychology, could hardly be asked for. Note too that Wundt assumes a developmental progression in history which interacts with individual development.

These ideas were by no means confined to Wundt. They represented a continuation of a line of German thought that reached back to the beginning of the 19th century, and earlier. Nor were they confined to the German intellectual tradition. Very similar ideas can be found in the writings of John Stuart Mill, who, like Wundt, conceived of psychology as a dual enterprise, one half of which studied elementary laws of mental life, the other half of which studied the "kinds of character produced in conformity to those general laws" (Mill, 1843/ 1948, p. 177).

A quite different program for psychology was developed by the philosopher of history, Wilhelm Dilthey, whose work influenced not only Wundt, but a vast range of scholarship in what came to be called the humanities and social sciences. Psychology, he believed, should be a special science of the mind which would serve as the foundation science *(grundeswissenschaft)* for all of the human sciences (philosophy, linguistics, history, law, art, literature, etc.). Without such a foundation science, he claimed, the human sciences, among which he included psychology, could not be a true system (Ermarth, 1978).

Early in his career, Dilthey considered the possibility that Wundt's experimental psychology might provide such a foundation science. However, he gradually came to reject this possibility because he felt that in attempting to satisfy the requirements of the natural sciences to formulate cause–effect laws between mental elements, psychologists had stripped mental processes of the real life relationships between people that gave the elements their meaning. He did not mince words in his attack on the academic psychology of the late 19th century:

> Contemporary psychology is an expanded doctrine of sensation and assocation. The fundamental power of mental life falls outside the scope of psychology. Psychology has become only a doctrine of the forms of psychic processes; thus it grasps only a part of that which we actually experience as mental life (quoted in Ermarth, 1978, p. 148)

His solution was to propose a completely different approach to the study of psychology. Psychology, he wrote, "must be subordinated to a developmental-historical approach which grasps mental processes in their coherence" (quoted in Ermarth, 1978, p. 183). He called this approach *descriptive* psychology, which was to be based on an analysis of real life mental processes in real life situations that include the reciprocal processes between people as well as the thoughts within individuals. As methods for carrying out this kind of analysis, Dilthey suggested the close study of the writings of such "life philosophers" as Augustine, Montaigne, and Pascal because they contained a deep understanding of full, experienced reality and disciplined application of empathetic understanding *(verstehen)* in which analysts place themselves in the concrete life situation of the person being analyzed.

Although differing from Wundt in important respects, Dilthey's thinking about the relation of individual thought to its sociohistorical context was similar to the cultural, supraindividual half of Wundt's system. In terms that have a very modern ring he defined culture as "the distilled summation of component and mental contents and the mental activities to which these contents are related" (in Ermarth, 1978, p. 12). Like Wundt, he denied the possibility of explaining cultural phenomena on the basis of psychological laws of the individual mind.

## THE FIRST SYNTHESIS

### Experimental Psychodynamics

Alexandr Romanovich's first attempt to forge a synthesis of the "two psychologies" drew its inspiration from the writings of Sigmund Freud and his followers. In emulation of the psychoanalytical writers, he conducted clinical research on free associations, but he mistrusted the results of such efforts, feeling that any conclusions he tried to reach about the flow of his subjects' thoughts were insufficiently grounded. In response to this dissatisfaction he created a methodology designed to embody a psychodynamic theory of mind in an objective set of laboratory practices. The centerpiece of this methodology was an experimental technique that he called *the combined motor method,* which, he hoped, would provide a way of rendering Freud's clinical methods accessible to experimental treatment. Simultaneously, he attempted to introduce the historical dimension by forging a synthesis between Marx and Freud, an attempt which he later judged a failure.

The fullest existing description of this work is contained in a monograph published in English in 1932 under the title *The Nature of Human Conflicts: Or Emotion, Conflict and Will.* In the first chapter he outlines his basic presuppositions and his experimental strategy. Following in the tradition shared by the psychoanalytical theorists, gestalt psychologists, and many others, Luria explicitly rejects mechanical determinism, declaring "The structure of the organism presupposes not an accidental mosaic, but a complex organization of separate systems . . . [that] unite as very definite parts into an integrated functional structure." (pp. 6–7)

Since this structure is the consequence of a long complicated development, and the parts are integrated into a whole functional system, how can it be possible to isolate elements in this system for purposes of psychological analysis? Phrased differently, how could one obtain valid evidence about the thought processes of another person? The answer that Luria provided was that other people's thoughts could not be observed directly; they could, however, be revealed *in*directly in so far as they could be reflected in a publicly displayable, voluntary behavior. He phrased his strategy as follows:

We should on the one hand, produce the central process of the disorganization of behavior; on the other hand, we should try to reflect this process in some system accessible and suitable for examination. The motor function is such a systematic, objectively reflected structure of the neuro-dynamic processes concealed from immediate examination. And there lies before us the use of the motor function as a system of reflected structure of hidden psychological processes. Thus we proceed along the path we call the combined motor method. (p. 18)

The first phase in his technique was to induce a well-coordinated, publicly available behavior as the medium for the psychological analysis to come. He used various devices for this purpose. Often the subject was requested to hold the left hand steady in a device that could record its movements, while simultaneously being asked to press a button or squeeze a bulb in response to verbal stimuli presented by the experimenter. Once this behavior became stable, the analyst sought to disrupt it *selectively* in line with his hypothesis about particular internal psychological states.

The combined motor method was applied to psychodiagnosis in a wide variety of real life circumstances consistent with his goal of demonstrating the possibility of a methodology powerful enough to reach beyond the laboratory to engage the kinds of long-term emotions which typically organize human behavior. The book is full of examples. In one case students waiting to be examined during a purge of potentially "undeserving" students in Moscow in 1924 (the term "purge" had not yet come into common use; Gant translated the term as "cleansing") were studied in order to demonstrate their preoccupations with the upcoming interrogation and aspects of their family backgrounds. Subjects were first instructed to squeeze a small rubber bulb each time they heard a word, to hold their other hand (which also held a rubber bulb) completely still, and to respond with the first word that came to mind in response to each word presented. "Neutral" words (common words that bore no known relationship to the interrogation) were interspersed with "critical" words such as "examination," "formula," to determine if they produced distinguishable responses. On the basis of subjects' free associations alone, responses to the two classes of words were indistinguishable, but the critical words markedly disturbed the ongoing motor responses, while the neutral ones did not, thereby verifying his technique.

The same method was used to study suspected criminals awaiting examination by a criminal prosecutor to demonstrate that it could be used as a kind of lie detector. In this case, critical words were selected that related specifically to known aspects of the crime ("knife," "handkerchief," etc.). The analysis on the basis of the combined motor method was then compared with evidence gathered during later investigations and the trial. Again, Luria reported success in identifying those subjects who had specific hidden thoughts which they did not want to reveal.

Nor did Luria neglect more purely experimental verifications of his techniques. He conducted experiments with normal adults who were first told various stories, which the analyst had to ferret out from the ways in which their motor behavior was selectively disrupted. He also conducted experiments with people suffering various neuroses and brain damage as a means of further verifying the effectiveness of his methods.

Work on the combined motor method is concentrated in the first two sections of the *The Nature of Human Conflicts* which was published in 1932 in English, but contains a record of research from 1923–1930. I find the book fascinating reading in part because I know that at the start of this period, Alexandr Romanovich was intent upon creating the combined motor method as a model system for the study of the psychodynamics of individual thought. By the end of this period, he was no longer using the combined motor method (although he did still record motor reactions in many of his experiments). Freudian ideas were declared completely unacceptable for a Soviet psychologist, and he had explicitly entered into the formulation of a new school of psychology founded on the principle that the mind is conditioned by its historical circumstances.

## THE SECOND SYNTHESIS

### *The Sociohistorical School of Psychology*

Among the ways in which the shifting underpinnings of his work are reflected in the book is a basic shift in research strategy. In the first half of the book the major technique is to study the selective disorganization of behavior among adults, the strategy for which the combined motor method was invented. In the last section, the combined motor method is no longer in evidence and the subjects are primarily children. The strategy now has shifted to study the genesis of organization instead of disorganization.

It is in this shift that the idea of cultural mediation comes to the fore. In the following section I will turn directly to writing which highlights the role of culture in mental development, but a brief treatment of this topic within the context of *The Nature of Human Conflicts* is worth at least passing attention, because it shows that the idea of cultural mediation was not external to his thinking about the cortical basis of voluntary behavior.

In the studies with children reported in *The Nature of Human Conflicts*, Luria would use very simple procedures, such as asking them to respond each time a signal was presented. Small children would respond correctly for a brief period, but soon they would respond in the intervals between signals. With increasing age, responses were confined more and more to the appropriate intervals, until, in adults, the task was so easy that the response appeared similar to a reflex. The specifics of the experimental results are less interesting than Luria's interpretation of them. First, he concluded that the young children were subject to diffuse cortical excitation because they lacked higher regulative neurodynamic functions. Second, he claimed that the change from child to adult was truly developmental in nature, that is, it entailed a qualitative shift in the functioning of the organism:

> The reactive process as we know it in the normal adult human is a complicated elaboration, in structure not having anything in common with those impulsive reactions which we observed in the child or the reflex activity of animals. The chief difference of the reactive process from those forms of activity in the child and animals is that in the former the direct character of the motor discharge is controlled. . . . It is thus incorrect to say that the stimulus directly provokes the reaction [in the adult — M.C.]. . . . The outstanding feature of the reactive process is the fact that the tendency of every natural reflex act to discharge its excitation directly is controlled by a complex reactive process. (1932, p. 394)

Luria called this complex reactive process which inhibits direct flow of cortical excitation into motor behavior a "functional barrier." Such functional barriers, he believed, arise from speech and symbolic mechanisms, the foundations of what he termed higher psychological functions.

Third, in an analytical move that harks directly back to Wundt, Luria claimed that the higher psychological functions manifested as functional barriers do not arise spontaneously in individual development. Rather, they are the internalized forms of culturally mediated, socially transmitted, forms of behavior. As he was fond of pointing out, this way of understanding human psychological functioning meant that:

> In order to explain the highly complex forms of human consciousness one must go beyond the human organism. One must seek the origins of conscious activity . . . not in the recesses of the human brain or in the depths of the spirit, but in the external conditions of life. Above all, this means that one must seek these origins in the external processes of social life, in the social and historical forms of human existence. (Luria, 1982, p. 25).

He was quite explicit about what he thought to be the link to his ideas about culture and the neurodynamics of simple choice reactions: "in the functional barrier we have not a natural mechanism, but one of cultural origin" (p. 394). He then went on to conclude: "The analysis of complex cultural mechanisms is the key to the understanding of the simple neurodynamical processes." (Luria, 1932, p. 428).

These ideas had begun to take root in Luria's work when, shortly after the work described in the early sections of *The Nature of Human Conflicts* was begun, he and his colleague Alexei Leontiev encountered Lev Vygotsky. The 10 years during which these men worked together fundamentally changed the terms in which Luria conceived his enterprise of creating a synthesis of the "two psychologies" formulated by Wundt, Dilthey, and their Western European colleagues. Among the many contributions of Vygotsky to Luria's thinking, perhaps the most crucial was that it provided a way for him to integrate his methodological resolution of the "two psychologies," which remained at the level of individual experience, with a broader conception of human mental life as culturally and historically conditioned.

The combined motor method provided a key link between to the two levels of analysis. Luria had conceived of mediation through a culturally shared medium of activity as the key methodological requirement for knowing another person's thoughts. In interaction with Vygotsky and Leontiev the idea grew that mediation through culturally shared objects is *the* central characteristic of human thought. In a remarkable series of articles published by the three men in *The Journal of Genetic Psychology* between 1928 and 1930, cultural mediation was raised to be the cornerstone of a new school of psychology. They based their new "sociohistorical," or "cultural-instrumental," psychology on the interlocking principles that human psychological processes are *culturally mediated,* that they are formed in the course of activities in which other human beings are essential participants, and that both the activities, their mediating means, and the kinds of functional mental systems they produced are *historically developing.*

Luria's opening statements on this topic make clear the basic postulates of the enterprise.

> Man differs from animals in that he can make and use tools. . . . the tools used by man not only radically change his conditions of existence, they even react on him in that they effect a change in him and his psychic condition. In the complicated interrelations with his surroundings his organization is being differentiated and refined; his hand and his brain assume definite shapes, a series of complicated methods of conduct are being evolved, with the aid of which man adapts himself more perfectly to the surrounding world. (Luria, 1928, p. 493)

This change, he argues, brings about a fundamental change in the structure of behavior.

> Instead of applying directly its natural function to the solution of a definite task, the child *puts in between that function and the task a certain auxiliary means* . . . by the medium of which the child manages to perform the task. . . . The direct, natural use of the function is replaced by a complex "instrumental" form. (Luria, 1928, p. 495)

For the next several years, the group conducted research aimed at demonstrating the general applicability of these ideas.

One of the basic techniques they used in their empirical work was to pose children a problem deliberately chosen to be somewhat too difficult to solve "bare handed." After allowing the child to struggle for a while, the investigator then presented potentially usable materials which, based on adult experience, could be used to solve the problem. This basic paradigm was explored in a wide variety of intellectual tasks, especially those involving memory and attention. In studies of memory, for example, the experimenter would ask young children to recall a list of names of common objects read aloud. Once it was established that the task was too difficult, the experimenter would provide different kinds of objects (potential memory "tools") to see if the child could invent mediated forms of memory. Properties of the potential mediators were systematically varied as means of distinguishing between children who could only use readily accessible mediating means from those who could make use of virtually any object as a mediator, ultimately reaching the point where they could create their own mnemonics.

Luria himself specialized in the study of language and thought, particularly the relation between voluntary movement and speech (a theme which finds its earliest expressions in *The Nature of Human Conflicts*). In 1929 he traveled to New Haven, Connecticut, where he delivered a paper coauthored with Vygotsky, on the nature of egocentric speech. Piaget had earlier stimulated interest in the way small children seem to talk to themselves when playing alongside other children, suggesting that this egocentric speech is a halfway house between an early autistic stage when children fail totally to consider others in the way they behave and a later time when speech becomes properly "for another" and therefore, socialized. Such speech, because it is egocentric, was thought to be functionless, a mere indicator of underlying cognitive immaturity. Luria and Vygotsky had quite the opposite view. In their opinion, egocentric speech is rather the middle stage in a transition from speech that controls another to speech that controls oneself; it is social in its origins and functional in the role it plays in helping the child to master the problem at hand.

The experimental procedure they invented in reaction to Piaget's interpretation of egocentric speech is a good example of their general methodological strategy: Children were put in problem-solving situations that were somewhat too difficult for them, and as their theory suggested it should, egocentric speech (speech not directed specifically to another), increased.

In a different application of this technique, which he referred to as the study of the "prehistory of writing," Luria (1978) studied children's developing ability to make marks on paper as means of remembering material presented by the experimenter. Urged on by Luria, very small children would, for example, make four marks on the paper to help them remember "four houses," but when time came for recall, they failed entirely to use their marks in remembering. At a later stage, but long before they could write, children could learn make marks that were, in fact, instrumental in their recall.

## THE CROSS-CULTURAL STRATEGY

Simultaneously with their studies of the developing ability of children to mediate their mental activity using means provided by their culture, Luria and his colleagues engaged in a broad investigation of the historical development of cultural forms of mediation, since their theory posited an interaction between the means provided by the culture and the forms of mediated activity children develop.

These connections are brought out clearly in Leontiev's article on voluntary attention, published as part of the series in the *Journal of Genetic Psychology*. (Leontiev, 1932). Leontiev illustrates the history of voluntary attention using reports from the anthropological literature:

> Already the tribal hunts which were the earliest instances of collectivism in man entailed the necessity of controlling the attention of the hunting group; this was an indispensable condition for organized hunting. The function of the leader here was to submit the behavior of the collective to a common end, which meant that first of all the aim had to be *indicated*, that is, attention had to be drawn to it. (Leontiev, 1932, p. 58)

Starting from such crude beginnings, indicatory behaviors were said to undergo a process of development in which they become differentiated and specialized, evolving into conventional signs, that is, into psychological tools. This historical level is then linked explicitly by Leontiev to the individual development of the child:

> The history of one man's mastery over the regulation of behavior of another repeats in many points the history of his mastery over tools. It presupposes a change in the structure of behavior, which turns behavior directed to an end into behavior directed circuitously. (Leontiev, 1930, p. 59)

During the latter half of the 1920s, the founders of the sociohistorical school scoured the anthropological literature for evidence in support of their belief in the interaction of cultural and individual development. The attraction of this line of thinking for Luria is obvious; it provided the link he was seeking between the two visions of psychology which he had sought to unite at the start of his career.

## THE EXPEDITIONS TO CENTRAL ASIA

Aware of the shortcomings of secondary data, in the early 1930s Vygotsky and Luria organized two field trips to Central Asia, subsequently conducted by Luria. The purpose of this research was to obtain firsthand empirical evidence concerning the historical development of cognitive functions in place of the secondhand reports upon which they had relied up to that time. The sites were rural locations undergoing rapid socioeconomic and cultural change as a consequence of the agricultural collectivization movement in the late 1920s.

Our knowledge of the thinking that went into this research comes mostly from the report which Luria wrote more than 30 years later. So far as I know, no report was made of the first expedition, and only a brief report of the results of the second expedition was published in English (Luria, 1934). Writing in 1934, Luria characterized the goal of the research as the study of:

> The system of thinking of primitive societies, the development of the psychological functions in their thinking, and the pointing out of those changes which this thinking undergoes in social and cultural transformation connected with socialist growth. (Luria, 1934, p. 255–256)

Luria's (1976) characterization of the goal of the research demonstrates both continuity with the original formulation and a greater subtlety with respect to characterization of the developmental comparisons intended. He writes that he seeks to demonstrate that "many mental processes are social and historical in origin . . . [and] that important manifestations of human consciousness have been directly shaped by the basic practices of human activity and the actual forms of culture" (Luria, 1976, p. 3).

The 1976 monograph presents many interesting results in support of this thesis; in the areas of classification (colored threads, geometrical figures, and various objects), logical deduction, and self-evaluation (roughly equivalent to what is now referred to as metacognition), Luria observed that traditional people respond to his tasks in ways systematically different from their neighbors who have been involved in collective agriculture and/or schooling.

Simplifying greatly, the following conclusions are most central: In the change from traditional agricultural life to collectivized labor in literate/industrialized circumstances

1. "Direct graphical-functional thinking" is replaced by at least the rudiments of "theoretical thinking."
2. The basic forms of cognitive activity go beyond mastery and reproduction of individual practical activity, cease to be purely concrete and situational, and become a part of more general, abstractly coded, systems of knowledge.
3. These changes give rise not only to new forms of reasoning, restricted to logical premises free of immediate experience, but new forms of self-analysis and imagination as well.

Until the 1960s this research represented, along with the research of W. H. R. Rivers and his colleagues at the turn of the century (Rivers, 1901), one of the most extensive attempts to investigate the nature of cultural differences in cognition. It was also important in the overall development of the research program of the sociohistorical school because the conclusions provided support for Vygotsky, Luria, and Leontiev's basic hypothesis that higher psychological functions, being cultural in origin, will differ according to the culture in which they are formed. However, this line of work also suffered from shortcomings, and in the context of the times, it could not be properly followed up.

As I have discussed elsewhere (Cole, 1988), while providing basic support for his thesis that human mind is historically and culturally contingent, Luria's research methods, and the conclusions they generated, are open to two principled kinds of scientific criticism. First, Luria neither studied nor modeled in his experiments the practical activity systems of the Uzbek and Kazakh peoples and their psychological processes; hence, his interpretations were not grounded in an analysis of indigenously organized culturally organized activities. Instead, for purposes of psychological diagnosis, he introduced distinctly Western European activity systems, in the form of psychological tests and interviews, which did not model local reality, but served instead as measurements of generalized psychological tendencies for which there was a developmental interpretation in Western European societies.

Using this approach, Luria found that contact with European culture either through schooling or participation in Soviet-run collective enterprises increased the likelihood that traditional peasants would respond appropriately to his intellectual puzzles in Russian terms, but these results are basically silent with respect to possible analogues in indigenous practices. Such analogues might or might not exist, but the research Luria engaged in would, in principle, not be able to tell us which case fits reality.

The second, closely related problem, which becomes the focus when the sociocultural tradition is taken up in cross-cultural research by modern investigators (Laboratory of Comparative Human Cognition, 1983), was Luria's failure to restrict his conclusions to particular domains, instead appearing to claim that *in general* there is a change in the complexity of cognition brought about by the socioeconomic change from pastoral agricultural to industrial modes of production. Too often he seems to be concluding that the results he reports are independent of problem content and activity context, representing generalized cognitive changes. This kind of conclusion simultaneously undermines his own established principle that psychological processes depend on living activity systems, and renders adults who display such behaviors childlike in inappropriate terms.

My overall assessment is that the Soviet experience with cross-cultural research in the service of building a sociohistorical theory of psychological processes provides an uneven picture. On the one hand the sociohistorical school is the only extant theoretical approach for which the cultural organization of activity and mind are central postulates. On the other hand, in moving from the realm of ontogeny to the realm of history, the school's essential insights about the crucial nature of culture as the unique medium of all human activity is obscured; its place is taken by a characterization of historical change based on political economy in which cultural organization is subordinate and a form of uniformitarian stage theory appears in its stead, vitiating the power of the theory.

Had the times been different, these problems might have been addressed by continued scientific work. In particular, it would have been possible, in principle, for Luria to join with Soviet ethnographers to develop an approach to cross-cultural work that fulfilled the methodological criteria that they applied to their intracultural research program. But the times were very difficult indeed. In the Soviet Union of the mid-1930s, the work was attacked on political grounds for insulting the intellectual capacities of the builders of socialism in Soviet Central Asia (Razmyslov, 1934). Simultaneously, Vygotsky and his colleagues came under heavy criticism for their involvement in psychological testing of schoolchildren, and their insufficiently critical stance toward "bourgeois" psychologies of Western Europe and the United States. In these circumstances, it was out of the question for Luria to become expert in ethnography and the allied disciplines that would have been needed to develop properly the cross-cultural line of their work.

In 1934 Vygotsky succumbed to tuberculosis. Leontiev, who along with Vygotsky and Luria had set up a new department of psychology in Kharkov, in the Ukraine, remained there to develop his own line of work on learning and development. Luria spent some time in Kharkov but then returned to Moscow and embarked on the specialization that eventually brought him world fame. He entered medical school. When he graduated from medical school in 1937 he did a 2-year internship in neurology at the Bourdenko Neurosurgical Institute, where be began to develop psychological techniques for the diagnosis of local brain lesions. From that time to the end of his life, he devoted the bulk of his energies to this line of work which made him world famous as a neuropsychologist.

My essential point, to which I return in the remainder of this chapter, is that the move into problems of medical psychology was not a repudiation of the prior decade and a half's effort to create a synthetic, comprehensive, school of psychology. Rather, it was a pragmatic strategy for continuing to pursue the scientific program that was already present in the 1920s.

## THE FINAL SYNTHESIS

### Cultural Theory of Mind and the Brain

If the cross-cultural research is seen as but one strategy of research within a program that emphasizes the cultural mediation of all complex human psychological processes, and instead one focuses on the kinds of research that Luria, Vygotsky, Leontiev, and their colleagues were conducting in Moscow in the late

1920s, it becomes clear that the forms of diagnosis and remediation that became well known in such books as *The Role of Speech in the Regulation of Normal and Abnormal Behavior* (1961), *Restoration of Function After Brain Injury* (1963), or *Traumatic Aphasia* (1970) were already present long before Luria began his medical education in earnest and before he obtained extensive experience working with the mentally retarded.

Proof of their bold claim that they had found a way to overcome the endemic "crisis in psychology" required the originators of the sociohistorical school to apply their ideas across the full range of problems which psychologists considered their domain. During the late 1920s and early 1930s, their writings and the writings of their students did indeed reach across an amazing proportion of the key areas of psychology and their subjects included aphasics, Parkinson's patients, the mentally ill, as well as children from varying regions of the country and of varying mental abilities.

The basic principle in all of this work remained the same. When a subject's natural attempts to fulfill a task are inadequate (either because they are young and have failed to develop the requisite means, or because their normal mediated forms of behavior have been disrupted owing to disease or injury) the deficits can be overcome by literally remediating their activity. As Luria phrased it, when direct attempts to control behavior lead to negative results, mastery can be achieved by indirect (e.g., mediated means). The challenge of psychological diagnosis is to discover the weak links which are the proximate cause of behavioral difficulties, and then to come up with ways to remediate the individual's behavior using, where necessary, external means, mental prostheses, to enable them to cope more effectively with the demands they face.

These basic propositions had both theoretical and practical implications for the domain of neuropsychology, Luria's preoccupation in the later part of his career. Theoretically, it meant that the functional cortical systems underpining specifically human forms of behavior involve "extracortical" components, external supports, including cultural objects in the world (which, for Luria, included human language). Leontiev dubbed these external cultural elements that become an intrinsic part of human cognitive functioning "functional organs," emphasizing the belief that in the process of development, the mastery of new tasks occurs as much by the creation of new, flexible, functional systems as by the creation of new morphological organs.

As a single example of such thinking I can note Luria's work on disturbances of writing and their remediation, in which he emphasized that writing, as an historically recent form of human behavior, could not be ascribed to a particular brain center, but rather, had to be analyzed in terms of the particular "functional organ" that it constituted. In practical terms, these ideas led to an entire system of remedial practices, each tailored to take account of both the location of the brain lesions and the particular functions that the therapist was attempting to restore.

The close link between the early formulations of the mediated nature of human activity and between early and later work on restoration of functions can be illustrated by one of Luria's favorite examples (described first, so far as I know, in *The Nature of Human Conflicts),* the way in which patients suffered from Parkinson's disease could gain control of their movements.

Having noted that patients who could not walk across a level floor could nonetheless walk up stairs, Vygotsky and Luria hypothesized that, in some way, higher, mediated forms of behavior were brought into play in the latter situation. Luria describes the verification of their hypothesis:

> Vygotsky . . . placed a series of small paper cards on the floor and asked a patient to step over each of them. . . . A patient who had been able to take no more than two or three steps by himself walked through the room, easily stepping over each piece of paper as if he were climbing a staircase. We had helped the patient to overcome the symptoms of his disease by getting him to reorganize the mental processes he used in walking. He had compensated for his defect by transferring the activity from the subcortical level where his nerves were damaged to the cortical level which was not affected by the disease. (Luria, 1979, p. 129)

It is clear that Luria used this same strategy in attempts to restore intellectual functions to patients suffering from local lesions. For example, although their deficits have almost the precise opposite structure from parkinson's patients, this is the strategy he used for patients with frontal lobe lessions, whose motor behavior is intact, but who are cut off from the possibility of control by "higher" areas of the brain central to voluntary action. Luria describes the difficulty that frontal lobe patients have when attempting to make transitions from one thought to another, and among whom cause–effect thinking is severely disturbed (described more fully in Luria, 1963). In one such case, a patient who was unable to recount a familiar narrative story was provided with external prompts for transitions between parts of the story, cards upon which were written such words as "however," "whereas," "after," "since," and so on. With the aid of the crucial transition formulas in external form, the patient was able to recount the narrative. With repeated experience, the patient eventually was able to dispense with the external props, further evidence, to Luria, of the principle that with development, external means are replaced by internal, psychological means.

Throughout Luria's publications of the 1960s and 1970s (many of which were written many years before) these same themes and methods surface again and again. Similar examples could be given from his work on mental retardation, comparisons of fraternal and identical twins, and many areas of neuropsychology. However, I hope that I have succeeded in making my general point. All of this later writing has its roots in the theoretical and empirical work done during the 1920s.

## Romantic Science

In the last decade of his life, as ill health began to take its toll, Alexandr Romanovich began to spend more time in the book-lined studies in his Moscow apartment and at his dacha. As the end grew near he returned to the pre-occupations of his youth, attempting in his writing to communicate his vision of his life's work.

It was during this period that he wrote two small books, each a special kind of case study: *The Mind of a Mnemonist* and *The Man With a Shattered World*. Each of these books enjoyed immediate and widespread popularity when they appeared in English. The story of the man with a phenomenal and peculiarly constructed memory and the man who regained the ability to write and com-municate the experience of shattering brain damage were sufficiently dramatic to engage the imagination of many people who had little idea of the theoretical import which Luria attached to this work. Nor did Alexandr Romanovich himself indicate in the books themselves the way in which they fit into his life's work. Instead each was treated by author and audience alike as case studies revealing important aspects of human nature.

It was only in his autobiography, which he was still revising at the time of his death, that he drew the various threads of his career together in an attempt to communicate the pattern that he had been seeking to weave. Here he returns explicitly to the dichotomy between a nomothetic, generalizing, natural science of humankind and an ideographic, humanistic, clinical study of individual people, or as he phrased it, the attempt to "preserve the spirit of clinical analysis while using laboratory aids as a means to meaningful scientific achievement."

Unimagined portraits he called them. He encountered Shereshevsky, the mnenomist, early in his career, when the ideas of the sociohistorical school were still in their infancy. He was fascinated by the very general implications of the man's way of knowing and remembering, for the personality as a whole, and for his theory that normal adults have so thoroughly mastered cultural forms of remembering, that "direct," "synesthesic" memory, such as Shereshevsky dis-played, have long since disappeared. From Luria's written record, it is clear that he studied Shereshevsky on and off for many years.

In the case of Zasetsky, too, it was more than a matter of the doctor doing the best he could for the patient and then sending him into the world to fare as fate ordained. The stack of schoolchildren's notebooks in which Zasetsky pain-stakingly reconstructed his experience and developed mental prostheses for dealing with his incurable affliction (the notebooks were on the bookshelfs of the Luria family archive) attest to the doctor's enduring concern with one of the few people to be able to describe the phenomenology of brain damage.

His last unimagined portrait, his own autobiography, provides the last testament to his belief in the principles upon which his life's work were based. In this portrait, he wrote:

There is no subject with exceptional abilities—I have none. Nor is there a specific capacity or a specific disaster. But there is a unique atmosphere of a life, beginning at that unique time which was the start of the Revolution. (Luria, 1979, p. 188)

From beginning to end, Alexandr Romanovich Luria was a man who believed that human beings are created by other human brings, in the special medium of human culture. He knew that many of his specific ideas were incorrect, but he believed to the end that the general theory developed with his colleagues was correct and would live on— as it does do, in his students and the tens of thousands of people who have found in his vision a basis for their understanding of themselves and human nature.

## REFERENCES

Cole, M. (1988). Cross cultural research in the socio-historical tradition. *Human Development, 31,* 137–152.

Ermath, M. (1978) *Wilhelm Dilthey: The critique of historical reason.* Chicago. U. of Chicago Press.

Laboratory of Comparative Human Cognition (1983). Culture and cognitive development. In P. Mussen (Ed.), *Handbook of child psychology* (Vol. 1). New York: Wiley.

Leontiev, A. N. (1932). Studies of the cultural development of the child, II. The development of voluntary attention. *Journal of Genetic Psychology, 40,* 52–83.

Luria, A. R., (1928). The problem of the cultural development of the child. *Journal of Genetic Psychology, 35,* 493–506.

Luria, A. R. (1932). *The nature of human conflicts.* (reprint 1976). New York: Liveright.

Luria, A. R. (1934). The second psychological expedition to Central Asia. *Journal of Genetic Psychology, 41,* 255–259.

Luria, A. R. (1961). *The role of speech in the regulation of normal and abnormal behavior.* New York: Irvington.

Luria, A. R. (1963). *Restoration of function after brain injury.* New York: Pergamon.

Luria, A. R. (1970). *Traumatic aphasia.* The Hague: Mouton.

Luria, A. R. (1976). *Cognitive development.* Cambridge, MA: Harvard University Press.

Luria, A. R. (1978). *The selected writings of A. R. Luria.* White Plains, NY: M. Sharpe.

Luria, A. R. (1979). *Making of mind.* Cambridge, MA: Harvard University Press.

Luria, A. R. (1982) *Language and cognition.* New York: Wiley-Interscience.

Mill, J. S. (1943/1948). A system of logic. Reprinted in W. Dennis. *Readings in the history of psychology.* New York: Appleton-Century-Crofts.

Razmyslov, P. (1934). Vygotsky and Luria's cutlural-historical theory of psychology. *Knigii proletarskoi revolutsii, 4,* 78–86.

Rivers, W. H. R. (1901) Vision. *Reports of the Cambridge Anthropological Expedition to the Torres Straits.* (A. C. Haddon, Ed.). Vol. 2, Part 1. Cambridge, England: Cambridge University Press.

Wundt, W. (1921). *Elements of folk psychology: Outlines of a psychological history of the development of mankind.* London: Allen & Unwin.

# 2

# The Frontal Lobes and Language

*Donald T. Stuss*

*Rotman Research Institute of Baycrest Centre; University of Toronto*

*D. Frank Benson*

*Department of Neurology, UCLA School of Medicine, Los Angeles*

Over his long and fruitful career, the great psychologist, A. R. Luria, amassed a vast experience in both developmental psychology and neuropsychology. This background provided a rich data base upon which to construct theories of brain activities, including language function. In this chapter, Luria's influence on current concepts of those aspects of language and communication most influenced by the frontal lobe will be reviewed. To present this material, an abstract of Luria's published theory of overall brain organization and function will be presented, stressing frontal influence. Next, Luria's categorization of language disorders based on frontal lobe pathology and his concepts on the regulatory role of language on brain function will be reviewed. Following this, our own theory of brain function and a working draft of modern concepts of frontally derived language disorders will be presented. The influence of Luria's concepts on contemporary investigations of the frontal lobes and frontal language disorders will be obvious.

## LURIA'S CONCEPT OF BRAIN ORGANIZATION

Through numerous publications spanning several decades, Luria presented many ideas concerning brain activity (1958, 1967, 1970a, 1970b, 1973a, 1980) with particular emphasis on the influence of the frontal lobes. This mass of material can be abstracted by listing four major points postulated by Luria.

First, he posited a tripartite concept of brain organization, emphasizing the distinct yet integrated functioning of different brain regions.

> There are . . . *three principal functional units of the brain* whose participation is
> necessary for any type of mental activity . . . a unit for *regulating tone or waking,* a
> unit for *obtaining, processing and storing information* arriving from the outside
> world and a unit for *programming, regulating and verifying mental activity.* (Luria,
> 1973a, p. 43)

Each of these units is itself hierarchical and multilayered. The first unit,
based on the reticular activating system, interacts in a reciprocal manner with the
cortex to maintain the optimal level of cortical excitation necessary for efficient
brain functioning. The second unit is located in the posterior lateral convexity, in
particular the brain regions underlying the primary sensory and association areas
of vision, audition and general sensation—the occipital, temporal, and parietal
areas. These regions interact with the environment by receiving, coding, and
storing information. The third functional unit lies in the frontal brain regions,
primarily anterior to the precentral gyrus. It is this unit that gives human activity
its active, directive, conscious character. All three units, working together in a
coherent manner, are necessary for optimal human activity.

Second, against this model of brain organization, Luria stressed the importance of the active character of human brain functioning:

> Human behavior is active in character . . . determined not only by past experience,
> but also by plans and designs formulating the *future.* . . . the human brain is a
> remarkable apparatus which cannot only create these models of the future, but also
> subordinate its behavior to them. . . . Man not only reacts passively to incoming
> information, but creates *intentions,* forms *plans* and *programmes* of his actions,
> inspects their performance, and *regulates* his behavior so that it conforms to these
> plans and programmes; finally, he *verifies* his conscious activity . . . correcting any
> mistakes he has made. (Luria, 1973a, pp. 13, 79–80).

While he acknowledged that a vast amount of brain activity could be carried
on with automatic responses that did not necessitate formal learning and monitoring, the latter properties were present and were an important aspect of higher
brain function.

Third, Luria emphasized the functions of the frontal lobes in the active
planning, creating, anticipating, and controlling role, noting the complexity of
this activity:

> Although the frontal lobes do not participate in the performance of the simplest and
> most usual actions, they can and must play a decisive role in . . . the programmes of
> all complex forms of activity; they maintain the dominant role of the programme and
> inhibit irrelevant and inappropriate actions. (Luria, 1980, p. 293)

"The functional organization of the human frontal lobes is one of the most
complex problems in modern science . . .," he wrote. (Luria, 1973a, p. 225).

Thus, Luria not only considered the directing, control functions to be crucial to human brain function but clearly localized these higher neural functions as frontal lobe activities.

Fourth, Luria, perhaps more than any researcher in history, drew attention to the intimate relationship between speech and the frontal lobes; he posited ". . . the *tertiary portions of the frontal lobes are in fact a superstructure . . . so that they perform a far more universal function of general regulation of behavior. . . .*" (Luria, 1973a, p. 89). "The chief distinguishing feature of the regulation of human conscious activity is that this regulation takes place with the close participation of *speech . . . higher mental processes are formed and take place on the basis of speech activity. . . .*" (Luria, 1973a, pp. 93–94). This close relationship was the basis for many of Luria's elaborations in language disturbances following frontal damage and the role of the frontal lobes in human behavior.

These four major points are the cornerstones upon which Luria's concepts of anterior language disturbances and the regulatory role of language can be presented in greater detail.

## ANTERIOR LANGUAGE DISTURBANCES

To understand the classification of frontal language disturbance, a further breakdown of Luria's major principles is important. First, speech and language are not unitary concepts, but can be divided into levels (Luria, 1973a). Speech, with the word as the basic unit of language and the sentence as the basic unit of narrative expression, represents the level of communication. At another level, speech is important in abstraction and categorical thinking, as it is essential for analysis and generalization of incoming information. At a third, even higher level, speech is a method of regulating, controlling, and organizing human mental processes in behavior by formulating decisions, fixing intentions, and drawing conclusions.

A second important concept is Luria's separation of speech and language according to the anterior and posterior functional zones (Luria, 1958, 1977). Posterior (parietal-occipital) brain regions are important in the simultaneous synthesis of incoming information; damage in these areas leads to particular syndromes, including deficits in decoding phonetic elements and in grasping logical, grammatical relations in language. Anterior cortex, on the other hand, including both frontal and frontal-temporal zones, is relevant in the synthesis of successive elements into a single continuous sequential series. Disturbance of "successive synthesis" may be observed in the reproduction of rhythms, movements, words or numbers, and series of actions. Anterior brain damage may cause a deterioration in the smooth flow from subject to verb (Luria, 1958, 1977). Luria (1974, 1977) described this as a failure in syntagmatic organization, a deficit of internal speech, eventually resulting in telegraphic style. In the

Vygotsky/Luria approach, the term "inner speech" indicated a transition state between the preliminary thought or idea and the extended verbal phrase, a linkage between personal thinking and formal communication.

In a more detailed classification, Luria divided anterior language disturbances into two major categories, motor aphasia and dynamic aphasia (Luria, 1977). Within the motor aphasias, he noted two forms. One, afferent or kinaesthetic motor aphasia, most commonly following lesions in the lower post-central region of the left hemisphere, occurs when movements of the articulatory muscles lose their afferent input, resulting in an inability to determine with accuracy the positions of the lips and tongues necessary to articulate motor speech (Luria, 1973a, 1977). The second form, efferent or kinetic motor aphasia due to a lesion in premotor (Broca's) area, causes loss of modulatory influence on motor cortex with a subsequent disturbance in the serial organization of skilled movements. While single movement articulations may be performed without problem, movement from one articulation to another is impaired. The disturbance may vary considerably in severity. When mild, a disturbance of the kinetic melody of speech is described; when severe, the result is a full efferent motor aphasia with telegraphic output (Luria, 1969). The differences noted by Luria resemble the variations called aphemia, little Broca and big Broca aphasia to be described later. If the lesion extends to subcortical motor ganglia, dysarthria and perseveration of separate elements is frequent (Luria, 1977).

Luria's second major form of frontal language disturbance was called dynamic aphasia (Luria, 1973, 1977), usually based on a left frontal lesion, most often the third frontal convolution. Characteristics include a lack of spontaneity of speech, particularly if long narratives are required, and a disturbance of the predicative component of speech necessary for the formation of complete thoughts and sentences. The basis for the disorder is found in the mechanism of narrative speech, which requires an intention to speak and the creation of a plan to follow, both dependent on intact frontal lobe functioning.

Luria states that dynamic aphasia can produce a telegraphic style. If the lesion is massive, the patient cannot even construct a simple phrase, even when given separate words. When less severe, the impairment is best elicited by less structured tests, such as narrative speech, telling a story, or describing a situation. If asked to tell a story, the patient tends to present minimal information, a loss of the "linear scheme of the phrase" posited as due to an impairment of inner speech with shortened form and decreased predicative function (Luria, 1977). Complete, organized phrases, and paragraphs become virtually impossible. If asked concrete questions, if someone else starts a phrase, or if other cues are given, that is, if structure is provided, the performance improves, sometimes dramatically.

Luria differentiates the described dynamic aphasia from a more general aspontaneity and adynamia, a state in which there is little spontaneous output and responses are passive and monontonous (Luria, 1973a). He also suggests that dynamic aphasia is a subtype of the classical transcortical motor aphasia (Luria, 1973a, 1977).

Several additional comments about Luria's views on language and the frontal lobes are relevant. First, Luria (1973a) states that, in general, there is insufficient knowledge concerning the status of the right hemisphere in language, but that no direct connection of the right frontal lobe with the speech organization of behavior is obvious. Second, with lesions in the left medial frontal zones that extend to the right frontal regions, "pre-aphasic" signs are noted, including intrusions of irrelevant associations, a disturbance of selectivity affecting language and resulting in perseverative errors, lack of suppression of inappropriate alternatives, and confabulation (Luria, Homskaya, Blinkov, & Critchley, (1967). Finally, he noted that frontal damage may result in comprehension problems, particularly when complex narratives are offered. He postulated that this was due to impaired frontal lobe functions of searching, selecting the meaningful aspects, and verifying the meaning (Luria, 1973a).

Through his many writings describing neuropsychological deficits following brain lesions, Luria wrote extensively on the effects of frontal damage on language. He specifically noted consistent language syndromes and the neuroanatomical sites of damage associated with these problems. Although couched in different names and emphasizing somewhat different aspects of language disorder, Luria's descriptive entities can be generally matched to types of aphasia described in the classical syndromes of aphasia. Luria went beyond pure phenomenological description, however, and stressed the frontal functions crucial to language as a tool in the organization and direction of all human behavior, a topic that can be discussed under the title of the regulatory role of language.

## THE REGULATORY ROLE OF LANGUAGE

Luria (1967) differentiated the nominative, semantic, and syntactical aspects of language, the commonly accepted functions of language, from its pragmatic or directive role. This directive or regulatory function was primarily associated with the frontal regions of the brain. While frontal lesions do not impair the phonetic, lexical or logical—grammatical functions of speech,

> They give rise to a severe disturbance of a *different function of speech, namely its regulatory function;* the patient can no longer direct and control his behavior with the aid of speech, either his own or that of another person. (Luria, 1973a, p. 211)

Indeed, this regulatory function ranks with the highest functions of psychology, since conscious purpose of action, systematic thought, voluntary memory, and regulation of the reticular activating system and cortex can all be linked to the regulatory function of speech. Discovery of the directive role played by the frontal cortex "should be considered among the most important achievements of neurological science" (Luria, 1977, p. 40).

These concepts were derived to a large degree from Vygotsky (1962), particularly the developmental aspect of self-regulation (Luria, 1967, 1977; Luria & Homskaya, 1964). The adult regulates a young child's behavior by command, inhibiting irrelevant responses. As the child learns to speak, the spoken instructions shared between the child and adult are taken over by the child, who uses externally stated and often detailed instructions to guide his or her own behaviors. By the age of 4 to 4½, a trend toward internal and contracted speech (inner speech) gradually appears. The child begins to regulate and subordinate his behavior according to this inner speech. Speech, in addition to serving communication and thought, becomes a major self-regulatory force, creating systems of connections for organizing active behavior and inhibiting actions irrelevant to the task at hand.

Association of this verbal self-regulation with the frontal lobes has derived primarily from research in patients with frontal lobe lesions. Numerous clinical examples illustrate the deficit. For instance, frontal lobe patients may easily verbalize task requirements but fail to use this information to guide behavior. Ackerly and Benton (1947) described a frontal lobe patient as having "an excellent sense of right and wrong when talking about it in an abstract manner, but [showing] no such sense in his actions." (p. 490). Milner (1964) described patients who could verbalize the sorting requirements of the Wisconsin Card Sorting Test but who were seemingly incapable of using this knowledge to complete the task successfully. Our patient (Alexander, Stuss, & Benson, 1979) with the Capgras Syndrome had recovered intellectually from bifrontal and right temporal damage, was aware of the impossibility of having two similar but separate families, but could never use this knowledge to alter his belief. The dissociation between the directive pragmatic role of the word and the actual behavior was further confirmed by this patient who never initiated even the smallest practical step toward return to work, despite verbal insistence that this was his avid desire.

Luria drew attention to this regulative role of language and published striking examples. First, he demonstrated that patients with posterior cerebral lesions do not lose the ability to use speech in a determining, directive role, in striking contrast to frontal lobe patients who may show a dissociation between what they say and what they do (Luria, 1969, 1973b; Luria & Homskaya, 1964). If the lesion is massive, the patient fails to carry out even the simplest in- structions, although repeating them accurately. Such patients will not demon- strate a restabilization of the orienting response with verbal instructions (Luria & Homskaya, 1964). If asked to press a bulb with the right hand when a red light is flashed and with the left hand to a blue light, frontal lobe patients respond stereotypically, with no relation of the response to the signal. If the examiner repeats the command to each stimulus, a "conditioned connection" might begin to assist responses, but even this would be lost in time.

Delayed responses clearly demonstrate this deficit in frontal lobe patients, as the responses are directly tied to the verbal command. For example, if asked to raise his or her hand in 15–20 seconds when the examiner knocks, or when the second hand of the watch reaches 20, the patient will do nothing or perhaps mimic the examiner. The failure is not a memory deficit since the patient can repeat the instructions. The verbal command stays in memory but has no regulatory or controlling influence. In contrast, Luria notes that verbal regulation can be effective in patients with subcortical motor processes such as Parkinson's disease, and in those patients with lesions in posterior cortical areas, limbic zones, or with limited premotor pathology (Luria, 1973a, 1980).

Luria's writings (Luria, 1973a, 1977) support a differentiation within the frontal lobe. The loss of activation with spoken instructions is most obvious with massive bilateral medial frontal lobe lesions. If the lesion is lateral, verbal instructions may help, but only after frequent repetitions (Luria, 1973). Even so, the benefit is not stable. If the pathology is less severe, verbal regulation can benefit simple tasks but be ineffective for more complex demands (Luria, 1967, 1973; Luria & Homskaya, 1964). Luria and colleagues (Luria, 1969; Luria, Pribram, & Homskaya, 1964), suggested that the left dorsal-lateral convexity plays an important role in verbal control of behavior.

Further lesion specificity regarding the regulatory functions of speech in the frontal lobes seems possible. First, significant verbal regulation deficit was not noted in patients after orbital frontal white matter damage (leucotomy) (Benson & Stuss, 1982). Second, left frontal pathology appears to have the most direct influence on this function, as Luria suggested. Stuss, Delgado, and Guzman (1987) described two patients with right anterior pathology and motor impersistence who could be taught to use self-initiated verbal self-commands to control some aspects of their impersistence, suggesting a left-hemisphere dominance for this function. Goldberg, Mayer, and Toglia (1981), however, reported that examiner-initiated commands could interrupt abnormal behavior in two patients with focal left supplementary motor area (SMA) damage. Third, Petrides (1985) and Milner (1982) suggest that frontal lobe patients have a more general deficit in the use of external cues to aid behavior with verbal cues being only one type. Nonverbal cues may serve as a right-hemisphere counterpart in guiding behavior.

In summary, Luria outlined at least three types of aphasia based on relatively circumscribed frontal pathology and, in addition, clearly outlined an important function of language, that of regulation of action. The superordinate control of both overt and covert human behavior, at least partly mediated by language, represents a frontal function of considerable importance. To examine the association of language and the frontal lobes further, we will present our own theory of brain function and describe a number of language disorder syndromes. Some of these syndromes have become apparent only with the advent of novel testing methods and advanced imaging techniques. They validate Luria's more phenomenological descriptions.

## A BEHAVIORAL/ANATOMICAL MODEL

We have proposed a model of brain organization that emphasized the role of the frontal lobes (Stuss & Benson, 1986). Several principles underlying this model had their origin in or are elaborations on the writings of Professor Luria.

First, psychological functions and brain-behavior correlates can be fully understood only in terms of an interactive organization of the entire brain. Second, the brain neither works in a mass action manner, nor are its functions strictly localized. Rather, abilities such as language must be understood as complex functional systems with different cortical and subcortical zones playing different, independent, and specific roles, the quality of breakdown of the function varying with the localization of the brain lesion. ". . . mental functions . . . must be *organized in systems of concertedly working zones, each of which performs its role in complex functional systems* . . . which may be located in completely different and often far distant areas of the brain." (Luria, 1973a, p. 31)

Third, although the brain is an integrated unity, there is a conceptual separation between frontal and nonfrontal cortical regions. The frontal lobes are dynamic, active, and controlling, bringing the rest of behavior (cortical tone; basic gnostic zones) into accordance with conscious goals and motivations (Luria, 1969, 1973a, 1977).

With these basic principles, a general model of brain organization can be presented. First, conceptually, the brain can be divided into frontal and nonfrontal segments with the latter comprised of posterior and basal brain regions. The posterior-basal regions comprise a series of *organized integrated fixed functional systems* with the frontal lobes playing an integral part in each functional system. Nevertheless, the general "gnostic" and/or "tonal" roles of the posterior-basal and frontal influences can be viewed as independent. Each *functional system* refers to a general mental activity such as memory or visual-spatial ability. Nine possible posterior/basal functional systems are graphically listed in relation to overall behavior in Fig. 2.1. As noted earlier, Luria had divided the posterior-basal functions into two major units: (1) A tonal unit, situated in upper brainstem and limbic regions, responsible for tone and vigilance of the cortex; (2) A gnostic unit, located in posterior cortical regions (temporal-parietal-occipital), responsible for the reception, elaboration, and storage of external information for basic cognition. Our model includes functional systems of both types within these regions.

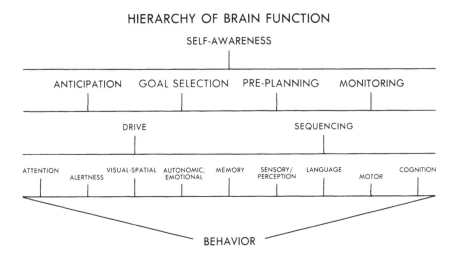

**FIGURE 1.** This figure depicts the proposed model of brain functioning. Organized, integrated, fixed functional systems such as attention underlie external behavior. These are hypothesized to be based, in relation to the frontal lobes, in more posterior/basal regions. The next three levels are more intimately associated with the frontal lobes. Reprinted with permission from Stuss and Benson, *The Frontal Lobes,* Raven Press, New York, 1986.

The posterior-basal systems should not be viewed as hard-wired independent modules, although they can be conceptualized as having some of the characteristics of such modules. They appear to be interactive, with certain neural zones playing a role in more than one system, their role dependent on the function of the entire system. For example, intact vision is important for language, as well as visual-spatial abilities.

In the descriptive phrase "organized integrated fixed functional system," the term *organized* reflects the concept that different parts of a complex functional system play separate but integral roles in the successful functioning of the entire system. Lesions in different regions associated with a particular function will influence the general function in a manner specific to the region damaged. "Organized" also implies that each posterior/basal functional system, at the level of routine knowledge or behavior, can function efficiently in well-rehearsed situations. Novel or complex situations extend beyond this level of organization and necessitate frontal lobe input, as will be described.

*Integrated* implies that the separate anatomical regions must be connected to generate the function. Based on present knowledge of these systems, integration is both lateralized and hierarchical, demanding participation of both hemispheres, selected subcortical structures, and interconnecting pathways. Luria consistently stressed that this integration should not be seen in a strict localizationist or connectionistic manner. While pathways exist, they connect "centers" and "zones" and the mode of integration is uncertain; spreading excitation, biochemical, and/or structural pathways are all possible methods of communication.

*Fixed* suggests that, in the normal adult human, the function and its relation to neuroanatomical zones is relatively constant across and within individuals, allowing for scientific investigation.

Thus, major psychological functions can be separated into a number of basic functional systems (also called schemas, faculties, and modules). These are complex combinations of various subsystems that are organized, integrated, and operating in relatively fixed anatomical portions within the posterior and basal sectors of the brain. The influence of the frontal lobe on these functional systems is crucial to understanding frontal language disorders.

Luria described a third functional unit, responsible for programming, regulating, and verifying mental activity, located primarily in the frontal lobes anterior to the precentral gyrus. Luria's terminology suggests that this unit was indivisible but his descriptions indicate a multiplicity of subfunctions within the frontal lobe. Moreover, he clearly stated that the frontal lobes were not homogeneous but heterogeneous (Luria, 1970, 1973a, 1980; Luria, Homskaya, Blinkov, & Critchley, 1967). Our conceptualization focuses on this diversity of frontal lobe function. Three separate divisions within the profrontal cortex are proposed, each conceptually more abstract and hierarchically "superior." Functionally, however, they must be viewed as working in a tightly knit and interactive manner in normal adult human functioning.

## Frontal (Anterior) Functional Systems

At least two systems having the characteristics described have partial localization in the more caudal regions of the frontal lobes. These frontal systems are functionally linked to each of the posterior/basal functional systems, most often interacting in a superordinate manner. The two functions, drive and sequencing, interact with all posterior/basal functional systems.

## Sequencing

Maintaining fragments of data as meaningful sequences is dependent to a great degree on the frontal lobes and is of obvious importance to higher cognitive activities. Luria (1970, 1973a), Albert (1972), Milner and Petrides (1984; Petrides and Milner, 1982) and Fuster (1980), using different tasks, concluded that, for both higher primates and humans, the ability to maintain serial order of behavior is dependent on intact frontal lobes. In particular, the more caudal frontal convexity regions appeared essential for this activity. In addition, Fuster (1980) and Stuss and Benson (1986) emphasize that the integration of temporally ordered information with prior knowledge demands frontal activity.

## Drive

A change in drive, either an increase (impulsivity, agitation) or decrease (apathy), is commonly described as a functional alteration following frontal lobe damage (Luria, 1973a) and anatomical localizations for altered drive has been suggested (Blumer & Benson, 1975). Medial saggital frontal structures are important in the initiation of behavior; damage in this area produces apathy. Orbital frontal regions, in contrast, appear relevant to the ability to inhibit drive. Again, the consequences of altered drive are manifested through the posterior-basal functional systems, the frontal functional systems acting as a superordinate factor.

## Executive Functions

Luria (1970, 1973a, 1980) emphasized the importance and diversity of prefrontal function, using discrete terms such as planning, intending, programming, regulating, and verifying. Luria, and others, have made almost universally acceptable the fact that the controlling or executive function of human behavior is associated with the prefrontal cortex. This control function provides conscious direction to the frontal and posterior/basal functional systems; information processing of novel or complex data is dependent on the posited submodules of the executive control function. Anticipation, goal selection, planning, monitoring—and perhaps others submodules—describe the unique activities of this superordinate prefrontal control function. The ability to take information from other brain regions, to anticipate problems, select goals, plan means to achieve these goals, experiment with behaviors and ideas, and modify responses according to anticipated reactions provides a totally integrated goal-directed human behavior. Executive control ranks among the highest of human mental accomplishments, a supervisory role that appears dependent on the action of intact prefrontal lobes.

## Self-awareness and Self-consciousness

Self-awareness (self-reflectiveness, self-consciousness) ranks highest as an attribute of human behavior and also appears to be a prefrontal function. While Luria was not specific, he did state that the role of the frontal lobes was to bring behavior into accordance with conscious goals and motives and clinical observations strongly suggest that self-consciousness depends on the prefrontal cortex (Stuss & Benson, 1986). Self-awareness appears necessary to control, via a feedback loop, a discrepancy between what a person "perceives" and what actually is (Carver & Scheier, 1982). This aspect of self-control appears similar to the cognitive psychology concept of "metacognition," a general term relating to the superordinate psychological ability to reflect on one's mental functions (Yussen, 1985) and implies an organized, deliberate acquisition and use of knowledge (Brown, 1978; Cavanaugh & Borkowski, 1980). Metacognition, as described, is considered the basis of truly intelligent behavior and clearly resembles the self-reflective functions attributed to the frontal lobes.

In our own conception (Benson and Stuss, in preparation), the self is subdivided into three functionally distinct aspects: *self-knowledge, self-control,* and *self-analysis*. The first refers to the unique body of knowledge, both personal and formal, acquired by an individual; in general this aspect of self is a basal/posterior brain function. The second, *self-control,* reflects the individual's ability to manipulate the body of knowledge to accomplish novel activities. The final aspect, *self-analysis,* defines the psychologically vague but clearly crucial human functions of introspection, retrospection, future planning, fantasy, imagination, and so on, the ability to construct mentally and analyze problems, both personal and scholarly. *Self-control* and *self-analysis* appear to be prefrontal functions although they depend on and act through the integrated sensory/motor information of the basal/posterior brain.

In summary, our model of brain/behavior organization is clearly derivative from Luria's (as well as others) conceptualizations. Subdivision into different hierarchic modules should only be interpreted in an integrated model of brain functioning, with different roles being evoked as required by the situation. In routine, overlearned situations, the frontal lobes play no active role; the posterior-basal systems are sufficient for response. We (1986) summarized the literature and concluded that, for all functions such as memory, visual-spatial abilities, and so on, the frontal lobes are essential only in novel and/or complex situations.

## FRONTAL LOBES AND LANGUAGE

To correlate the hypothesized frontal function with *in vitro* language disorders, a rather rigid anatomically based structure will be presented. It is immediately recognized that real life problems are less specific (and less clear) than idealized syndromatic descriptions. Also, it will be presumed that the left hemisphere is dominant for language. Finally, it must be accepted that work in this area is recent and far from complete; alterations and improvements of the proposed disorders can be anticipated. With these caveats, language disorders following damage in several distinct areas in both the left and the right frontal lobes can be discussed.

## Frontal Language Disturbances—The Left Frontal Lobe

### Inferior Motor Cortex/Posterior Operculum

Damage to the posterior operculum (area 44; Broca'a area proper), or a subcortical undercutting, results in a well-defined syndrome of speech impairment without language deficit frequently called aphemia (Bastian, 1898; Dejerine, 1914/1977; Lichtheim, 1885). Acute mutism without primary laryngeal pathology is the initial sign. As verbal output recovers, a hypophonic, slow output evolves, with a fragmented melodic transition between phonemes, syllables and words. The altered speech pattern may resemble a foreign accent, first described as dysprosody by Monrad–Krohn (1947). A difficulty in making the transition from one articulation to another appears similar to the "apraxia of speech" described by others (Darley, 1968; Johns & Darley, 1970).

Cortical articulation disturbances have also been more specifically described. The posterior inferior frontal gyrus, involved in aphemia, does not appear to be necessary for well-articulated speech (Levine & Mohr, 1979). Damage to the inferior motor cortex proper, on the other hand, appears to cause a defect in articulation (Tonkonogy & Goodglass, 1981).

### Broca Aphasia

One widely accepted sign of left-hemisphere involvement is the syndrome called Broca aphasia. Common clinical signs include right-sided motor weakness, ideomotor limb apraxia testable in the left hand, nonfluent verbal output, short phrase length, agrammatical verbal content, impaired repetition in naming, and relatively preserved comprehension (Benson, 1979; Benson & Geschwind, 1971; Kertesz, 1979; Lecours, Lhermitte, & Bryons, 1983).

Although traditionally considered to be due to pathology in the dominant posterior-inferior frontal lobe, in particular the pars triangularis and pars orbitalis of the inferior frontal gyrus, the full permanent syndrome of Broca aphasia requires deep extension of the lesion to the insula, adjacent white matter, and possibly the basal ganglia (Brunner, Kornhuber, Seemuller, Suger, & Wallesch, 1982; Naeser, Hayward, Laughlin, & Zatz, 1981).

Infarction of Broca's area alone or its immediate surroundings does not produce a permanent syndrome of Broca aphasia (Foix, 1928; Mohr, 1973; Mohr et al., 1978). A "little Broca" lesion is similar in location, but not in size, to the lesion causing aphemia. Signs include initial mutism, rapid improvement and some degree of language impairment in both spoken and written language.

Neurological changes may include mild transient right-sided weakness, often limited to the face. Evolution into aphemia, with slow speech and difficulty in transferring from one articulation to another, is common.

## Transcortical Motor Aphasia

Lichtheim (1885) considered transcortical motor aphasia (TCM aphasia) to be a separation of conceptual brain processes from the motor output area. Lesions are typically located in midfrontal areas, anterior or superior to Broca's area, although the exact regions involved have not been decisively delineated. The syndrome varies, probably dependent on size and location of the lesion.

The clinical syndrome of TCM aphasia may resemble Broca aphasia superficially. Right motor signs are common but not obligatory; if present, they tend to be transient. Conjugate eye deviation toward the side of the lesion indicates involvement of the frontal eye field. Initially the patient is mute. As speech returns, articulation is normal, but the verbal output is sparse and slow, with a striking difficulty in initiation of speech, particularly detailed narrative discourse. Attempts to generate word lists reveal significant decrease with hesitancy and disorganization. Sentence structure is short but grammatically competent. Comprehension is relatively intact. Repetition of individual words and phrases is good to excellent; it is the key differentiating feature. In general terms, TCM aphasia is Broca aphasia with relative preservation of repetition. There are many similarities with Luria's dynamic aphasia.

## Supplementary Motor Area (SMA) Language Disturbance

Originally, the supplementary motor area (SMA) language disturbance, based on damage in the medial frontal area in the distribution of the anterior cerebral artery, was considered a subtype of TCM aphasia (Kertesz, 1979) but the characteristics are sufficiently discrete to warrant its recognition as an independent syndrome (Alexander & Schmitt, 1980; Alexander, Benson & Stuss, in press; Goldberg et al., 1981; Masdeu, 1980; Masdeu, Schoene, & Funkenstein, 1978; Rubens, 1975; Stuss & Benson, 1986). Neurological findings include weakness and sensory loss of the contralateral lower limb, mild weakness of the shoulder (Fisher, 1975) and a grasp reflex.

As in TCM aphasia, there is an initial muteness, followed by decreased verbal output. Echolalia may be prominent early. The striking feature is a lack of spontaneous initiation of speech, although speech when produced, is well articulated. There are few aphasic symptoms, although hesitations are common. Even when speech recovers into more elaborate and less hesitant responses, attempts to elicit a sustained narrative still fail (Damasio & Van Hoesen, 1983). With extension of the lesion into more inferior medial frontal regions, additional features such as personality changes, apathy, slowness, and unconcern may be observed (Alexander et al., in press).

## Subcortical Aphasia

Only one syndrome of subcortical aphasia extends into subcortical frontal regions (Alexander, 1984; Damasio, Damasio, Rizzo, Varney, & Gorsh, 1982; Naeser, 1983; Naeser et al., 1982). Damage to the putamen, caudate, and/or anterior internal capsule with extension into left frontal lobe white matter will initially resemble Broca aphasia with onset of mutism and right hemiparesis. With recovery, good comprehension but seriously impaired articulation becomes evident. The output shows a longer phrase length than Broca aphasia with relatively intact syntactical structure.

## Prefrontal Language Disturbances

When frontal lobe damage extends more anteriorly, two additional frontal language disorders may be observed, possibly in combination with other language disturbances, dependent on lesion location and extent. The most commonly recognized is a disturbance of verbal self-regulation. Less commonly described is an impairment in organization and planning through the medium of language. The latter is observed in tasks demanding manipulative language usage when the material is complex or novel (e.g., explaining metaphors, abstractions, or proverbs, arranging of linguistic information, verbalizing complex narratives in an organized, directed manner and comparing actual utterances with the intention) (Alexander et al., in press; Kaczmarek, 1984). These disorders are neither language nor cognitive problems; rather they represent a disturbance of the executive planning and monitoring functions of the prefrontal cortex exhibited through the medium of complex language situations (Stuss & Benson, 1986; Stuss et al., 1983).

In summary, recent advances in brain–behavior correlation techniques have opened new vistas in understanding the left frontal lobe's participation in language. Two areas appear key to these advances, both presaged by the observations of Luria: first, improved clinical differentiations reflecting specific symptomatology in the more precise anatomical localizations have been made possible by the newer imaging techniques; second, the influence of more general prefrontal functions can be documented. In this respect, the contribution of the right frontal lobe also deserves attention.

### *Frontal Language Disturbances—The Right Frontal Lobe*

Although the left hemisphere is dominant for speech and language in most humans, many neurobehavioral researchers acknowledge Hughling Jackson's (1878) claim that the right hemisphere controls the emotional aspects of speech. A speech and language organization in the right hemisphere for emotional expression parallel to the left-hemisphere activity in propositional speech has been postulated (Ross, 1981). This association can be probed by a specific comparison of the effects of right and left frontal lobe damage on verbal output (Alexander et al., in press). Certain of these parallels have yet to be confirmed experimentally.

## Inferior Motor Cortex/Posterior Operculum

"Affective motor dysprosody" (Ross, 1981; Ross & Mesulam, 1979) parallels aphemia after left frontal pathology. Patients with lesions in this region are impaired in the expression of emotion through speech and gesture. They have difficulty placing the melodic contours into speech to communicate the underlying emotional feelings. Their speech is flat and the ability to reflect sadness, surprise, sarcasm, and other indirect aspects of communication (paragrammatical) are impaired. Singing is without melody. Visual-spatial disorders, if present, are transient or not severe. Left-sided motor deficits are transient and not pronounced. Intact emotions are dissociated from their expression, resulting in a "pure affective dumbness."

## Larger Opercular/Inferior Motor Cortex Pathology

In parallel with the larger left frontal lesion producing Broca's aphasia, a comparable lesion in the right hemisphere appears to cause a distinct symptom complex. Left hemiparesis is common, particularly left facial weakness. The primary disturbance is affective motor dysprosody. While verbalizations expressing sarcasm, anger, and so on, can be produced, speech intonations to reflect these intentions cannot. There may also be a difficulty in understanding higher-level metaphors, particularly if affective in content. Comprehension of affective prosody is intact but repetition of affective prosody is impaired. Visual-spatial disturbances are noted, particularly with complex material. With this lesion, affective motor dysprosody is combined with a more extensive deficit in emotional expression.

## Dorsolateral Frontal Verbal Output Disorder

Damage to the middle and superior right frontal gyri and underlying white matter, similar to that producing TCM aphasia, produces only mild affective motor dysprosody but the spontaneous use of the melodic component of prosody is decreased (Alexander et al., in press). Imitation of affective prosody is intact. The primary deficit is one of activation. Verbal fluency may be impaired, and there is a suggestion that nonverbal fluency is more severely affected (Jones–Gotman & Milner, 1977). Left motor signs are transient if present, but there may be conjugate eye deviation to the right.

A syndrome based on anterior extension of the lesion responsible for the right prefrontal verbal output disorder can be proposed, although lesion documentation for the symptoms is lacking. A piecemeal, disorganized narrative style producing vague and rambling narratives lacking organization and coherence are seen. The ability to make inferences, that is, see a relationship between two apparently unrelated statements, is disturbed. Discourse is socially inappropriate, lacking attention to the interpersonal implications of the communication context. With extension of the lesion medially, content may become extremely disordered, lacking both self-monitoring and the ability to inhibit associations; confabulation is present.

In summary, although the comparisons are not ideal and current knowledge is insufficient to make an exact parallel, there appears to be an active bilateral involvement of the frontal lobes in speech and language, with a parallel organization in each hemisphere. The left and right frontal areas appear to be active according to their respective roles in cerebral activity. In each hemisphere, the following subdivisions appear relevant. First, each hemisphere has a syndrome associated primarily with the motor output. Second, each has a more elaborate syndrome, involving motor output problems plus additional deficits, likely due to involvement of brain regions other than frontal. Third, activation deficits appear more intimately linked with SMA and anterior cingulum, with extension of problems in activation related to the connections between the SMA and the premotor-motor output area. Fourth, formulation/organization problems are evident, related more to the prefrontal regions.

As has been noted, these contemporary descriptions can be compared with Luria's earlier presentations. Luria observed, recorded, and interpreted many cases with frontal lobe damage and from this experience formulated basic functions of the frontal lobes and their effect on language. More recent works amplify and clarify Luria's presentations. While there are some areas of disagreement, particularly in the correlation of phenomenological details, the major premises proposed by Luria have been confirmed. His diligent labors in the evaluation of brain-damaged individuals, his ability to integrate individual symptom combinations into a larger picture and, from this composite, to isolate pertinent brain functions and their neuroanatomical bases have led the way into contemporary neurobehavioral investigations of frontal lobe function. We can confidently anticipate future advances in understanding of frontal language functions but the basic structure on which these advances will stand has been provided by Luria's contributions.

## SUMMARY

Historically, there have been many reasons to understand why certain researchers considered the frontal lobes as the silent zones of the cerebral cortex (Luria, 1980). Today, however, the emphasis on the study of active behavior has renewed the interest in the study of frontal lobe functioning. We have postulated a behavioral/anatomical model of brain organization that attempts to integrate current clinical and brain-behavior research, while emphasizing the diversity, specificity, and directive role of the frontal lobes. Language was selected as perhaps the best function to highlight the distinction between frontal and "non-frontal" (posterior/basal) functions, emphasizing the active, directive character of the frontal lobe. While many authors have added to these basic concepts, Luria's contributions remain as one of the most important. His teachings serve as an example of the directive and controlling function of speech, since his published writings and his disciples continue to this day to guide neuroscientists. Considering Luria's emphasis on monitoring and verifying, he would agree that research and advancement of knowledge in the functions of the frontal lobes and language must continue.

## REFERENCES

Ackerly, S. S., & Benton, A. L. (1947). Report of a case of bilateral frontal lobe defect. *Research Publications–Association for Research in Nervous and Mental Disease, 27,* 479–504.

Albert, M. L. (1972) Auditory sequencing and left cerebral dominance for language. *Neuropsychologia, 10,* 245–248.

Alexander, M. P. (1984, October). *Frontal language disorders.* Presentation to a neurobehavioral seminar, UCLA School of Medicine, Los Angeles.

Alexander, M. P., Benson, D. F., & Stuss, D. T. (in press). Frontal lobes and languages. *Brain and Language.*

Alexander, M. P., & Schmitt, M. A. (1980). The aphasia syndrome of stroke in the left anterior cerebral artery territory. *Archives of Neurology, 37,* 97–100.

Alexander, M. P., Stuss, D. T., & Benson, D. F. (1979). Capgras syndrome: A reduplicative phenomenon. *Neurology (NY), 29,* 334–339.

Bastian, H. C. (1898). *Aphasia and other speech defects.* London: H. K. Lewis.

Benson, D. F. (1979). *Aphasia, alexia, and agraphia.* New York: Churchill Livingstone.

Benson, D. F., & Geschwind, N. (1971). Aphasia and related cortical disturbances. In A. B. Baker & L. H. Baker (Eds.), *Clinical neurology.* New York: Harper & Row.

Benson, D. F., & Stuss, D. T. (1982). Motor abilities after frontal leukotomy. *Neurology (NY), 32,* 1353–1357.

Benson, D. F., & Stuss, D. T. (in preparation). *Self and the frontal lobes.*

Blumer, D., & Benson, D. F. (1975). Personality changes with frontal and temporal lobe lesions. In D. F. Benson & D. Blumer (Eds.), *Psychiatric aspects of neurologic disease* (Vol. 1, pp. 151–170). New York: Grune & Stratton.

Brown, A. L. (1978). Knowing when, where, and how to remember: A problem of metacognition. In R. Glasser (Ed.), *Advances in instructional psychology* (Vol. 1, pp. 77–165). Hillsdale, NJ: Lawrence Erlbaum Associates.

Brunner, R. J., Kornhuber, H. H., Seemuller, E., Suger, G., & Wallesch, C.–W. (1982). Basal ganglia participation in language pathology. *Brain and Language, 16,* 281–299.

Carver, C., & Scheier, M. F. (1982). Self-awareness and the self-regulation of behavior. In G. Underwood (Ed.), *Aspects of consciousness. Vol. 3: Awareness and self-awareness* (pp. 235–266). New York: Academic Press.

Cavanaugh, J. C., & Borkowski, J. G. (1980). Searching for metamemory-memory connections: A developmental study. *Developmental Psychobiology, 16,* 441–453.

Damasio, A. R., Damasio, H., Rizzo, M., Varney, N., & Gorsh, F. (1982). Aphasia with nonhemorrhagic lesions in the basal ganglia and internal capsule. *Archives of Neurology, 39,* 15–20.

Damasio, A. R., & Van Hoesen, G. W. (1983). Emotional disturbances associated with focal lesions of the limbic frontal lobe. In K. M. Heilman & P. Satz (Eds.), *Neuropsychology of human emotion* (pp. 85–110). New York: Guilford Press.

Darley, F. L. (1968). *Apraxia of speech: 101 years of terminological confusion.* Unpublished paper presented at the annual meeting of the American Speech and Hearing Association.

Dejerine, J. (1914/1977). *Sémiologie des affections du systéme nerveux* (Vol. 2, 3rd ed). Paris: Masson.

Fisher, C. M. (1975). The anatomy and pathology of the cerebral vasculature. In J. S. Myer (Ed.), *Modern concepts of cerebrovascular disease* (pp. 1–42). New York: Spectrum.

Foix, C. (1928). Aphasies. In G. Roger, F. Widal, & P. J. Teissier (Eds.), *Nouveau traité de médecine* (Vol. 18, pp. 135–213). Paris: Masson.

Fuster, J. M. (1980). *The prefrontal cortex. Anatomy, physiology, and neuropsychology of the frontal lobe.* New York: Raven Press.

Goldberg, G., Mayer, N. H., & Toglia, J. U. (1981). Medial frontal cortex infarction and the alien hand sign. *Archives of Neurology, 38,* 683–686.

Jackson, H. (1878). Remarks on non-protrusion of the tongue in some cases of aphasia. *Lancet, 1,* 716. In J. Taylor (Ed.), (1932) *Selected writings of Hughlings Jackson,* Vol. 2. London: Hodder & Stoughton.

Johns, D. F., & Darley, F. L. (1970). Phonemic variability in apraxia of speech. *Journal of Speech and Hearing Research, 13,* 556–583.

Jones–Gotman, M., & Milner, B. (1977). Design fluency: The invention of nonsense drawings after focal cortical lesions. *Neuropsychologia, 15,* 653–674.

Kaczmarek, B. L. J. (1984). Neurolinguistic analysis of verbal utterances in patients with focal lesions of frontal lobes. *Brain and Language, 21,* 52–58.

Kertesz, A. (1979). *Aphasia and associated disorders: Taxonomy, localization and recovery.* New York: Grune & Stratton.

Lecours, A. R., Lhermitte, F., & Bryons, B. (1983). *Aphasiology.* London: Baillière, Tindall.

Levine, D. N., & Mohr, J. P. (1979). Language after bilateral cerebral infarctions: Role of the minor hemisphere in speech. *Neurology (NY), 29,* 927–938.

Lichtheim, L. (1885). On aphasia. *Brain, 7,* 463–484.

Luria, A. R. (1958). Brain disorders and language analysis. *Language and Speech, 1,* 14–34.

Luria, A. R. (1967). The regulative function of speech in its development and dissolution. In K. Salzinger & S. Salzinger (Eds.), *Research in verbal behavior and some neurophysiological implications* (pp. 405–422). New York: Academic Press.

Luria, A. R. (1969). Frontal lobe syndromes. In P. J. Vinken & G. W. Bruyn (Eds.), *Handbook of clinical neurology* (Vol. 2, pp. 725–757). Amsterdam: North Holland.

Luria, A. R. (1970a). The functional organization of the brain. *Scientific American, 222,* 66–78.

Luria, A. R. (1970b). *Traumatic aphasia: Its syndromes, psychology and treatment.* The Hague: Mouton.

Luria, A. R. (1973a). *The working brain. An introduction to neuropsychology* (B. Haigh, Trans.). New York: Basic Books.

Luria, A. R. (1973b). The frontal lobes and the regulation of behavior. In K. H. Pribram & A. R. Luria (Eds.), *Psychophysiology of the frontal lobes* (pp. 3–26). New York: Academic Press.

Luria, A. R. (1974). Language and brain. Towards the basic problems of neurolinguistics. *Brain and Language, 1,* 1–14.

Luria, A. R. (1977). *Neuropsychological studies in aphasia.* Amsterdam: Swets & Zeitlinger.

Luria, A. R. (1980). *Higher cortical functions in man.* New York: Basic Books.

Luria, A. R., & Homskaya, E. D. (1964). Disturbance in the regulative role of speech with frontal lobe lesions. In J. M. Warren & K. Akert (Eds.), *The frontal granular cortex and behavior* (pp. 353–371). New York: McGraw–Hill.

Luria, A. R., Homskaya, E. D., Blinkov, S. M., & Critchley, M. (1967). Impaired selectivity of mental processes in association with a lesion of the frontal lobe. *Neuropsychologia, 5,* 105–117.

Luria, A. R., Pribram, K. H., & Homskaya, E. D. (1964). An experimental analysis of the behavioral disturbance produced by a left frontal arachnoidal endothelioma (meningioma). *Neuropsychologia, 2,* 257–280.

Masdeu, J. C. (1980). Aphasia after infarction of the left supplementary motor area. *Neurology (NY), 30,* 359.

Masdeu, J. C., Schoene, W. C., & Funkenstein, H. (1978). Aphasia following infarction of the left supplementary motor area. *Neurology (NY), 28,* 1220–1223.

Milner, B. (1964). Some effects of frontal lobectomy in man. In J. M. Warren & K. Akert (Eds.), *The frontal granular cortex and behavior* (pp. 313–334). New York: McGraw–Hill.

Milner, B. (1982). Some cognitive effects of frontal lobe lesions in man. In D. E. Broadbent & L. Weiskrantz (Eds.), *The neuropsychology of cognitive function* (pp. 211–226). London: Royal Society.

Milner, B., & Petrides, M. (1984). Behavioural effects of frontal-lobe lesions in man. *Trends in Neuroscience, 7,* 403–407.

Mohr, J. P. (1973). Rapid amelioration of motor aphasia. *Archives of Neurology, 28,* 77–82.

Mohr, J. P., Pessin, M. S., Finkelstein, S., Funkenstein, H. H., Duncan, G. W., & Davis, K. R. (1978). Broca aphasia: Pathologic and clinical aspects. *Neurology (NY), 28,* 311–324.

Monrad–Krohn, G. H. (1947). Dysprosody or altered "melody of language." *Brain, 70,* 405–415.

Naeser, M. A. (1983). CT scan lesion size and lesion locus in cortical and subcortical aphasias. In A. Kertesz (Ed.), *Localization in neuropsychology* (pp. 63–119). New York: Academic Press.

Naeser, M. A., Alexander, M. P., Helm-Estabrooks, N., Levine, H. L., Laughlin, S. A., & Geschwind, N. (1982). Aphasia with predominantly subcortical lesion sites: Description of three capsular/putaminal aphasia syndromes. *Archives of Neurology, 39,* 2–14.

Naeser, M. A., Hayward, R. W., Laughlin, S. A., & Zatz, L. M. (1981). Quantitative CT scan studies in aphasia. I. Infarct size and CT numbers. *Brain and Language, 12,* 140–164.

Petrides, M. (1985). Deficits on conditional associative-learning tasks after frontal- and temporal-lobe lesions in man. *Neuropsychologia, 23,* 601–614.

Petrides, M., & Milner, B. (1982). Deficits on subject-ordered tasks after frontal- and temporal-lobe lesions in man. *Neuropsychologia, 20,* 249–262.

Ross, E. D. (1981). The aprosodias: Functional-anatomic organization of the affective components of language in the right hemisphere. *Archives of Neurology, 38,* 561–569.

Ross, E. D., & Mesulam, M.–M. (1979). Dominant language functions of the right hemisphere? Prosody and emotional gesturing. *Archives of Neurology, 36,* 144–148.

Rubens, A. B. (1975). Aphasia with infarction in the territory of the anterior cerebral artery. *Cortex, 11,* 239–250.

Stuss, D. T., & Benson, D. F. (1986). *The frontal lobes.* New York: Raven Press.

Stuss, D. T., Benson, D. F., Kaplan, E. F., Weir, W. S., Naeser, M. A., Lieberman, A., & Ferrill, D. (1983). The involvement of orbitofrontal cerebrum in cognitive tasks. *Neuropsychologia, 21,* 235–248.

Stuss, D. T., Delgado, M., & Guzman, D. A. (1987). Verbal regulation in the control of motor impersistence: A proposed rehabilitation procedure. *Journal of Neurologic Rehabilitation, 1,* 1–6.

Tonkonogy, J., & Goodglass, H. (1981). Language function, foot of the third frontal gyrus, and rolandic operculum. *Archives of Neurology, 38,* 486–490.

Vygotsky, L. S. (1962). *Thought and language* (E. Hanfmann & G. Vakar, eds. and trans.). Cambridge, MA: MIT Press.

Yussen, S. R. (1985). The role of metacognition in contemporary theories of cognitive development. In D. L. Forrest–Pressley, G. E. MacKinnon, & T. G. Waller (Eds.), *Metacognition, cognition, and human performance. Vol. 1. Theoretical perspectives* (pp. 253–283). Orlando, FL: Academic Press.

# 3

# The Case of Carolyn Wilson[1]— A 38-year Follow-up of a Schizophrenic Patient with Two Prefrontal Lobotomies

*Allan F. Mirsky*
*H. Enger Rosvold*

*Laboratory of Psychology and Psychopathology, National Institute of Mental Health*

## BACKGROUND

One of the major contributions made by Professor Luria during his extremely productive career was to the analysis of the role of the frontal lobes in the support of behavior. He described clearly how such functions as the execution of complex programs of activity, the formation of orienting behavior, and the matching of action to intention—when there is a mismatch between initial intention and the consequences of action—were impaired following frontal lesions. These functions could be labeled as the executive, attentional, and flexibility-shift aspects of human cognitive and problem-solving behavior. The impairment of these functions is illustrated in dramatic fashion in patients with lesions of the frontal lobes, of whom the following case is an example. Carolyn Wilson suffered from schizophrenia of for at least 11 years. After other known treatments had been tried without success, she received a prefrontal lobotomy on December 21, 1946, and then a more posterior section on July 26, 1947. She was able to return to her home after the second operation and although she has never been symptom-free, she has never been rehospitalized. This is an account of her

---

[1]The name and other possibly identifying facts about this patient have been changed. A brief precis of this case has been presented by Valenstein (1986) and the identifying facts conform with those used by him.

life since the surgery, a reconstruction of the events leading to the surgery, and a summary of the neuropsychological studies conducted over the past 40 years. The report concludes with a discussion of the case as if it had been contributed by Professor Luria.

The surgeon's notes regarding the first procedure are presented in their entirety:

12/21/46    *Operation:*   Prefrontal lobotomy
            *Operator:*   Dr. Gorman
            *Anaesthesia:*   I.V. pentothal; local trephine openings were made
            bilaterally 3 ½ cm. to rt. and left of the mid-skull; just in front of the
            coronal sutures. The dura was incised and the dissection carried out by
            electrocautery and suction down to the orbital surface on both sides. The
            lobotomy was thus performed. Very little bleeding was encountered and
            when proper hemostasis was secured, the dura was closed, the bone
            buttons replaced, and the galea and skin closed with interrupted black silk
            sutures. The patient withstood the operative procedure well and was
            returned to the ward in good condition.

The reasons for reoperating Carolyn within a year are not documented, but probably reflect the failure of the first procedure to produce the desired clinical result. There is no record of her being released after the first procedure, and it is presumed that she spent the time in several private sanatoria. Some of the postoperative nursing notes (excerpts to follow) suggest the type of interoperative (and most likely preoperative) behavior that led to the grave decision to perform the second (as well as the first) lobotomy.

12/24/46    (3 days post surgery)
12:00:      (Midnight): Very irritable, noisy. "Breathe, get your eyes out, sit on her,
            you dirt! Quit your dirt and sit on her! You look like a dove. Use your
            brain and stop your poetry. I'm sick of your rosetta stone."
12:45:      Began to sing to the tune wedding bells combining such lines as, "gener-
            als, swords, marriages, crucifixion" . . . Also sang parodies in French
            and German.
3:00 A.M.:  Began to screech at top of voice again and used abusive language. Made
            ugly looking faces with grinding teeth.
6:20 A.M.:  No temperature or blood pressure was taken as I could not handle patient
            alone. Refuses very necessary mouth care. Spits in nurse's face and tries
            biting.

This excerpt is typical of the florid psychotic behavior Carolyn displayed in the hospital, including flight of ideas, mania, verbal and physical aggression, incontinence of urine and feces, and refusal to eat, drink, or to care for herself. A considerable part of the time she was in the hospital, she was in restraint, and was considered dangerous.

The surgeon's notes regarding the second procedure are as follows:

*Date:* 7/26/47
*Operator:* Dr. Gorman
*1st Assistant:* Dr. Hall
*Anesthesia:* I.V. pentothal and endotracheal nitrous oxide, oxygen.
*Procedure:* The forehead was shaved posteriorly to a line between the ear tips and the scars of the previous pre-frontal lobotomy were seen. The area was prepared and draped in the usual manner and the incision was made through the previous lobotomy incision ·on the right side and carried down to the periosteum. The periosteum was densely adherent to the bone and thus was carefully elevated by means of a periosteal elevator. The incision was similarly made and carried down to the periosteum on the left side and the previous bone buttons were removed. The dura was incised in a semicircular fashion and retracted medially. The place of the previous dissection was identified. A ventricular needle was introduced until it hit the floor of the anterior fossa. A new section was made at an angle some 15° posterior to the previous angle. The section was carried in an infero-medial direction to the falx and laterally as well as far as possible with the straight leucotome. However, no sections were made in the superior medial or superior lateral quadrant. A similar section was made on the left side some 15° posterior to the previous place in a similar manner. When hemostasis was adequate, slightly less than lcc of pantopaque was introduced into the left tract and about lcc of pantopaque into the right tract. The dura was closed with interrupted sutures of black silk, several strips of gelfoam were placed along the slightly gaping margins of the dura which had retracted somewhat. The galea was closed with interrupted sutures of black silk and the skin was closed in a similar manner with interrupted sutures of black silk.

The description of the two procedures indicates that both operations used the Lyerly–Poppen procedure, a modification of the standard technique developed by Freeman and Watts. Figure 1 illustrates the Lyerly–Poppen technique.

Clearly, the cumulative effect of the two surgical procedures was to disconnect the majority of the patient's prefrontal regions, particularly in the inferior parts, from the rest of her brain.

The behavior that led to this radical treatment, at least in the immediate inter- and postoperative periods, was as described. We now present a brief resumé of the essential details of the patient's history before the surgery.

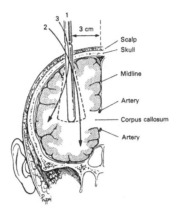

**FIGURE 1**   The Lyerly "open" lobotomy as later modified by James Poppen: (1) The spatula was inserted and then swung laterally; (2 and 3) a suction tube was inserted to extend the damage more deeply and laterally as well as to clean the area of the wound. (From Valenstein, *Great and Desperate Cures,* 1986). The lesion in Carolyn was at least as extensive as shown here, since it was extended medially to the falx (i.e., to the midline) and (at least in part) ventrally to the floor of the anterior fossa. It is possible that there was some damage to the olfactory bulb and tract.

## Premorbid History[2]:

Carolyn Wilson was born into a wealthy family on December 23, 1909. She went to private preparatory schools, as did Claire, her older sister and only sibling. She attended Vassar College and the University of Pennsylvania Medical School, where she completed the first year of studies successfully. Carolyn was enrolled in her second year of medical school when she was hospitalized for a severe psychiatric disorder, not long after her parents broke up a brief and impetuous marriage. The available data do not support entirely the view that the onset of Carolyn's illness was sudden and abrupt; more likely, it represented an exacerbation of moderately severe difficulties that may have been in evidence for some years prior to her hospitalization. Possibly of some bearing is the fact that Carolyn and her mother quarreled bitterly and often, as early as Carolyn's grade-school days.

There are many reports of Carolyn's trying to establish independence from her mother, who was herself quite dependent on her own older sister, Carolyn's aunt. Mrs. Wilson visited her sister in Chicago as often as she could, and took

---

[2]Many of these details were provided to H. E. Rosvold by friends and acquaintances of the Wilson family.

Carolyn with her, willy-nilly. In fact, Carolyn was born in Chicago because her mother did not trust the physicians or hospital facilities in the Grosse Pointe area. Carolyn found Chicago and her mother and aunt tiresome and quarreled with them often. Often, as a teen-ager, she would "disappear" between Grosse Pointe and Chicago; no one would know her whereabouts for days at a time. Whether these episodes were due entirely to adolescent rebelliousness, or whether, in fact, she might occasionally have been in some confused, psychotic-like state for short periods cannot be established. There are a number of reports, however, that she was hospitalized briefly on several occasions, from at least her college days onward, for emotional difficulties. But these were probably labeled physical illnesses, since her first obviously psychiatric hospitalization took place during her second year of medical school.

Therefore, although this hospitalization came shortly after the breakup of Carolyn's brief marriage, the latter event appears to have only served as a trigger rather than a major contributing cause of the illness.

From the period of approximately 1935[3] through 1946, Carolyn was hospitalized at a number of exclusive private psychiatric facilities, most of which were located in the northeastern part of the United States. Available data suggest that she met the diagnosis of a chronic schizophrenia (or possibly schizoaffective disorder) with the classical symptoms of delusions, incoherence, bizarre, and illogical behavior, including obsessions, compulsions, depression, and cognitive deterioration. The symptoms she displayed in the hospital, where her psychosurgery was performed, indicate that there was a strong, manic-like, almost affective coloration to her syndrome, as well. Although we sought to obtain hospital records of her treatment during the period 1935–1946, this effort was almost entirely unsuccessful; consequently, we do not know whether there were extensive or even occasional periods of remission. That there was at least one partial remission is suggested by a note from a private sanitarium dated May 15, 1937. The note reads:

Hawthorne Hill

Wilson, Miss Carolyn

Carolyn's greeting was natural, spontaneous, and friendly. She was clear and fairly definite in her statements, at times showed a little hesitancy and abstraction but not extended nor did it increase during the half hour's interview. There was no sign of fatigue. She did not exhibit any pressure of ideas or feelings, any evidence of depression or delusions. The mild complaints about lack of young people for companions, other patients talking of their ills, and seeing several different doctors

---

[3]Although 1935 would have meant that she was 26 in her second year of medical school rather than 23 or 24 (as the usual chronology would suggest), this is probably due to the interruptions in her schooling occasioned by her hospitalization for "physical" illnesses.

without continuity seemed based on a general sense of dissatisfaction without reference to self, or any discrimination against herself.

Wants a change (in the hospital) or home with a nurse. Agrees that she did not do well with greater freedom, and needs more feeling of security than at present, also that going away now would be such a marked change that it would not be easy to handle. She was urged to accept her present situation, to realize that the doctors are considering what is best for her, that her condition requires time to change, and to stay where she is, gradually working up through the hospital facilities to wider activities and freedom till she can make satisfactory adjustments outside. To join her sister abroad, even with a nurse, would hardly seem a wise move at this time. Before such a change, she should be at a much better level.

Returning home would have been difficult, since both of Carolyn's parents had died in the interim between her first (obvious) psychiatric hospitalization and the prefrontal lobotomy. Her sister would have been a poor companion, let alone caretaker, since her primary interests were in the gay life of an aspiring, albeit well-heeled, artist in the romantic capitals of Europe. Over the years, her sister Claire, and her husband, Dr. Miller, made repeated attempts to have Carolyn join them or at least to have her live with them. This was actually attempted for a brief time after Carolyn's discharge following her second lobotomy. The experience was a disaster. It served temporarily to discourage Claire's attempts to take control of Carolyn's life (and, possibly, her half of her father's estate?). (This issue needs some discussion. Since Mr. Wilson had received the prophetic advice that his daughter was in for a long siege of illness, he arranged for half of his substantial estate to be kept in trust for her. An old friend, who was a former judge of the Michigan probate court, agreed to serve as executor, and later was named conservator of Carolyn's estate. Claire's sisterly efforts to enter and control Carolyn's convalescence and life must be viewed in the light that she had probably spent the bulk of her own half of the Wilson estate before Carolyn's release from the hospital.)

We must therefore conclude, that from the period 1935 through 1946, despite the best available psychiatric care, Carolyn's illness became steadily worse. ECT was used, undoubtedly because it was one of the treatments of choice for manic behavior during this era. Probably it was used rather sparingly, since the treatment network into which Carolyn was directed was psychoanalytical, rather than biological, in orientation. The presumption is that her downhill course during the decade or more of active psychiatric care was not obviously iatrogenic in any sense that we currently understand the term, except for the experience of 11 years of institutionalization. Further, she did not present the picture of a blunted, obtunded, anergic patient. We conclude that as a result of the schizophrenic disorder, the unhappy but still reasonable young patient described in the clinical note from Hawthorne Hill became the delusional, driven, deteriorated, and dangerous wretch for whom psychosurgery was performed twice in a 7-month period in 1946–1947.

## CAROLYN'S POSTOPERATIVE COURSE

### The Early Period

Since, so far as can be determined, there was no substantial change in Carolyn's behavior after the first lobotomy (as well as no available documentation of her interoperative course), we will consider both procedures as a single, radical prefrontal lobotomy. Within several months after the procedure performed on July 26, 1947, Carolyn was ready for discharge. Her assaultive, destructive, and delusional behavior had largely disappeared, and she was tractable and approachable.[4] Although some cognitive abilities seemed grossly intact, she exhibited major impairment in memory, judgment, foresight, and affect and was unable to attend to her personal needs. She was a prime candidate for a nursing home; but, after pressure from sister Claire, the decision was made by her conservator to release her to the custody of her sister in the huge, virtually empty family home in Grosse Pointe. All concerned totally underestimated the amount of care required by a postlobotomy patient. Claire had planned on holding elegant soirees, visits to museums, shopping expeditions to charming boutiques, and trips to Cannes or Deauville; instead, she had to cope with a disoriented woman who could barely anticipate her own bladder and bowel needs, who would eat everything on the dinner table, whether or not it was dinner time, and who could scarcely remember the events of the day. As a result of her overeating, she became noticeably overweight.[5]

Carolyn was taken in hand within a few months after her discharge by a private nurse, Mrs. Church, who (with her husband) happened to be renting rooms in the Wilson mansion. As a nurse, Mrs. Church had had extensive surgical experience, and was very knowledgeable about postoperative management of patients. She had observed the difficulties that Claire was experiencing with Carolyn and felt that she could provide the proper training and care for her. The conservator gave Mrs. Church the opportunity to assume the management of

[4]For some years after the lobotomy, Carolyn was observed occasionally to grimace in such a way as to bare her teeth. The circumstances that would lead to this behavior are obscure, although they sometimes seemed to be related to frustration of a desired goal. Nevertheless, it seems reasonable to assume that this might represent a pallid, primitive remnant of the aggressive biting that made Carolyn so difficult to care for in her late preoperative period.

[5]It is interesting to speculate whether Carolyn's bulimic behavior, in which she appeared not to have distinguished among foods, and ingested large amounts of food, is related to surgically induced damage to the orbital surface of the frontal lobe and/or to the olfactory bulb and tract. Potter and Butters (1980) reported significant impairment of odor-quality discrimination in patients with prefrontal lesions.

the case; this she did with great assurance, and succeeded in civilizing Carolyn to such an extent that she could go out (accompanied) to public places such as restaurants and theaters.

The following is excerpted from a report to the conservator by Dr. Burness Moore, a psychiatric consultant who participated in Carolyn's treatment in the early postoperative period. The report was based on two visits to the patient in which he was accompanied by Dr. Rosvold in April, 1949. The document was stimulated in part by pressure from indefatigable sister Claire, who still wished to make Carolyn part of her own bohemian life.

## *Appearance and Behavior*

At the time of our visit to her residence, Miss Wilson answered the door and greeted the examiner by name. She had been told approximately an hour earlier that we would visit. She was attractively dressed and neat and cleanly in appearance. She led the visitors into the living room but neglected to introduce us to her nurse, Mrs. Robert Church, who had come forward meanwhile. Miss Wilson was smiling and pleasant, and responded readily to the questions which were asked of her. She claimed to remember very little about her illness before her operations, but on questioning answered with information which was approximately correct, although it was apparent to the examiner, under whose care she had been at the time of her operation, that her memory was defective for many details. For example, she said she had had her first mental breakdown after she had graduated from medical school and while she was serving an internship. It is known to the examiner that the patient's breakdown occurred during her second year of medical school and that she never completed medical school. She was unable to recall any of the names of her professors. Her account of her hospitalizations was somewhat mixed up. During the interview she frequently turned to Mrs. Church as though asking her to help her out. When Mrs. Church voluntarily retired from the room, Miss Wilson went on to answer questions as best she could without any show of anxiety. Later, while the examiner and Dr. Rosvold inspected the house and talked with Mrs. Church upstairs, the patient remained in the living room. . . . At the time of our departure she again behaved appropriately and made the usual parting courtesies.

Mrs. Church informed us that Miss Wilson was somewhat irritable when she first came under her care, but during the past few months she has become more pleasant and contented. She is at all times cooperative and obediently follows Mrs. Church's instructions. She would, however, wear the same dress day after day and would tend to be careless about personal cleanliness if it were not for Mrs. Church's surveillance. She plays at cards and children's games with Mrs. Church's children aged 8 and 6 and never becomes disturbed or irritable with them. At mealtime she tends to rapidly eat all food of one type, before going on to other foods. Under Mrs. Church's directions, however, she had dieted and has lost considerable weight. She enjoys looking at the television programs with the rest of the family and seems to laugh and react appropriately to the content of the programs. She reads considerably, but is unable to tell any stories which she has read. If left alone she tends to look at the pictures of men in magazines and giggles in a silly fashion. She goes downtown shopping and to the movies with Mrs. Church, but is suggestable and cannot be trusted entirely to make her own purchases.

## Emotional Status

On both occasions that she was examined, Miss Wilson was smiling most of the time in a somewhat vacuous way. She laughed when a remark properly called for this emotional display, but there were a few occasions when her laughter was inappropriate. At no time did she appear to become serious. On the other hand, she did not appear to be overly euphoric and denied that she has any depression. There was little evidence of any tension or anxiety during either of the interviews.

## Mental Functions

Both recent and remote memory are obviously and seriously impaired. On the second occasion she stated that we had seen her previously in February, but when this statement was questioned she modified it to 2 or 3 weeks ago. Orientation was correct except that she missed the day of the week by 2 days. Immediate recall of 5 objects was failed almost completely. She was able to remember an address but gave the number incorrectly, was unable to remember a flower, a date or a number immediately after these had been repeated to her twice and she had repeated them after the examiner. Five minutes later she could not recall any of the objects given. She was able to perform a few simple arithmetical problems, but failed when more than 2 manipulations were required. She subtracted 7 from 100 serially with normal rapidity but with 4 failures. She was able to paraphrase proverbs, but obviously missed the abstraction required in proper understanding of the proverbs. She gave the correct responses to 3 questions about behavior in social situations, but apparently recognized her lack of judgment in responding that the population of New York City was a million, 20 million, 300 million and Grosse Point has a population of 300 thousand. Throughout this examination her attention was good and she cooperated well in tasks despite previous psychological examination by Dr. Rosvold. Throughout her speech was relevant and she responded coherently.

## Conclusions

Since the patient was last seen by this examiner in November 1947, approximately 5 months after her second lobotomy operation, it is apparent that she has undergone marked improvement in behavior and mental functioning. In November, 1947, the patient was still quite retarded in motor activity and was still disoriented and untidy, even though her assaultive intractable behavior disappeared. She now presents a quite acceptable appearance, is healthy physically, and gives every evidence of being happy and contented. There are still defects in her mental functioning, in the way of memory defect and somewhat poor judgment in reasoning ability, *but this is to be expected in the light of her prolonged mental illness and the 2 lobotomy operations* (emphasis added). However, it seems likely that her present good condition is in part largely attributable to the excellent care which she is receiving. This care is definitely of a superior sort, and the cost of approximately $91.00 per week is exceptionally reasonable. The patient is quite dependent on Mrs. Church, and in the opinion of this examiner it would be unwise to disturb her present excellent adjustment by any change whatsoever. The patient is able to accept only limited responsibilities, and the stresses and strains of too much travel and social contacts in which she would feel inferior to others should be avoided.

The underlined sentence in the last paragraph epitomizes the difficulty in interpreting the behavioral deficits seen in Carolyn: How is it possible to disentangle the effects due to the schizophrenic illness, to the 11 years of (possibly) deleterious institutional care, and to the extensive frontal lobe damage produced by the two psychosurgical procedures? This April, 1949 report (when Carolyn was nearly 40 years of age) could be substituted virtually word for word for a description of Carolyn's mental capacities and functioning 39 years later, in 1987; there has been no striking change in her condition in the 37 years she has been followed. At present she would pass unnoticed in any gathering and appears to be what she is: a well-bred and well-behaved lady who is approaching her 80th year. We return to the psychological assessment in a subsequent section of this report.

## Carolyn's Postoperative Course: 1949–1987

Carolyn's behavior is in some ways unchanged by the passage of time, and in other ways has been modified in the direction of greater socialization. She still has the tendency to buy the first item she sees in a store, using little discretion as to size, color, or style. In drugstores her chief interest is the magazine rack and in viewing pictures of males which she strokes and fondles. Gradually Carolyn learned to walk around her own block unattended and, with special relish, the two blocks to church. Earlier, on two of these occasions she started small fires which she extinguished of her own accord. In the process, however, she sustained minor burns. In the past she learned to type but had difficulty composing a letter and in generating content. The total production generally was very simple and childlike and rarely exceeded 150 words. As a rehabilitative effort she worked in the local public library, where she filed cards tirelessly and without error.

Under the care of Mrs. Church, the two caretakers who succeeded her, and a succession of tutors and companions, Carolyn has maintained a stable, uneventful, and placid existence. The current caretaker is Mrs. Swanson. Carolyn rises early in the morning, so as to have breakfast with the family, bathes, makes her bed, selects her clothing for the day, and reviews the activities planned for the day. In summer, she might swim laps in the pool (observed by Mrs. Swanson) behind the house, or help pick some of the vegetables for the day's meals from the vegetable garden grown by Mr. Swanson. Earlier, when living with the Church family, she spent summers with them at the beach, where she enjoyed swimming, an activity which she does well. She is treated by the Swansons much like an elderly aunt who is somewhat senile: with loving care and attention, but little chance for independent action, and with constant vigilance lest she injure herself. On one occasion more than 30 years earlier, she stepped into a scalding hot tub and burned herself seriously. She has little sense of how hot water is, and whether it is at an injurious temperature.

Twice a week, the Swansons are spelled in their care of Carolyn by Mrs. Cermak, a retired nurse, who takes Carolyn on excursions to local restaurants, dinner-theaters or movies. Stimulation has always been part of the regimen for Carolyn; it was recommended to the original conservator, and to his successor. There was early a concerted effort, generally instigated by sister Claire, to elevate Carolyn to activities and "cultural experiences" appropriate to one of her station, that is, a member of one of the most prominent Grosse Pointe families. This has taken various forms, including piano lessons, art lessons (which seemed to eventuate mostly in the preparation of scrap books), and physical activities such as swimming and tennis and trips. Carolyn bowls passably well and has participated with a bowling "team" of other middle-aged and elderly persons.

The early attempts to allow her some independence and freedom of action were unsuccessful. For example, to receive her art lessons, she had merely to take a designated bus from a bus stop a short distance from her caretaker's home. Although she was well rehearsed in the number of the bus, and her eventual destination, she would invariably take the first bus to come along and end up lost. Trips unsupervised by Mrs. Church appeared to be occasions to eat enormous amounts of food in a restaurant, with relatively little appreciation of the setting or the countryside. If given her own choice, Carolyn would order the first two or three things on the menu and then proceed to eat them ravenously. What follows is a note from a visit that Rosvold made to Grosse Pointe in 1953, during which he had lunch with Carolyn at a restaurant and allowed her to order unsupervised.

> She was in very good spirits today and quite jovial about everything. We went to Hofheimer's and she enjoyed it. Again she ordered the first thing on the menu—and this time she amazed even the waitress. "Potato pancakes, macaroni and french fries;" the waitress looked at her as much as to say 'Good Lord! How do you keep so

*TABLE 1*

Wechsler IQ scores for Carolyn Wilson Selected Scores, 1948–1984

| Age | 39 | 41 | 43 | 45 | 49 | 52 | 74 | 75 |
| --- | --- | --- | --- | --- | --- | --- | --- | --- |
| Date | 11/17/48 | 4/20/50 | 7/11/52 | 2/27/54 | 9/27/58 | 4/29/61 | 10/5/81[a] | 8/29/84[b] |
| Full Scale IQ | 103 | 108 | 119 | 119 | 124 | 125 | 117 | 101 |
| Verbal IQ | 103 | 106 | 121 | 109 | 119 | 119 | 115 | 100 |
| Performance IQ | 102 | 110 | 115 | 127 | 127 | 125 | 116 | 103 |
| Information | 11 | 11 | 11 | 13 | 11 | 13 | 12 | 10 |
| Comprehension | 5 | 8 | 13 | 10 | 13 | 12 | 9 | 8 |
| Digit Span | 13 | 14 | 14 | 11 | 11 | 10 | 10 | 8 |
| Arithmetic | 10 | 10 | 13 | 7 | 12 | 10 | 9 | 6 |
| Similarities | 9 | 3 | 8 | 8 | 12 | 11 | 11 | 9 |
| Vocabulary | 13 | 14 | 14 | 15 | 14 | 15 | 12 | 9 |
| Picture Arr. | 4 | 6 | 9 | 11 | 6 | 8 | 6 | 4 |
| Picture Compl. | 8 | 6 | 6 | 12 | 9 | 10 | 8 | 5 |
| Block Design | 11 | 12 | 12 | 13 | 18 | 14 | 12 | 10 |
| Obj. Assemb. | 12 | 12 | 14 | 16 | 15 | 15 | 8 | 7 |
| Digit Symbol | 9 | 12 | 11 | 10 | 12 | 11 | 8 | 6 |

[a]Wechsler Adult Intelligence Scale (WAIS); [b]WAIS—Revised Form
All other tests are from the Wechsler–Bellevue scale.

Subsequent tests have shown a resumption of Carolyn's energy and abilities following Mrs. Swanson's successful convalescence.

The tests generally show a substantial increase in abilities about 5 years postsurgery (1952), which has been maintained more or less intact until the recent temporary decline. Carolyn's strengths have been in information, vocabulary, and in the perceptual-cognitive problem-solving skills tapped by the Block Design and Object Assembly Subtests. Although the Block Design test (in particular) is often thought to be a sensitive indicator of frontal lobe or cerebral damage, it has not proven to be so in this case. Weaknesses over the years have been in Picture Arrangement and Picture Completion (possibly reflecting her inability to manage more than routine, superficial social tasks), with occasional low scores in Comprehension and Similarities.

Aside from Carolyn's pervasive remote memory deficit, the most striking of her cognitive losses is seen in tasks requiring a flexible approach to problem solving and the ability to modify her behavior adaptively as the situation requires. This is revealed most vividly in the Wisconsin Card Sorting Test (WCST), (Grant & Berg, 1948). This task is particularly sensitive to dorsolateral frontal cortical damage. It requires the subject to sort a set of test cards that depict symbols (triangle, cross, circle, star) varying in number and color, in accordance with a set of samples. Since the test cards may not match the samples, the subject has to choose the attribute (color, form, number) with which to sort. The examiner calls a sort "right" or "wrong" and, once the subject has sorted 10 in row correctly, changes the category. The usual order of sorting calls for the subject to go through color-form-and number, and then to repeat, until 128 cards have been sorted. Carolyn has been administered this test approximately 50 times since 1950 and has been unable to solve it.

One of the methods of scoring this test involves tallying the number of errors, which are classified in several ways including total errors, perseverative errors, nonperseverative errors, unique errors and so on. Carolyn typically will fixate on either color or number and make 80 or more perseverative errors. Another method of scoring involves counting the number of categories achieved, with one category defined as sorting by color, form, or number for 10 trials in a row. Normal subjects may achieve 9 or 10 categories in sorting 128 cards. On occasion over the years, Carolyn has been able to achieve one category, but has never been able to shift independently to a second category. Table 2 presents samples of four administrations of the WCST when Carolyn was 41, 51, 61, and 73 years old respectively. C. N, or F indicates the nature of the particular sorting principle on a given trial. Two or three letters (e.g., CN, CF, or CNF) means that the test card matched the sample on two or more categories. U indicates a unique match, not in accordance with C, F, or N. An X indicates an incorrect placement. On the December 3, 1960, test, Carolyn began with numbers, switched after one trial to color, and proceeded to sort the remaining 120-plus cards on the basis of color; this occurred despite the fact that on the next 87 trials the sort by color was called incorrect. On the October 23, 1970, test, Carolyn chose number; she was called correct for this choice and was then able to achieve 10 correct trials in a row. She was unable to shift to another category, however, and made 118 perseverative "number" choices in a row, of which 85 were called wrong. On numerous occasions, the examiner, in attempting to test the limits of her impairment, discussed the general idea of the test (i.e., to shift from one sorting principle to another) and by guiding her performance on a trial-by-trial basis, was able to get her to achieve 2 or 3 categories. Without such guidance, Carolyn would immediately lapse into a perseverative number or color sort. A variety of other tests were administered to Carolyn over the years, some of them repeatedly. The test results will not be reviewed here. In the main, if a test suggested a cognitive loss in 1948, 1949, or 1950, it has remained in the impaired range. Similarly, capacities that appeared to have been intact or spared or that showed substantial recovery from 1948 to 1950 have for the most part remained intact. As Carolyn approaches her 80th year, however, some waning of cognitive skills, particularly those dependent on speedy performance, would not be unexpected.

In 1981, a full-scale neuropsychological and neurological evaluation of Carolyn was conducted at the National Institute of Mental Health. An abbreviated summary of the neuropsychological examination is presented in Table 3.

## *Psychophysiological Recording—Evaluation of P300*

As part of a complete evaluation of central nervous system functioning, it was our purpose to evaluate whether the P300 component of the event-related brain potential could be recorded in Carolyn Wilson. The P300 has been shown in numerous investigations to be a sensitive measure of the deployment of attention (Duncan–Johnson & Donchin, 1977). To this effect, a go/no-go reaction time task was used to elicit P300, in which the target stimulus was a rare tone. The choice of a paradigm to elicit P300 was based on previous work, which has shown that large P300s can be elicited by rare stimuli in schizophrenic (e.g., Verleger & Cohen, 1978; Duncan–Johnson, Roth & Kopell, 1984) as well as normal control subjects (e.g., Duncan–Johnson & Donchin, 1982).

Tone bursts (500 Hz, 60-msec. duration) were presented binaurally through earphones (TDH-39) at the rate of one every 1.5 sec. The tones were either "loud" or "soft" and were delivered in a Bernoulli sequence. (Intensity ratings were made by the experimenters and confirmed by the subject.) The probability of occurrence of the soft tone on any trial was .10 in the first and third trial blocks and .30 in the second block. The loud tone was presented at the complementary probability, .90 or .70.

The EEG was recorded from FPz, Fz, Cz, Pz, and Oz referred to linked mastoids. EOG was recorded from electrodes in the orbital region. Stimulus presentation and data collection were controlled by a PDP-11/34 computer.

*TABLE 2*

Representative Wisconsin Card Sorting Test Performances: 1950–1982

| | Apr. 20, 1950; Age 41 | Dec. 3, 1960; Age 51 | Oct. 23, 1970[a]; Age 61 | Oct. 6, 1982; Age 73 |
|---|---|---|---|---|
| 1 | F | N | CFN | N |
| 2 | N | N | CN | N |
| 3 | F | NC | CN | CN |
| 4 | F | NC | C | CN |
| 5 | N | N | CN | N |
| 6 | C | NC | CN | CN |
| 7 | F | NC | C | CF |
| 8 | N | NF | CN | CN |
| 9 | CN | NC | C | N |
| 10 | C | N | CN | FN |
| 11 | U | NF | CF | N |
| 12 | U | FC | CN | CN |
| 13 | N | NC | C | CF |
| 14 | CNF | N | CF | CFN |
| 15 | CN | N | CF | CN |
| 16 | N | N | C | N |
| 17 | NF | NF | C | FN |
| 18 | N | N | CN | N |

| | | | | | | | | | | | | | | | | | | | | | | |
|---|---|---|---|---|---|---|---|---|---|---|---|---|---|---|---|---|---|---|---|---|---|---|
| 19 | N | NC x | N | NC x | N | N | CF | CF x | C | N | N | N | NC | N | N | N | N | CN | CN x | CN | N x | CN x |
| 20 | NF | N x | N | C x | NF x | N | CF x | C | CF | N | N | N | N | N | N | N | N | N | N x | N | N | N x |
| 21 | CN | NF x | N | N x | NC | NF | CN | CN x | CNF | N | N | NFC | NFC | FN | FN | CFN | CN | FN | FN x | FN x | CFN | CFN |
| 22 | CN | NC | NFC | NFC x | NC | NC | CN | CN | C | NC | NC | NFC | NC | CN | CN | C x | CFN | CN x | CN | CFN x | CN | N x |
| 23 | N | N | N | N x | C | C | C | C x | C | NC | NFC | N | NFC | N | N | N | CN | N | N | N | N | N x |
| 24 | N | N | C | C x | N | NF | C | C | C | NF | NF | NF | NF | N | N x | NF | NF | NF | NF x | NF | N x | NF x |
| 25 | NF | NF | U | C x | NF x | N | C | C x | C | NF | NF | NF | NF | FN | FN | FN | FN | FN | FN x | FN | NF x | NF x |
| 26 | N | N | FN | FN x | N | NF | CF x | CF | C | N | N | N | NF | N | N | N | FN | FN | FN x | FN | N x | N x |
| 27 | C | NF | N | N x | NF | N | CFN | CFN | CFN | NF | NF | NF | NF | N | N | N | N | N | FN x | FN x | FN | FN x |
| 28 | CFN | NFC x | U | U x | NFC | NF | C | C | C | NFC | NFC | NFC | NFC | CNF | CFN | CFN | FN | CFN | CFN x | CFN | CFN x | CFN |
| 29 | F | N x | FN | C x | N | FN | CFN x | CF | CFN | N | N | N | N | N | N | N | N | N | N x | N | CFN x | N x |
| 30 | N | FNC x | N | NCF x | N | N | CF | CF x | CF | N | N | N | N | N | N | N | N | N | N x | N | N x | CFN x |
| 31 | N | FC x | N | N x | N | N | CNF x | CF | CF | N | N | N | N | N | N | N | N | N | N x | N | N x | CFN x |
| 32 | NC | FC x | NC | N x | NC | NC | C | C x | C | NC | NC | NC | NC | CN | CN | CN | CN | CN | N | CN x | N | N x |
| Number Correct: | 46 | | | | 40 | | | | | 43 | | | | 35 | | | | | | | | |
| Number of Errors | 82 | | | | 88 | | | | | 85 | | | | 93 | | | | | | | | |
| Number of Categories | 0 | | | | 1 | | | | | 1 | | | | 0 | | | | | | | | |

ᵃIn this administration, Carolyn was reinforced for sorting by number, although the test calls for starting with color before shifting to number. The examiner's intent was to see whether she could shift to color after the experience of being rewarded for sorting according to her spontaneous choice—number. The effort failed and she perseverated on number for an additional 118 trials.

## TABLE 3

Neuropsychological Evaluation of Carolyn Wilson, October 1981 (Age 72) Wechsler Adult Intelligence Scale[a]

| | | |
|---|---|---|
| | Verbal IQ: | 115 |
| | Performance IQ: | 116 |
| | Full Scale IQ | 117 |

Wechsler Memory Scale

Memory Quotient (MQ):                  100 (somewhat impaired, compared with IQ)

Memory Testing

Generally, mild to moderate impairment on all tasks; increases with effortfulness of task. Substantial, but erratic impairment of remote memory.

Attention Testing

Reaction time: moderate impairment for age (20–50 msec)
Continuous Performance Test (Rosvold, Mirsky, Sarason, Bransome, & Beck, 1956):
              X task: 79% correct (Impaired)
              AX task: 97% correct (Nonimpaired)
Wisconsin Card Sorting Test: Failed to achieve one category on two examinations; 80+ perseverative errors
[b]Stroop Test (Stroop, 1935): impairment seen on interference index
[b]Trail Making Test (Reitan, 1958): (Nonimpaired)

Special Tests

| | |
|---|---|
| Luria–Nebraska (Golden et al. 1980): | All scores within normal limits |
| Gorham's Proverbs (Gorham, 1956): | Moderately Impaired |
| [c]Pattern Perception[d] | Moderately Impaired |
| [c]Raven's Progressive Matrices (Raven, 1960): | Moderate Impaired |
| [c]Porteus Maze Test (Porteus & Kepner, 1944): | Normal performance; Maze IQ: 122 |

Summary:    The most noteworthy aspects of this performance are as follows:
1. Relatively well-preserved psychometric intellectual skills.
2. Moderate to severe loss on special tests of cognitive ability, especially those measuring "executive" functions.
3. Moderate to severe impairment on all tests of memory.
4. Variable losses in tests of attention or vigilance, ranging from impaired (WCST, CPT-X task) to intact (CPT-AX task; Trail Making Test).
5. No impairment as assessed by Trail Making, Luria–Nebraska, or Porteus Maze Tests.

[a]The subtest scores appear in Table 1.
[b]Administered at an earlier date and included here for completeness.
[c]These tests were also administered earlier to Carolyn (i.e., during the period 1950–1975) with similar results.
[d]The Pattern Perception Test, a visual-perceptual task similar to the Raven's Progressive Matrices, measures adequacy of visual-perceptual capacities.

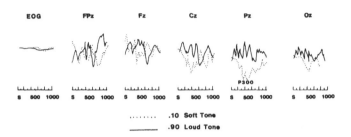

**FIGURE 2** Average event-related brain potentials elicited by the soft (.10) and loud (.90) tones, superimposed for the EOG and EEG leads. The rare and frequent averages are composed of two and four trials, respectively. Stimulus occurrence is indicated by an S on the time scale. Positivity at the scalp electrode with respect to the reference electrodes is plotted as a downward deflection.

The subject was instructed to listen to the series of tones and to press a button as quickly as possible following each soft tone. The subject was cautioned to avoid blinking or looking down at her hand when she pressed the button. Trials were automatically excluded from the average if, contaminated by artifacts.

Performance was 100% correct in each trial block. However, due to consistent eye blinks time-locked to presentation of the tones, data from the first two trial blocks had to be totally discarded. In the third block, the data were recorded with the subject's eyes closed. Our technique of EOG editing eliminated most of the contamination due to eye movement. The number of trials included in the averages of the soft (.10) and loud (.90) tones were two and four, respectively. The averages based on these trials are presented in Figure 2.

Whereas the low signal-to-noise ratio in our data makes any interpretation ambiguous, the pattern of results suggests that the rare stimulus elicited a P300 that was absent in the event-related potential elicited by the frequent stimulus. This statement is based on the latency of the positive peak seen in the Cz and Pz waveforms elicited by the rare stimulus. The averages associated with the rare and frequent stimuli are superimposed at the five EEG leads in Figure 2 to facilitate comparison. It is notable that the scalp distribution of the P300, with a parietal maximum, is not typical of a 72-year-old. In elderly subjects, P300 is typically of equal amplitude at Fz, Cz, and Pz (Ford, Roth, Mohs, Hopkins, & Kopell 1979). The atypical distribution may be a consequence of the extensive damage to prefrontal cortex.

## Neurological Evaluation

Carolyn was also given a full battery of neurological tests, including a CT scan and PET scan (based on 2-fluoro-deoxyglucose). The lesions caused by the psychosurgical procedures were clearly evident in the CT scan, in areas of massive destruction of the tissue of the frontal lobes (Figure 3). The results of the PET scan were similarly quite dramatic: the anterior 30–40% of the entire cerebrum, comprising primarily the prefrontal regions, was severely, if not totally, hypometabolic (Figure 4). This suggests that the prefrontal areas of Carolyn's brain are largely nonfunctional.

## Affective Behavior, Emotion and Personality

In a number of places in this account there has been mention of Carolyn's affective behavior. Aside from the grimacing and teeth baring that she shows on occasion, the meaning of which is uncertain, Carolyn's demeanor is markedly placid and unruffled. A recent instance of grimacing is provided by Mrs. Cermak. Carolyn tends, on occasion, to keep her coat on even when the indoor temperature does not warrant it. When told to remove it, she will do so but bares her teeth while so doing. Strong affect or emotion is rarely (if ever) observed, and she appears to have no close emotional or affective ties to any person or thing. She will laugh in a shallow but appropriate way in interpersonal contexts but appears to take her cue as to whether or not to laugh from what others are doing. This underlines the extent to which she is sensitive to what we might call "positive" social cues. However, this sensitivity does not extend to "negative" social cues. A striking example of the absence of emotional involvement is provided by her behavior after the death in 1963 of Mr. Church, the husband of her first caretaker. Although she had known this man well for more than 15 years, she was unmoved by his death and showed no sign or expression of grief, despite the fact that Mrs. Church and her two sons were much affected. More recently Mrs. Cermak hit a dog while driving with Carolyn to a restaurant. Carolyn was unperturbed by this event.

An MMPI test administered to Carolyn as part of her 1981 evaluation at NIMH showed a high score on the schizophrenia scale, a residual of her prior illness. The test did not reveal much else, except for a tendency to classify many cards in the "can't say" category. The high schizophrenia score was also seen in a 1984 MMPI administration.

## CAROLYN WILSON AS EVALUATED BY LURIA

Although Carolyn was never seen by Professor Luria, we might speculate as to what he might have said about her, based on his writings, especially in *Higher Cortical Functions in Man* (Luria, 1966).

"This is indeed a most interesting case, and the 40-year followup is remarkable. Interpretation of the symptoms is of course complicated by the fact that she suffered from severe psychiatric problems prior to the frontal lobe lesion result-

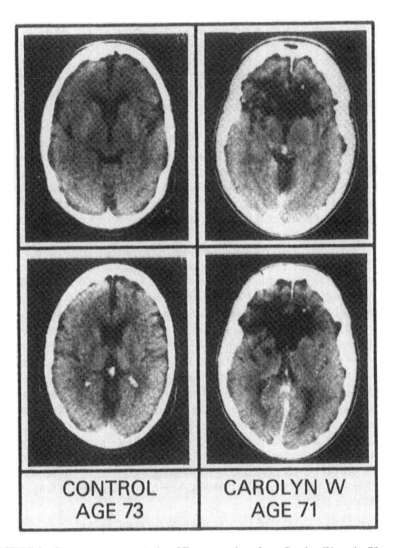

**FIGURE 3** Shown are representative CT-scan sections from Carolyn W. and a 73-year-old female control subject free of obvious neurological disorder. Carolyn's scan shows evidence of massive damage to the prefrontal areas and increased ventricular size following introduction of the leucotome and suction tube. Evidence of the first (more anterior) and second (more posterior) sections can be seen in the more anterior and posterior darkened regions, indicative of tissue loss.

ing from her lobotomies. We also used lobotomy treatment in the Soviet Union for difficult cases, prior to the introduction of the neuroleptic medications. Some have written recently that schizophrenia is a disease of the frontal lobes; this is not exactly a new idea. My student, Goldberg, has recently pointed out some of the problems with this concept (Goldberg, 1985). If we took it seriously, it would make it difficult, if not impossible, to decide which of her symptoms can be attributed to which cause. Nevertheless, I believe that many of Miss Wilson's behaviors are quite typical of those seen in patients with frontal lobe disease and can be unambiguously attributed to the lesion, whatever coloration may have been added by her psychiatric problems. I have often noted in cases of frontal lobe injury or disease, that aside from the disturbances of organized, goal-directed behavior (which this woman shows clearly), there can be profound emotional changes. Failure does not cause any prolonged emotional reaction (as in being told "wrong" for 90 choices on the card-sorting task). She shows indifference to her surroundings and, unlike other persons with brain lesions, will not show any marked emotional conflicts. So her behavior after the death of her caretaker's husband and the incident with the dog are not unexpected.

"Concerning her most interesting pattern of intellectual deficits, I am not surprised that her IQ tests are in the normal or superior range. Hebb, some years ago, described a case with a superior IQ despite the presence of a complete hemispherectomy. Special tests are needed to reveal how the patient solves the problem. I have developed such tests and find sympathetic to my own view the tests developed by Goldstein, Scherer, and Weigl of the impaired abstract, categorical behavior. The card-sorting test shows nicely the tendency of such patients to perseverate on one particular link of a perceptual-motor act. It reminds me of a patient who, in working in the carpenter's shop, kept on planing a plank until he began to plane the bench itself. This behavior shows also the failure of the regulating function of speech in such lesions. Although she may have verbalized to herself, "This is wrong. I should sort the next card by form," she cannot form the necessary system of verbal connections to regulate this motor sequence. Such cases are untrainable. She will never again regain the regulating function of a plan or intention over her behavior even if you test her for 100 years!

"The problems with attention that this woman shows, as in the X task of the CPT, reaction time and the Stroop test, remind us of the important connection between the reticular formation and the analyzers of the frontal lobes. The procedure developed by Ivanov–Smolensk is much like the CPT and has been used to illuminate this fundamental symptom of the frontally injured person. Homskaya and I have also described similar findings, which we have identified as failure of the regulating function of speech in these subjects. Miss Wilson can surely say "X—I press" or "Y—I do not," but to translate this into an efficient motor sequence is difficult for her. The additional reminder or alerting stimulus provided by the A in the AX task enables her to overcome this defect to a large

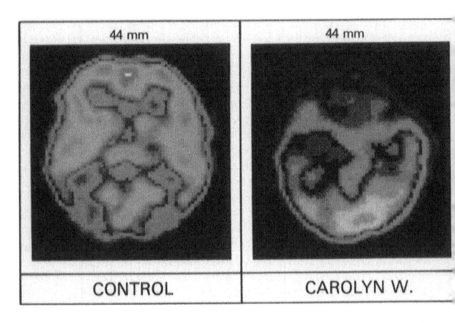

**FIGURE 4** PET Scan of Carolyn Wilson and a control subject, 2-fluoro-deoxyglucose administration. Carolyn's scan shows evidence of a massive area of hypometabolic cortex in the prefrontal regions of the brain. Dark blue indicates low or absent glucose utilization; lighter colors indicate greater glucose utilization. Thus, whites and reds indicate greatest utilization, orange and yellow moderate utilization, and so on.

extent. If her lesion were larger, even this compensatory action would be denied her.

"I should like to point out another aspect of her frontal disability. I note with interest her rather consistent and persistent failure on those Wechsler subtests requiring the placement of a series of pictures into a correct sequence (Picture Arrangement) or the identification of the missing element of a pictorial gestalt (Picture Completion). These defects point again to her inability to develop an overall scheme requiring a sequence of actions or to observe the lack of a key missing element. The overall integrative-conceptual drive provided by the frontal lobes is gone.

"Two last points. One concerns the memory deficit this woman shows. Rosvold, Pribram and Mishkin (following the earlier lead of Finan, Harlow, and Jacobsen) developed sophisticated animal models in monkeys of problem-solving behavior—the delayed response and delayed alternation tasks—and showed how vulnerable these behaviors are to frontal lobe injury. This is certainly a vivid demonstration of that defect.

"And finally, I applaud the use of the psychophysiological procedure, the P300 method, to show the failure of attention to be manifest in the frontal and central analyzers, as seen in the respective leads. I was especially interested to note that the patient was unable to restrain her eye-blinks during the P300 recording procedure, according to the description provided. I have presented some examples of failure to exhibit normal eye-movement patterns in frontal-lobe cases (Luria 1966); this I believe is fundamental to the general gnostic failure seen in these patients. It is a pity that more such studies could not have been done with this patient. However, the P300 phenomenon reminds me of the theorizing of my colleague, W. Kohler, about the accumulation of positive hydrogen ions during perceptual operations.

"To summarize, I believe that these symptoms are clearly attributable to the frontal lesion that this woman sustained in 1946–1947; the multiplicity of symptoms also attests to the numerous functions that are supported by the prefrontal cortex and bring into sharp relief the major organizing, executive, affective, and mnestic capacities dependent on the analyzers in the frontal lobes of the brain.

## CONCLUSION

We have presented the data on Carolyn Wilson in this volume honoring Professor Luria because we believe that it is a case that would have interested him greatly; moreover, it is a case that displays many of the symptoms of frontal lobe injury that he described so clearly and dramatically in his writings.

Carolyn's life is as decent as it is because of the availability of the resources left her by her father and the dedication and wisdom of her conservators, caretakers, and companions. The decision to perform psychosurgery in 1946–1947 did result in an enormous reduction of her psychiatric symptoms, but at the cost of major cognitive losses. It did provide her with an opportunity to participate in some of the good things in life. Whether she would have ever recovered spontaneously (as some recent longterm follow-up studies of schizophrenic patients by M. Bleuler suggests) or would have died in a psychiatric hospital cannot be known. We think that the decision was correct at the time.

The case we have presented is, we believe, no less interesting than cases such as Henry, who sustained a permanent memory loss after a bilateral medial temporal lobe resection (Milner, 1966). The data demonstrate what is possible to achieve with a severely brain-injured person, given almost unlimited resources.

## ACKNOWLEDGMENTS

Thanks are due to the following persons who assisted in the examination of Carolyn Wilson during her stay at the clinical center of the National Institutes of Health (NIH) in 1981 and who allowed us to use some of their information in the preparation of this case history: Drs. Connie C. Duncan, Monte Buchsbaum, Henry Holcomb, Herbert Lansdell, Theodore P. Zahn and Herbert Weingartner; also Pamela Schwerdt and Sheila Smallberg Cohen, and Lee Mann. Thanks are also due to Carolyn's conservator, who permitted her to visit NIH so that we could conduct some of the examinations described in this report.

## REFERENCES

Duncan–Johnson, C. C., & Donchin, E. (1977). On quantifying surprise: The variation of event-related potentials with subjective probability. *Psychophysiology, 14*, 456–467.

Duncan–Johnson, C. C., & Donchin, E. (1982). The P300 component of the event-related brain potential as an index of information processing. *Biological Psychology, 14*, 1–52.

Duncan–Johnson, C. C., Roth, W. T., & Kopell, B. S. (1984). Effects of stimulus sequence on P300 and reaction time in schizophrenics: A preliminary report. In R. Karrer, J. Cohen, & P. Tueting (Eds.), *Brain and information: Event related potentials*. New York Academy of Science, pp. 570–577.

Ford, J. M., Roth, W. T., Mohs, R. C., Hopkins, W. F., & Kopell, B. S. (1979). Event-related potentials recorded from young and old adults during a memory retrieval task. *Electroencephalography & Clinical Neurophysiology, 47*, 450–459.

Goldberg, E. (1985). Akinesia, tardive dysmentia, and frontal lobe disorder in schizophrenia. *Schizophrenia Bulletin, 11*, 253–263.

Grant, D. A., and Berg, E. A. (1948). A behavioral analysis of degree of reinforcement and ease of shifting to new responses in a Weigl-type card sorting problem. *Journal of Experimental Psychology, 38*, 404–411.

Luria, A. (1966). *Higher cortical functions in man*. New York: Basic Books.

Milner, B. (1966). Amnesia following operation on temporal lobes. In C. M. W. Wittey & O. L. Zangwill (Eds.), *Amnesia*. London: Butterworth.

Potter, H., & Butters, N. (1980). An assessment of olfactory deficits in patients with damage to prefrontal cortex. *Neuropsychologia, 18*, 621–628.

Reitan, R. M. (1958). Validity of the Trail Making Test as an indication of organic brain damage. *Perceptual Motor Skills, 8*, 271–276.

Rosvold, H. E., Mirsky, A. F., Sarason, I., Bransome, E. D., & Beck, L. H. (1956). A continuous performance test of brain damage. *Journal of Consulting Psychology, 20*, 343–350.

Stroop, J. R. (1935). Studies of interference in serial verbal reactions. *Journal of Experimental Psychology, 18*, 643–662.

Valenstein, E. (1986). *Great and desperate cures*. New York: Basic Books.

Verleger, R., & Cohen, R. (1978). Effects of certainty, modality shifts and guess outcome on evoked potentials and reaction time in chronic schizophrenics. *Psychological Medicine, 8*, 81–93.

# 4

# The Frontal Cortex—A Luria/Pribram Rapprochement

*Karl H. Pribram*

*Neuropsychology Laboratories, Stanford University and Center for Brain Research and Informational Sciences, Radford University*

## INTRODUCTION

When I began research on the functions of the anterior frontal cortex I found that neurobehavioral considerations related this part of the brain to the functions of the limbic part of the forebrain, not to the motor functions of the precentral cortex. The peri-Rolandic cortex, on the basis of neurobehavioral analysis, belonged with the remainder of the cerebral convexity. Thus a major distinction was made between the functions in behavior of the frontolimbic formations and those of the posterior cerebral convexity (see reviews by Pribram 1954, 1958a, 1958b, and the initial part of this chapter).

Alexandr Romanovich Luria conceived of the anterior frontal cortex in a different fashion. He emphasized the proximity of the anterior frontal cortex to those parts of the cortex which were electrically excitable in terms of motor functions (including those my colleagues Kaada, Epstein, and I had discovered in 1949 on the medial and basal surfaces of the hemisphere). This proximity to motor systems continued to be of considerable concern to me as well, but only recently have I hit upon an idea around which this concern can be precisely formulated.

It is this formulation which forms the core of this chapter dedicated to the memory of Luria.

The idea is simple. There is an important attribute by which the systems of the central part of the cerebral mantle differ from others: the peri-Rolandic systems are the only forebrain systems by which the organism can manipulate his or her environment. The systems of the posterior cerebral convexity primarily process sensory input in terms of "local sign", i.l. "epicritic" spatiotemporal perceptual organization for which there is no direct expression. The systems of the limbic forebrain primarily process input from chemical, pain and temperature receptors in terms of steady state "protocritic" sensibilities (see Pribram 1977; Chin, Pribram, Drake, & Greene, 1976) which provide the basis for passion rather than action. Thus, only by relationship to the peri-Rolandic systems can perceptual organization and sensibility be effectively utilized.

As I hope to demonstrate, the idea of *relating* protocritic to epicritic processing via the peri-Rolandic somatic systems clarifies ambiguities that have hitherto plagued conceptions based on either type of processing alone. Perhaps the most important clarification has to do with the view that anterior frontal lobe function is critical to planning. There is no doubt but that this is so (see, e.g., Penfield, 1948). For years I held to the idea that the deficit in planning that follows frontal lobe damage are due to the connections with the limbic forebrain which, when disrupted, lead to interference with the serial ordering of behavior. Interference was conceived to originate in heightened distractibility. This turns out to be only a part of the story.

Joaquin Fuster, in the initial edition of his volume on frontal lobe function, also forwards "the disruption of serially ordered behavior" view (1980). However, every experimental test of this hypothesis performed in my laboratory failed to confirm it (Barrett, 1969; Kimble & Pribram, 1963; Pribram, 1961; Brody & Pribram, 1978). In part this is due to the fact that all behavior, by virtue of restrictions in the final common path (Sherrington, 1911) is serially ordered and thus brain damage that does away with ordered behavior must indeed be sizable. Nonetheless, something about seriality and temporal order is disturbed by anterior frontal damage and it is that something which needs to be identified.

In the second edition of Fuster's publication the problem is recognized and handled in a sophisticated fashion: Fuster concludes that anterior frontal damage disrupts the processing of "cross temporal contingencies."

This same something is labeled "temporal tagging" by Brenda Milner and Michael Petrides (1984, 1988). These investigators have shown that, after frontal damage, recalling the *relative* recency of serially ordered events is disturbed.

In my own work, experimental results indicated that deficiencies in processing sequences of events could be overcome by providing monkeys with a "cognitive prosthesis" which "parsed" or "chunked" what would otherwise be an uninterrupted flow of sensory inputs. This prothesis can be thought of as providing tags for maintaining and recalling "serial position" within a sequence (Pribram & Tubbs, 1967; Mishkin, 1973).

However, as was reviewed in detail in a previous publication (Pribram, 1987) it is not only the processing of cross temporal contingencies or temporal tagging that is disupted by anterior frontal damage: the processing of spatial relations, i.e. the processing of cross spatial and spatiotemporal contingencies is also impaired. As in the case of processing serial position, the difficulty becomes manifest whenever an input must be processed within a context established on the basis of prior experience.

Clarification of these ideas comes when the anatomical and functional relationships between anterior frontal and other forebrain systems is delineated. Three different subdivisions based on different arrangements can be discerned: an orbital, a ventrolateral and a dorsolateral. Anatomically, the orbital subdivision, by way of the uncinate fasciculus, is related to the paleopallium; (especially the amygdala); the ventrolateral subdivison to the sensorymotor systems of the posterior convexity; and the dorsalateral, to the archipallium (especially the hippocampus). Functionally, the orbital subdivision will be shown to process *proprieties* based on limbically formulated sensibilities; the ventrolateral subdivision will be shown to be involved in *praxis* by way of processing sensory load, and the dorsolateral subdivision will be shown to deal with establishing *priorities*.

## SUBDIVIDING THE FRONTAL CORTEX

### *Thalamocortical Definition of Subdivisions*

The frontal cortex of primates can be divided into three major divisions each of which is made up of subdivisions. The three major divisions are the precentral (including pre- and supplementary motor), the anterior (also called prefrontal, orbitofrontal, or far frontal), and the cingulate (also called limbic). These major divisions are defined on the basis of their thalamic projections: the precentral deriving its thalamic input from the ventrolateral group of nuclei, the anterior frontal from the nucleus medialis dorsalis, and the cingulate from the anterior group (for review, see Pribram, 1958a, 1958b).

The subdivisions of these major divisions can also be defined in terms of their thalamic input: the immediate precentral cortex receives an input from the nucleus ventralis lateralis, pars caudalis, and the nucleus ventralis posterior, pars oralis, which in turn are the major terminals of cerebellar projection. The premotor parts of this division receive an input from the nucleus ventralis lateralis, pars oralis, which in turn is the major termination of input through the globus pallidus of the lateral nigrostriatal system. A further subdivision can be made between the lateral premotor and the supplementary motor systems in that the more laterally placed systems deal more with orofacial and the supplementary motor systems with the axial muscular projections (Goldberg, 1985).

The subdivisions of the cingulate cortex follow the subdivisions of the anterior thalamic nuclei: Nucleus anterior medialis projects to the anterior cingulate cortex; nucleus anterior lateralis, to the posterior cingulate cortex (Pribram & Fulton, 1954). The nucleus lateralis dorsalis (which ought to be classified as part of the anterior group) projects to the retrosplenial part of the cingulate gyrus.

Finally, the primate anterior far frontal cortex can be subdivided according to subdivisions of the nucleus medialis dorsalis: The microcellular part projects to the dorsolateral frontal cortex, the perilamminar magnocellular part to the periarcuate cortex, and the midline magnocellular part to the orbitofrontal cortex (Pribram, Chow, & Semmes, 1953).

## A Frontolimbic vs. Cortical Convexity Distinction

There are additional, hitherto ignored, interesting and important (for understanding the functional relationship to psychological processing) findings regarding the thalamocortical projections. The thalamus is a three-dimensional structure while the cortex is (from the standpoint of thalamic projections) essentially a two-dimensional sheet of cells. Thus, the projections from thalamus to cortex must "lose" one dimension. When one plots the precisely arranged "fan" of projections from each thalamic nucleus one can readily determine which dimension is eliminated.

With regard to the projections from the anterior nuclear group and the nucleus medialis dorsalis, the eliminated dimension is the anterior–posterior. An anterior–posterior file of cells in the thalamus projects to a single locus of cortex. Thus, for example, one finds degeneration of such an extended row of thalamic cells, ranging from the most anterior to the most posterior part of the nucleus medialis dorsalis after a resection limited to the frontal pole (Pribram, Chow, & Semmes, 1953).

With regard to the ventrolateral group of nuclei the situation is entirely different. Here the anterior–posterior dimension is clearly maintained: The front part of the nucleus projects to the forward parts of the cerebral convexity; as one proceeds back in the thalamus the projections reach the more posterior parts of the cortex, curving around into the temporal lobe when the projections of the pulvinar are reached. On the other hand, a file of cells extending, more or less, dorsoventrally (but angled somewhat laterally from its medial edge) projects to single locus on the cortex (Chow & Pribram, 1958).

This distinction between the anterior and medial nuclei on the one hand and the ventrolateral group of nuclei on the other, is endorsed by the fact that the internal medullary lamina separates the two classes of nuclei. Clearly, therefore, we should seek for commonality among the functions of the anterior, far frontal parts of the cortex and the limbic formations, and commonality of functions between the precentral and postcentral portions of the cerebral mantle (Pribram, 1958a, 1958b).

The close anatomical relationship of the far frontal cortex and the limbic medial forebrain is also emphasized when comparative anatomical data are reviewed. In cats and other nonprimates, gyrus prorius is the homologue of the far frontal cortex of primates. This gyrus receives its projection from the midline magnocellular part of the nucleus medialis dorsalis. This projection covers a good share of the anterior part of the medial frontal cortex; gyrus proreus on the lateral surface is limited to a narrow sliver. It is as if there has been a rotation of the medial frotal cortex laterally (just as there seems to have occurred a rotation medially of the occipital cortex, especially between monkey and humans) during the evolution of primates.

## A Rolandic vs. Extra-Rolandic Distinction

A further lesson can be learned from an analysis of the precise arrangement of thalamocortical projections and from comparing nonprimate with primate cortical anatomy. In tracing the thalamic projections to the precentral cortex, a surprising finding came to light. The dorsoventral arrangement of terminations, both pre-and postcentrally, is diametrically opposite to the arrangement of the projections farther forward and farther back. The dorsoventral terminations of the Rolandic projections reflect a lateral-medial origin from the thalamus; the dorsoventral terminations both forward and back of the peri-Rolandic cortex reflect a medial to lateral origin (Chow & Pribram, 1956).

Again comparison of nonprimate with primate cortical anatomy clarifies this surprising finding. In nonprimate species such as the carnivores, the suprasylvian and ectosylvian gyri extend the full length of the lateral surface of the cerebral convexity. The cruciate sulcus, the homologue of the Rolandic fissure, is mainly found on the medial surface of the hemisphere with only a minimal extension onto the lateral surface. It is as if in the evolution of primates this sulcus has migrated laterally to become the prominent central fissure (that becomes so intimately related to the cerebellar system).

Such a migration has split the supra- and ectosylvian gyri into anterior and posterior segments. That such a split has occurred is supported by the fact that terminations of thalamocortical projections to the anterior and posterior segments originate in adjacent parts of the ventrolateral nuclei. Should this conjecture regarding a split be correct, it would go a long way toward accounting for the difficulty in making a differential diagnosis between apraxias that are due to frontal, and those that are due to parietal damage.

## Skill vs. Praxis

Jason Brown (1987) in a review of frontal lobe syndromes, defines apraxia as "a substitution or defective selection of partial movements with lesions of the left premotor cortex [which] is due to an alteration of motor timing or a change in the kinetic pattern for a particular motor sequence" (p. 37).

In order to test whether in fact damage to both parietal and frontal (premotor) systems can produce apraxia and to pin down in a quantitative fashion just what changes in timing, in the kinetic pattern of movement occurs in apraxia the following (Pribram 1986) was performed: Monkeys were trained (using peanuts as reinforcements) to move a lever in a T-shaped slot beginning at the juncture of the arms of the T with its stem. The movements were then to be directed to the right, to the left, and finally down and up, in that order. Records were kept of the monkeys' ability to perform the movements in the correct order and the number and duration of contacts with the sides of the slots that formed the T. (This was done by having the sides and the lever lined with copper and wiring them so that contact could be recorded.)

Resections were made of precentral cortex, of the cortex of the inferior parietal lobule and of the premotor cortex, and of the latter two lesions combined. Precentral resections led to many more and briefer contacts along the path of the lever within the T slot, a loss of fine motor skill. No change in overall sequencing occurred. Both the parietal and the premotor resections produced a breakdown in the sequencing of the movements but only insofar as the same movement was carried out repetitiously, interpreted as evidence of apraxia. There was no observed difference between the effects of the anterior and those of the posterior resection and the overall order of the act was not disturbed. When the parietal and premotor resections were combined this deficit was enhanced; still there was no change in overall ordering of the action. More on this distinction between the systems that deal with skill and with praxis in the summary and synthesis.

## ANTERIOR FRONTAL SUBDIVISIONS

When lesions occur in the Rolandic and premotor parts of the frontal lobe neurological signs and symptoms occur which are relatively easy to spot. By contrast, the lesions of the anterior frontal cortex are essentially "silent" unless specific and sophisticated inquiries are addressed to the organism. Such inquiry has been greatly aided by the deployment of nonhuman primate models of anterior frontal lesion-produced deficits in behavior.

### Description of Tasks

The tasks which have been found most useful in delineating the deficit following anterior frontal damage are all characterized by a delay between stimulus presentation and the opportunity for a response to occur. During this delay distractors are introduced and the cue to the correct response disappears. The tasks fall into two main categories: delayed response and delayed alternation. Further, variations in the tasks have produced several subcategories of each category, variations which have been found to be extremely useful both as tools for subdividing the anterior frontal cortex and for understanding the nature of the deficit.

The delayed response task, in its direct form, involves hiding within sight of the subject, a reward in one of two identical-looking boxes set side by side, bringing down a distracting opaque screen for at least 5 seconds and then raising the screen to provide the subject with a single opportunity to locate the reward. The boxes are immediately withdrawn beyond the subject's reach and the next trial begun. Should the subject have failed to find the reward on the just-completed trial, the trial is repeated (correction technique), that is, the reward is again hidden within sight of the subject in the same box as in the previous trial. Should the subject succeed in finding the reward on the previous trial, the location (i.e., the box) for the hiding of the reward is chosen according to a pseudorandom table.

The indirect form of the delayed response task is more often called a delayed matching from sample. In this task a cue is presented instead of the reward during stimulus presentation; at the time of choice this cue and some other are available and the subject must choose the same cue as that initially presented in order to obtain the reward. A further variant of this task is the delayed nonmatch, in which the subject must choose the cue which was not present at the time of stimulus presentation. This version combines the attributes of the delayed response task with those of the delayed alternation procedure.

In the delayed alternation task the subject is not shown where the reward is located, he is simply given the opportunity to choose between two boxes. On the first trial both contain a reward. After the choice has been made, a distracting opaque screen is interposed between the boxes and the subject for at least 5 seconds and the next opportunity for choice is given. On this second trial the subject will find the reward in the box other than the one he chose initially and if he continues to choose successfully he will do so by adopting a win-shift strategy. Should the subject choose the empty box, the trial is repeated (correction technique). Unless this correction procedure is used, monkeys when they are the subject fail to learn the alternation task (at least in 5,000 trials, Pribram, unpublished data).

Three variants of delayed alternation which have proved especially useful are a go/no-go version, the object alternation procedure and discrimination reversals. In the go/no-go task the subject must alternately go to fetch the reward on one trial and withhold his response on the subsequent trial. Failure to go or failure to withhold result in the repetition of the trial (correction procedure). In the object alternation procedure the reward is alternated between two different objects rather than between two different locations. In this variant the spatial aspect of the task is reduced, a reduction which is enhanced when the objects are placed among 6, 8, or 12 locations, according to a random number table (Pribram, 1961b). Discrimination reversals are, in fact, alternations which vary the numbers of trials that occur between the shift of reinforcement that signals the alternation. There is a gradual transition between alternation, double alternation, triple alternation, and so on, and the ordinary nonreversal discrimination task.

The inflection point occurs at three nonalternation trials in normal subjects, but is raised to four to five such trials after frontal lobe damage. (Pribram, 1961b).

## Description of Lesion Sites

Earlier an anatomical rationale for subdividing the anterior frontal cortex was given in terms of the thalamic projections which terminate in different parts of this cortex. Unfortunately all of the investigators involved in pursuing the parcellation experiments did not adhere to this particular mode of subdividing: Many experimenters simply divided the anterior part of the frontal lobe into a dorsal part centered on the sulcus principalis and a vertral part, which included both the lip of the lobe and the entire orbital surface. Furthermore, surgical result does not always match surgical intent. The fibers in the depth of the sulci (medial, orbital, and principal) in the anterior part of the frontal lobe are separated by only millimeters and can be differentially spared only by exercising the greatest care and skill.

Despite this, meaningful conclusions can be teased out of the results of such experiments, provided the various lesions are kept clearly differentiated by appropriate labels. It is therefore necessary to adopt a uniform terminology for the resections that often differs from that used in the original reports because different investigators used the same term to describe different lesions or different terms to describe the same lesion.

The greatest problem arises from the use of the term "orbital." Here the convention will be followed that the term orbital refers to the general expanse of the ventral part of the lobe and that when specific parts of this cortex are referred to, orbital will be conjoined to a modifier. Thus posterior orbital refers to the agranular cortex located in the most posterior part of the orbital cortex (Area 13 of Walker, the projection of the midline magnocellular portion of nucleus medialis dorsalis of the thalamus). This cortex is intimately related through the uncinate fasciculus to the anterior insula, temporal pole, and amygdala.

The term medial orbital will be used to refer to the dysgranular cortex of the medial orbital gyrus, which is continuous with the cortex on the medial surface of the lobe and receives a projection from the anterior thalamic nucleus (Pribram & Fulton, 1954). In keeping with the agranular and dysgranular cytoarchitecture of the posterior and medial orbital cortex, it was found to be electrically excitable, that is, head and eye movements and a host of visceral responses (respiratory, heart rate, blood pressure) are obtained when this cortex (as well as that of the anterior cingulate gyrus with which it is continuous) is electrically stimulated (Kaada, Pribram, & Epstein, 1949). This finding gave rise to the concept of a mediobasal motor cortex, the existence of a limbic system motor cortex in addition to the more classical Rolandic and precentral systems (Pribram, 1961a).

The eugranular cortex on the lateral orbital gyrus is continuous with that forming the ventral lip and adjacent ventral gyrus of the frontal lobe. This cortex is part of the projection of the microcellular part of n. medialis dorsalis. When a lesion of this cortex is reported in conjunction with a lesion of posterior and medial orbital cortex the lesion is here labeled as orbitoventral. When a lesion of this cortex is made in isolation the lesion is referred to as ventral. When the resection extends laterally up to the gyrus adjacent to the sulcus principalis, the lesion is called ventrolateral.

Finally a dorsolateral resection is identified as including the eugranular cortex surrounding the sulcus principalis. Such lesions usually extend to and include the marginal gyrus. The dorsolateral cortex is the termination of the remaining projection of the microcellular part of nucleus medialis dorsalis.

When smaller lesions are reported, for example, periarcuate, around the arcuate sulcus; periprincipalis, around the sulcus principalis, and so on, the nomenclature is reasonably clear. When larger lesions are made they are simply referred to as lateral frontal when they excluded the posterior and medial orbital gyri. The resections are referred to as medial frontal when they are restricted to these gyri and the medial surface of the lobe. When the entire anterior frontal cortex is removed, the lesion is referred to as anterior frontal.

## The Orbital Contribution: Propriety

A good subject to begin with is the orbital contribution to psychological processing because it is so closely linked to that of the limbic forebrain. Damage limited to either the medial orbital (Pribram, Mishkin, Rosvold, & Kaplan, 1952) or the posterior orbital (Pribram & Bagshaw, 1953) does not produce any impairments in performance of the direct form of the delayed response task. Damage to both the medial and posterior orbital cortex does, however, produce a deficit in delayed alternation performance (Pribram, Lim, Poppen, & Bagshaw, 1966; Pribram, Mishkin, Rosvold, & Kaplan, 1952; Pribram, Wilson, & Connors, 1962). This deficit is due to the accumulation of many repetitive errors of both commission and omission which become apparent especially in the go/no-go version of the task. In fact these lesions produce a greater deficit in this variant of the task than on the right/left version (Pribram, 1973), a result which is opposite to that obtained when lateral frontal resections are made (Mishkin & Pribram, 1955).

Other effects observed after resections of the medial and/or posterior orbital damage are a decrease in aggression (Butter, Mishkin, & Mirsky, 1968; Butter, Snyder, & McDonald, 1970), and an increased tendency to put food items in their mouths (Butter, McDonald, & Snyder, 1969). Both of these effects had previously been observed when posterior orbital lesions are combined with those of the anterior insula, temporal pole and amygdala (Pribram & Bagshaw, 1953). It is such results which link the effects of orbital lesions on behavior to those of the limbic forebrain.

The question arises as to what such changes in behavior are due to? Brutkowski had argued that the orbital lesions in monkeys and dogs produce disinhibition of ordinarily present drive inhibition rather than the more obvious perseverative interference (see the extensive reviews of the conditioning literature by Brutkowski, 1964, 1965; and Konorski, 1972). The findings that monkeys with orbital resections continue to work harder than normals for nonfood items despite a normal preference for food items (Butter, McDonald, & Snyder, 1969), a result similar to that obtained with amaygdalectomized monkeys (Weiskrantz & Wilson, 1958), would seem to support Brutkowski's hypothesis, which was mainly based on work with dogs.

However, data showing that the response rates following orbital or lateral frontal resections are the same as those of normal monkeys during conditioning of an intermittently reinforced bar press response (Butter, Mishkin, & Rosvold, 1963) plus the additional data that monkeys with orbitoventral lesions stop responding for longer than do monkeys with dorsolateral frontal resections when novel stimuli are introduced during a similar bar pressing task (Butter, 1964) cast considerable doubt on a disinhibition hypothesis based solely on an increased drive for food.

The fact that failure in delayed alternation is characterized by proportionately as many errors of omission as of commission also indicates that the drive disinhibition hypothesis is untenable (Pribram, Lim, Poppen, & Bagshaw, 1966). Similarly damaging to a drive disinhibition hypothesis were the results of an experiment testing the object reversals using the go/no-go technique with monkeys who had sustained resections of orbital cortex (McEnaney & Butter, 1969). Once again the animals not only made more errors of commission than normals but also more errors of omission. They perseverated their refusal to respond to the previously negative stimulus.

Further evidence along these lines comes from the fact that monkeys with large orbitoventral lesions show a greater resistance to extinction of a bar press response even in the absence of food reinforcement (Butter, Mishkin, & Rosvold, 1963). These results confirmed and extended those obtained earlier with total anterior frontal and limbic (posterior orbital, insula, temporal pole, and amygdala) resections (Pribram, 1961a; Pribram & Weiskrantz, 1957) and are consistent with the finding that frontal and limbic lesions enhance the extinction of a conditioned avoidance response (Pribram & Weiskrantz, 1957).

These last results would readily fit a response disinhibiton hypothesis (one that plagued limbic system research for many years) were it not for the finding of errors of omission in the delayed alternation task. Also, monkeys with large orbitoventral resections take longer to habituate to novel stimuli (Butter, 1964), as do monkeys with total anterior frontal resections (Pribram, 1961a) and those with amygdalectomy (Schwartzbaum & Pribram, 1960). These results and those from a long series of conditioning experiments led Mishkin to propose that anterior frontal resections produce perseveration of central sets of whatever origin. Subsequent experimental results (Butter, 1969) showed, however, that monkeys with orbital resections do not perseverate in place or object reversal tasks. Furthermore, the definition of central set, when it is extended to include a failure to habituate to novelty, tends to lose its meaning.

The enhanced distractibility and sensitivity to pro- and retroactive interference, which accounts for the failure to habituate (see Malmo, 1942; Pribram, 1961b) may well be dependent on the organization of drive states, provided we understand by this that such states are composed of endocrine and other neurochemical systems (Estes, 1959). The limbic forebrain has been found to be a selective host to a variety of neuroendocrine and neurochemical secretions which can form the basis of a neural representation of the internal state of the organism by way of which neural control over peripheral endocrine and exocrine secretions is exerted (McGaugh et al., 1979; Martinez, 1983; Pribram, 1969b).

The import of this research for this review is that such neuroendocrine and neurochemical factors influence the organization of attention and intention. Habituation to novelty (registration and consolidation in the face of distraction) and therefore the organization of what is responded to as familiar is disturbed by the lesions. Experimental psychologists test for familiarity with "recognition" tasks and recently Mishkin (1982) has used the delayed nonmatching from sample as an instance of such a recognition procedure. Not surprisingly, he has found deficits with limbic (amygdala and hippocampus) resections and drawn the conclusion that these structures are involved with recognition memory. For those working in the neurological tradition where agnosias, since the time of Freud and Henry Head, have been related to lesions of the parietal convexity, this conclusion is confusing. The confusion is resolved when it is realized that the delay tasks, as do the "recognition" tasks used by experimental psychologists to test humans, test for the dimension "familiarity," not the identification of objects which is the neurologist's definition of recognition. In short, the orbital contribution based on processing both interoceptive and exteroceptive inputs to psychological processing is to provide a critical facility the evaluation of propriety, to the feeling of familiarity.

## The Lateral Frontal Cortex: Praxis and Priority

The results of attempts to subdivide the lateral frontal cortex have been reviewed recently in great detail (Pribram, 1986). As in the case of the orbitofrontal cortex reviewed above, much of the evidence appeared initially to be in conflict. To avoid undue repitition this detail is omitted from the current essay.

When the nuances of test procedures and lesion sites were carefully, analyzed the following conclusions emerged. (insert see pg (4–18)

The major part of the lateral frontal cortex centering on its ventral lip, influences all types of alternation performance and can be further subdivided according to modality by tests involving variants of alternation (e.g., object alternation, discrimination reversal). Using these variants, dorsal periarcuate auditory, anterior periarcuate visual, and posterior periarcuate kinesthetic subdivisions have been identified. The deficits produced by lesions in these subdivisions is sensitive to the *sensory load* imposed as a requirement for performing adequately. This suggests that some sort of sensory servocontrol feedback mechanism is involved. Connections between lunate (area 8) and arcuate (area 8) are well known (see e.g., Bonin & Baily 19XX). Goldman-Rakic (1979; Goldman-Rakic & Schwartz, 1982) has elegantly worked out the connections between frontal and parietal cortex and these with the corpus striatum, connections which can serve such a sensory servosystem. The ventrolateral subsystem is thus ideally situated to fine tune praxis especially where current action depends on the sensory consequences of prior actions (as in the variants of the alternation procedures).

Finally, there is a dorsolateral focus centering on the sulcus principalis which influences performance on both the spatial delayed response and the spatial delayed alternation task but *not* on the go/no-go or object versions of alternation. This suggests that a spatial factor important to task performance has been interfered with by the lesion of this cortex. However, the presumed kinesthetic basis for this spatial deficit proved not to be related to the spatial aspects of these and other tasks but rather to the temporal aspects (Pribram 1986). This left the spatial deficit unexplained.

Still, an explanation *can* be provided when connections between the cortex surrounding the sulcus principalis and the hippocampus (Nauta, 1964) are considered. It is this dorsolateral part of the anterior frontal cortex which has resisted fractionation with respect to sensory mode but which is especially sensitive to the "spatial" aspects of the delay task. This is exactly the situation with regard to hippocampal function. In fact the deficits produced by resections of the primate hippocampus and those produced by resections of the primate hippocampus and those produced by resections of the cortex surrounding the sulcus principalis mimic (with the critical exception that spatial delayed response remains intact after hippocampectomy) each other to such an extent that it is hard to distinguish between them.

I have extensively reviewed (Pribram, 1986) the evidence for considering the difficulty with "spatial" problems as due to an increase in sensitivity to distraction under certain specifiable conditions. Briefly, the essential evidence is that when such interference is minimized, as when the delay interval is darkened, monkeys with frontal resections can perform the delay task (Anderson, Hunt, Vander Stoep, & Pribram, 1976; Malmo 1942). Further, spatial cues have been found to be more distracting than visual and auditory cues for normal monkeys and especially so for monkeys with resections of the anterior frontal and to a somewhat lesser extent (thus the sparing of delayed response?) hippocampal cortices (Douglas & Pribram, 1969; Grueninger & Pribram, 1969). Whatever the interpretation of the "spatial" deficit the data are consonant with the conclusion that the cortex surrounding the sulcus principalis is derived from an archicerebral primordium.

The key to understanding the contribution of the lateral frontal cortex to processing is provided by the proposals made by Goldberg (1985, 1987) regarding the functions of the premotor systems which, in turn, are based on the concepts of Sanides (1966; which are also reviewed and extended by Pandya & Barnes, 1987). These proposals divide the premotor cortex into a medial, supplementary premotor region and a lateral, periarcuate premotor region. The medial region is, on the basis of evidence from comparative anatomical studies, shown to be derived from archicortical origins, the lateral region, from paleocortical primordia. The two regions are suggested to function differently: The medial is concerned in developing models which program behavior in feedforward fashion; by contrast, the lateral region programs behavior via a variety of sensory feedback mechanisms.

This analysis can be readily extended to the remainder of the motor cortex: The evidence regarding the difference in orientation of the projection fan of thalamocortical connections, presented in the initial part of this review, indicates that the primary somatosensorimotor cortex also derives from the medial surface of the hemisphere, perhaps from the cortex of the cingulate gyrus. Accordingly, it would seem that the supplementary motor cortex participates in the sketching the outlines of the model while the precentral cortex implements its finer aspects. Such a scheme is supported by the fact that the supplementary motor cortex receives an input from the basal ganglia (known to determine postural and sensory sets) while the precentral motor cortex, in its involvement with the cerebellum, provides the details necessary to carry out a feedforward regulated action. I have elsewhere (Pribram, Sherafat, & Beekman 1984) provided a review of the evidence and a mathematically precise model based on one developed by Houk & Rymer, (1981) by which such a feed-forward process operates.

The lateral premotor region is the one so intimately interconnected with the inferior-posterior parietal cortex as indicated by Schwartz and Goldman–Rakic (1984), Goldberg (1985), and the thalamocortical and comparative anatomical data reviewed in the initial parts of this chapter. As indicated, it is damage to this system that produces apraxias, which according to Goldberg's thesis should devolve on faulty feedback processing. It is not too farfetched to wonder whether the repetitions which the lesioned monkeys made in the task reported in the first section of this review might not have been due to the necessity for gaining additional sensory feedback before proceeding.

There is one further speculation regarding apraxia that is worth considering. Elsewhere (Pribram & Carlton, 1987) I have described the neural mechanism that is involved in the construction of objects from images. Essentially this mechanism operates to extract invariances, constancies, from sets of images by a process of convolution and correlation. An object is experienced when the resultant of the correlation remains constant across further transformation of the set of images.

When objects are constructed in the somatic sensorimotor domain they are of two kinds. One sort of object is the familiar external "objective" object. Damage to the peri-Rolandic cortex (including the superior parietal gyrus) results in object agnosia. When, however, the lateral premotor and inferior parietal cortex is damaged, apraxias and neglect syndromes develop. Could the apraxias be thought of as a mild form of neglect in the sense that the "object" which is constructed by this premotor-parietal system is the "self"? If this hypothesis is correct, apraxias result from a failure in the appreciation (based on feedback?) of self: an awkwardness more pervasive than the impairment of skills. Thus one can envisage a gradually increased impairment ranging from apraxia through Parkinsonian tremors at rest, and so on, to neglect. This syndrome can be clearly distinguished from the one produced by cerebellar-Rolandic damage which is characterized by loss of skill, intention tremor, and paresis.

A word of caution. The statements made above could be interpreted as a denial of distinctions between such syndromes as Parkinson's, neglect, and apraxia. This is definitely *not* what is meant. Even apraxias of frontal origin can be expected to differ subtly from those of parietal origin, and it may well be as Jason Brown (1985) suggests that the lesions which produces apraxia must invade the limbic forebrain as shown by the work of Terrence W. Deacon (personal communication). Parietal and frontal cortex, though reciprocally connected, show an upstream–downstream relationship to one another. According to Deacon, a downstream corticocortical connection terminates most heavily in layers iiic–iv; an upstream connection terminates in layer i and sometimes in bands in vb. Thus there is a clear hierarchical connectivity from anterior cingulate to anterior frontal to periarcuate to premotor and motor cortices. At the same time parietal cortex is upstream from posterior cingulate, as well as from all of frontal cortex.

What I *am* trying to convey is that a *class* of disorders due to damage of systems of paleocerebral origin can be discerned. Within that class a variety of syndromes traceable to differences in neuroanatomical and neurochemical substrates can be made out.

How does this approach to the problem help connect the functions of the anterior frontal cortex to those of the somatosensorimotor regions? As noted in this review, there seems to be a gradient of relationships of delay problem performance to sensory mode reaching from a periarcuate auditory and visual to a more anterior kinesthetic location. These relationships fit with the general hypothesis that the function of the anterior frontal cortex is to relate the processes served by the limbic forebrain to those of the somatosensorimotor systems, broadly as defined. Furthermore the results also support the suggestion that these relationships are of a feedback nature, viz Stamm's experiments in which kinesthetic feedback was manipulated (1987).

Furthermore there are the strong connections through the uncinate fasciculus with the structures of the temporal lobe which are derived from paleocerebral systems (amygdala, pyriform cortex, and adjacent temporal polar juxtallocortex) which indicate that these parts of the anterior frontal cortex are to be considered as relatives of the lateral premotor rather than as relatives of the precentral motor systems.

## CONCLUSION

One final word. Jason Brown (1987) has suggested that the mechanism for feedback and feedforward depends on the operation of sets of tuned relaxation oscillators that constitute the brainstem and spinal cord systems which are influenced by the various frontal lobe processes under consideration. The evidence for the existence of such tuned oscillators has been repeatedly presented from the time of Graham-Brown (1914) through von Holst (1937, 1948) and Bernstein (1967) and his group (Gelfand, Gurfinkel, Tsetlin, & Shik, 1971). This evidence has been thoroughly reviewed by Gallistel (1980). The mechanism whereby a cortical influence can be imposed on such systems of oscillators has also been worked out within the concept of an "image of achievement". Such "images" must operate within the spectral frequency domain. Pribram (1987) and Pribram et. al. (1984) have presented evidence that neurons in the motor cortex are tuned to different frequencies of movement (independent of velocity and acceleration). These authors also detail the mechanism whereby such tuned cortical cells can program the subcortical motor systems.

The profusion of data collected by hard labor over the past half century can thus be fitted into a tentative scheme. No longer are we stuck with vague concepts of frontal lobe function. The role of the anterior frontal cortex in emotion and motivation is seen as relating protocritic (interoceptive plus pain and temperature) to epicritic processes in the feedback mode. Evaluation (what Arnold, 1970 calls appraisal) of proprieties is the function of the periarcuate and ventrolateral portions of this cortex (Konow & Pribram, 1970). Evaluation is a sort of internal rehearsal, a feedback by way of which proprieties become refined, that is, more in keeping with current sensory input and with the consequences of actions.

The role of the anterior frontal cortex in processing priorities (planning) relates protocritic to epicritic processing in the feed-forward mode. This is the function of the dorsolateral frontal cortex. In the feed-forward mode current and consequent input form the context within which "models" are constructed in "fast time," models which in turn are used to modify subsequent behavior. One definition of praxis given by the Century Dictionary (1914) is "an example or collection of examples for practice; a model." Thus the role of the frontal cortex in one form of "short-term memory" is clarified: the close connection between the dorsolateral frontal cortex and the hippocampus; the similarity of the cytoarchitecture of the hippocampus and that of the cerebellum; the close connection of the peri-Rolandic cortex (which is most likely derived, as noted, from the archicerebrum as is the hippocampus) and the cerebellum; and the known function of the cerebellum as a feed-forward mechanism (see, e.g., Ruch, 1951; Pribram, 1971, 1981) all attest to the likelihood that the dorsolateral frontal cortex is indeed involved in such "projective" processes.

It is of course, these "models" obtained through praxis that allow the processing of serial position in a remembered sequence—and the extrapolation of serial position into the future. It is this aspect of planning which is impaired by anterior frontal damage. When combined with defective evaluation and appraisal of proprieties regarding projected action, the full-blown anterior frontal deficit becomes manifest.

A prodigious amount of research has been accomplished since the initial findings obtained with experiments on nonhuman primates in the Yale laboratories headed by John Fulton and Robert Yerkes led to the, to my mind unjustified, practice of leukotomy performed on thousands of human subjects (see Valenstein, 1986). This procedure and continued observations of patients such as those made by Luria has fired the curiosity of a dedicated group of neuropsychologists who continued the research begun in the Yale Laboratories until the present. Only now, with continued input from the clinic and the laboratory are we beginning to understand the effects of damage to the primate frontal lobe.

## REFERENCES

Anderson, R. M., Hunt, S. C., Vander Stoep, A., & Pribram, K. H. (1976). Object permanency and delayed response as spatial context in monkeys with frontal lesions. *Neuropsychologia, 14*, 481–490.

Arnold, M. B. (Ed.). (1970). *Feelings and emotions*. New York: Academic Press.

Barrett, T. W. (1969). Studies of the function of the amygdaloid complex in Macaca Mulatta. *Neuropsychologia, 7*, 1–12.

Battig, K., Rosvold, H. E., & Mishkin, M. (1962). Comparison of the effects of frontal and caudate lesions on discrimination learning in monkeys. *Journal of Comparative and Physiological Psychology, 55*, 458–463.

Bernstein, N. (1967). *The coordination and regulation of movement*. Oxford: Pergamon.

Brown, J. W. (1987). The microstructure of action. In, E. Perecman (Ed.), *The frontal lobes revisited* (pp. 251–272). New York: IRBN Press.

Brutkowski, S. (1964). Prefrontal cortex and drive inhibition. In J. M. Warren & K. Akert (Eds.), *Frontal granular cortex and behavior* (pp. 219–241). New York: McGraw-Hill.

Brutkowski, S. (1965). Functions of prefrontal cortex in animals. *Physiological Reviews, 45,* 721–746.

Brutkowski, S., Mishkin, M., & Rosvold, H. E. (1963). Positive and inhibitory motor reflexes in monkeys after ablation of orbital or dorsolateral surface of the frontal cortex. In E. Gutman & P. Hnik (Eds.), *Central and peripheral mechanisms of motor functions* (pp. 113–141). Prague: Czechoslovak Academy of Sciences.

Butter, C. M. (1964). Habituation of responses to novel stimuli in monkeys with selective frontal lesions. *Science, 194,* 313–315.

Butter, C. M. (1969). Impairments in selective attention to visual stimuli in monkeys with inferotemporal and lateral striate lesions. *Brain Research, 12,* 374–383.

Butter, C. M., McDonald, J. A., & Snyder, D. R. (1969). Orality, preference behavior and reinforcement value of nonfood object in monkeys orbital frontal lesions. *Science, 164,* 1306–1307.

Butter, C. M., Mishkin, M., & Mirsky, A. F. (1968). Emotional responses toward humans in monkeys with selective frontal lesions. *Physiology and Behavior, 3,* 213–215.

Butter, C. M., Mishkin, M., & Rosvold, E. H. (1963). Conditioning and extinction of a food rewarded response after selective ablations of the frontal cortex in rhesus monkeys. *Experimental Neurology, 7* (1), 65–75.

Butter, C. M., Snyder, D. R., & McDonald, J. A. (1970). Effects of orbital frontal lesions on aversive and aggressive behaviors in rhesus monkeys. *Journal of Comparative and Physiological Psychology, 72,* 132–144.

Chin, J. H., Pribram, K. H., Drake, K., & Greene, L. O., Jr. (1976). Disruption of temperature discrimination during limbic forebrain stimulation in monkeys. *Neuropsychologia, 14,* 293–310.

Chow, K. L., & Pribram, K. H. (1956). Cortical projection of the thalamic ventrolateral nuclear group in monkeys. *Journal of Comparative Neurology, 104,* 57–75.

Douglas, R. J., & Pribram, K. H. (1969). Distraction and habituation in monkeys with limbic lesions. *Journal of Comparative and Physiological Psychology, 69,* 473–480.

Estes, W. K. (1959). The statistical approach to learning theory. In S. Koch (Ed.), *Psychology: A study of a science: Vol. 2. General systematic formulations, learning and special processes.* New York: McGraw-Hill.

Fuster, J. M. (1980). *Frontal Lobe Symposium* (in press).

Gallistel, C. R. (1980). *The organization of action: A new synthesis.* Hillsdale, NJ: Erlbaum.

Gelfand, I. M., Gurfinkel, V. S., Tsetlin, M. L., & Shik, M. L. (1971). Some problems in the analysis of movements. In I. M. Gelfand, V. S. Gurfinkel, S. V. Fromin, & M. L. Tsetlin (Eds.), *Models of the structural-functional organization of certain biological systems.* Cambridge, MA: MIT Press.

Goldberg, G. (1985). Supplementary motor area: Review and hypotheses. *Behavioral and Brain Sciences, 8,* 567–588.

Goldberg, G. (1987). From intent to action. Evolution and function and of the premotor systems of the frontal lobe. In E. Perecman (Ed.), *The frontal lobes revisited* (pp. 273–306). New York: IRBN Press.

Goldman-Rakic, P. S. (1978). Neuronal plasticity in primate telencephalon: Anomalous projections induced by prenatal removal of frontal cortex. *Science, 202,* 768–770.

Goldman-Rakic, P. S., & Schwartz, M. L. (1982). Interdigitation of contralateral and ipsilateral columnar projections to frontal association cortex in primates. *Science, 216,* 755–757.

Graham-Brown, T. (1914). On the nature of the fundamental activity of the nervous centres; together with an analysis of the conditioning of rhythmic activity in progression, and a theory of evolution of function of the nervous system. *Journal of Physiology (London), 48,* 18–46.

Grueninger, W., & Pribram, K. H. (1969). The effects of spatial and nonspatial distractors on performance latency of monkeys with frontal lesions. *Journal of Comparative and Physiological Psychology, 68,* 203–209.

Houk, J. C., & Rymer, W. Z. (1981). Neural control of muscle length and tension. In V. B. Brooks (Ed.), *Motor control.* Bethesda, MD: American Physiological Society Handbook of Physiology.

Kaada, B. R., Pribram, K. H., & Epstein, J. A. (1949). Respiratory and vascular responses in monkeys from temporal pole, insular, orbital surface and cingulate gyrus. *Journal of Neurophysiology, 12,* 347–356.

Kimble, D. P., & Pribram, K. H. (1963). Hippocampectomy and behavioral sequences. *Science, 139,* 824–825.

Konorski, J. (1976). *Integrative activity of the brain: An interdisciplinary approach.* Chicago, IL: University of Chicago Press.

Konorski, J. (1972). Some hypotheses concerning the functional organization of prefrontal cortex. *Acta Neurobiologiae Experimentalis, 32,* 595–613.

Konow, A., & Pribram, K. H. (1970). Error recognition and utilization produced by injury to the frontal cortex in man. *Neuropsychologia, 8,* 489–491.

Malmo, R. B. (1942). Interference factors in delayed response in monkeys after removal of frontal lobes. *Journal of Neurophysiology, 5,* 295–308.

Martinez, J. L. (1983). Endogenous modulators of learning and memory. In S. T. Cooper (Ed.), *Theory in psychopharmacology* (Vol. 2, pp. 48–74). New York: Academic Press.

McEnaney, K. W., & Butter, C. M. (1969). Perseveration of responding and nonresponding in monkeys with orbital frontal ablations. *Journal of Comparative and Physiological Psychology, 69,* 558–561.

McGaugh, J. L., Gold, P. E., Handwerker, M. J., Jensen, R. A., Martinez, J. L., Jr., Meligeni, J. A., & Vasquez, B. J. (1979). Altering memory by electrical and chemical stimulation of the brain. *International Brain Research Organization Monograph Series, 4,* 151–164.

Milner, B., & Petrides, M. (1984). Behavioural effects of frontal-lobe lesions in man. *Trends in Neurosciences, 7*(11), 403–407.

Mishkin, M. (1982). A memory system in the monkey. *Philosophical Transactions of the Royal Society of London, Series B, 298*, 85–95.

Mishkin, M., & Pribram, K. H. (1955). Analysis of the effects of frontal lesions in monkey: I. Variations of delayed alternation. *Journal of Comparative and Physiological Psychology, 48*, 492–495.

Nauta, W. J. H. (1964). Some efferent connections of the prefrontal cortex in the monkey. In J. M. Warren & K. Akert (Eds.), *The frontal granular cortex and behavior* (pp. 28–55). New York: McGraw-Hill.

Oscar-Berman, M. (1975). The effects of dorsolateral and ventrolateral orbitofrontal lesions on spatial discrimination learning and delayed response in two modalities. *Neuropsychologia, 13*, 237–246.

Pandya, D. N., & Barnes, C. L. (1987). Architecture and connections of the frontal lobe. In E. Perecman (Ed.), *The frontal lobes revisited* (pp. 41–72).

Passingham, R. E. (1972a). Visual discrimination learning after selective prefrontal ablations in monkeys *(Macaca mulatta). Neuropsychologia, 10*, 27–33.

Passingham, R. E. (1972b). Non-reversal shifts after selective prefrontal ablations in monkeys *(Macaca mulatta). Neuropsychologia, 10*, 41–46.

Passingham, R. E., & Ettlinger, G. (1972). Tactile discrimination learning after selective prefrontal ablations in monkeys *(Macaca mulatta). Neuropsychologia, 10*, 17–26.

Penfield, W. (1948). Bilateral frontal gyrectomy and postoperative intelligence. *Res. Publ. Ass. Nerv. Ment. Dis., 27*, 519–564.

Pinsker, H. M., & French, G. M. (1967). Indirect delayed reactions under various testing conditions in normal and midlateral frontal monkeys. *Neuropsychologia, 5*, 13–24.

Pohl, W. G. (1973). Dissociation of spatial and discrimination deficits following frontal and parietal lesions in monkeys. *Journal of Comparative and Physiological Psychology, 82*, 227–239.

Pribram, K. H. (1954). Toward a science of neuropsychology: Method and data. In R. A. Patton (Ed.), *Current trends in psychology and the behavioral sciences* (pp. 115–142.) Pittsburgh, PA: University of Pittsburgh Press.

Pribram, K. H. (1958a). Comparative neurology and the evolution of behavior. In A. Roe & G. G. Simpson (Eds.), *Behavior and evolution* (pp. 140–164). New Haven, CT: Yale University Press.

Pribram, K. H. (1958b). Neocortical function in behavior. In H. F. Harlow & C. N. Woolsey (Eds.), *Biological and biochemical bases of behavior* (pp. 151–172). Madison: University of Wisconsin Press.

Pribram, K. H. (1961a). Limbic system. In D. E. Sheer (Ed.), *Electrical stimulation of the brain* (pp. 311–320). Austin: University of Texas Press.

Pribram, K. H. (1961b). A further experimental analysis of the behavioral deficit that follows injury to the primate frontal cortex. *Experimental Neurology, 3*, 432–466.

Pribram, K. H. (1969a). DADTA III: Computer control of the experimental analysis of behavior. *Perceptual and Motor Skills, 29*, 599–608.

Pribram, K. H. (1971). *Languages of the brain: Experimental paradoxes and principles in neuropsychology*. Englewood Cliffs, NJ: Prentice-Hall.

Pribram, K. H. (1973). The primate frontal cortex—executive of the brain. In K. H. Pribram & A. R. Luria (Eds.), *Psychophysiology of the frontal lobes*. New York: Academic Press.

Pribram, K. H. (1977). Peptides and protocritic processes. In L. H. Miller, C. L. Sandman, & A. J. Kastin (Eds.), *Neuropeptide influences on the brain and behavior* (pp. 213–232). New York: Raven Press.

Pribram, K. H. (1986). Subdivisions of the anterior frontal cortex revisited.

Pribram, K. H., & Bagshaw, M. H. (1953). Further analysis of the temporal lobe syndrome utilizing frontotemporal ablations in monkeys. *Journal of Comparative Neurology, 99,* 347–375.

Pribram, K. H., & Carlton, E. (1987). *Brain mechanisms in perception and cognition.* Hillsdale, NJ: Erlbaum.

Pribram, K. H., Chow, K. L., & Semmes, J. (1953). Limit and organization of the cortical projection from the medial thalamic nucleus in monkeys. *Journal of Comparative Neurology, 95,* 433–440.

Pribram, K. H., & Fulton, J. F. (1954). An experimental critique of the effects of anterior cingulate ablations in monkey. *Brain, 77,* 34–44.

Pribram, K. H., Gardner, K. W., Pressman, G. L., & Bagshaw, M. H. (1963). Automated analysis of multiple choice behavior. *Journal of the Experimental Analysis of Behavior, 6,* 123–124.

Pribram, K. H., Lim, H., Poppen, R., & Bagshaw, M. H. (1966). Limbic lesions and the temporal structure of redundancy. *Journal of Comparative and Physiological Psychology, 61,* 365–373.

Pribram, K. H., & McGuinness, D. (1975). Arousal, activation and effort in the control of attention. *Psychology Reviews, 82,* 116–149.

Pribram, K. H., & Mishkin, M., Rosvold, H. E., & Kaplan, S. J. (1952). Effects on delayed-response performance of lesions of dorsolateral and ventromedial frontal cortex of baboons. *Journal of Comparative and Physiological Psychology, 45,* 565–575.

Pribram, K. H., Plotkin, H. C., Anderson, R. M., & Leong, D. (1977). Information sources in the delayed alternation task for normal and "frontal" monkeys. *Neuropsychologia, 15,* 329–340.

Pribram, K. H., Sherafat, A., & Beekman, G. J. (1984). Frequency encoding in motor systems. In H. T. A. Whiting (Ed.), *Human motor actions: Bernstein reassessed* (pp. 121–156). Amsterdam: North-Holland.

Pribram, K. H., & Tubbs, W. E. (1967). Short-term memory, parsing and the primate frontal cortex. *Science, 156,* 1765–1767.

Pribram, K. H., & Weiskrantz, L. (1957). A comparison of the effects of medial and lateral cerebral resections on conditioned avoidance behavior of monkeys. *Journal of Comparative and Physiological Psychology, 50,* 74–80.

Pribram, K. H., Wilson, W. A., & Connors, J. (1962). The effects of lesions of the medial forebrain on alternation behavior of rhesus monkeys. *Experimental Neurology, 6,* 36–47.

Ruch, T. C. (1951). Motor systems. In S. S. Stevens (Ed.), *Handbook of experimental psychology* (pp. 154–208). New York: Wiley.

Sanides, F. (1966). The architecture of the human frontal lobe and the relation to its functional differentiation. *International Journal of Neurology, 5,* 247–261.

Schwartz, M. L., & Goldman-Rakic, P. S. (1984). Callosal and intrahemispheric connectivity of the prefrontal association cortex in rhesus monkey: Relation between intraparietal and principal sulcal cortex. *Journal of Comparative and Physiological Psychology, 226,* 403–420.

Schwartzbaum, J. S. & Pribram, K. H. (1960). The effects of amygdalectomy in monkeys on transposition along a brightness continuum. *Journal of Comparative and Physiological Psychology, 53,* 396–399.

Stamm, J. S. (1987). The riddle of the monkey's delayed-response deficit has been solved. In E. Perecman (Ed.), *The frontal lobes revisited* (pp. 73–90). New York: IRBN Press.

Valenstein, E. S. (1986). *Great and desperate cures: The rise and decline of psychosurgery and other radical illness.* New York: Basic Books.

von Holst, E. (1948). Von der Mathematik der nervoesen Ordnungsleistungen. *Experientia, 4,* 374–381.

von Holst, E. (1937). Vom Wesen der Ordnung im Zentralnervensystem. *Naturwissenschaften, 25,* 625–631.

Weiskrantz, L., & Wilson, W. A. (1958). The effect of ventral rhinencephalic lesions on avoidance thresholds in monkeys. *Journal of Comparative and Physiological Psychology, 51,* 167–171.

# 5

# Processes Underlying the Memory Impairments of Demented Patients

*Nelson Butters, David P. Salmon, William C. Heindel*

*San Diego Veterans Administration Medical Center and University of California School of Medicine at San Diego*

Luria's neuropsychology exemplified the enormous advantages of the process-achievement approach to clinical phenomena (Luria, 1966a). Rather than focusing on an easily quantifiable achievement or failure, Luria searched for the cognitive processes (and neurological substrates) that were responsible for patients' overall performance. This emphasis on underlying processes led to his descriptions of the various forms of perseveration associated with anterior cerebral damage and to his enumeration of the factors that can contribute to the impaired constructional abilities of left- and right-hemisphere patients (Luria, 1966b, 1976). In recent years, Kaplan and her associates (Albert & Kaplan, 1980; Milberg, Hebben, & Kaplan, 1986) have also championed the process-achievement approach to neuropsychological phenomena and have stressed that close scrutiny of error patterns is often vital to a full understanding of the cognitive factors involved in patients' impaired performances.

The purpose of the present chapter is to review recent studies from our laboratory in which the process-achievement approach has been used to differentiate the global memory impairments manifested by patients with various forms of amnesia and dementia. Although actuarial approaches to neuropsychology have suggested that the severe memory deficits of such patient populations are highly similar when assessed with standardized tests of memory, investigations applying the concepts and models of cognitive neuropsychology have often noted important differences among these superficially (i.e., quantitatively) comparable retention deficiencies. For example, two patients, both with memory quotients of 75, may be distinguished from each other by the roles that storage, retrieval, and encoding mechanisms play in their respective impairments. It is obvious that any extension of neuropsychology into the realm of cognitive rehabilitation and pharmacological therapies for memory impairments will require extensive knowledge about the status of such underlying processes.

To exemplify the utility of cognitive psychology to the study of impaired memory, Butters (1984) reviewed a series of studies comparing the memory disorders of patients with diencephalic (i.e., alcoholic Korsakoff patients) and basal ganglia (i.e., Huntington's disease patients) damage. It was noted that the anterograde amnesia of alcoholic Korsakoff (AK) patients involved a failure in storage due to an increased sensitivity to proactive interference and limited encoding, whereas the severe deficit of Huntington's disease (HD) patients on recall measures of learning was related to an inability to initiate systematic retrieval processes. The memory failures of AK patients, but not those of HD patients, could be attenuated by the introduction of procedures which reduced proactive interference (e.g., distributed rather than massed learning trials). However, only the HD patients performed at almost normal levels when recognition rather than recall measures of learning were employed.

Besides this distinction between storage and retrieval impairments, AK and HD patients appeared to differ in their ability to acquire a visuomotor skill (Martone, Butters, Payne, Becker, & Sax, 1984). Using the reading of mirror-reflected words as a measure of skill learning, Cohen and Squire (1980) had concluded that AK patients were capable of normal learning and retention of this skill (as measured by reduction in the temporal durations necessary to read mirror-reflected word triads) despite a severe inability to recognize the specific words used to train the skill. When Martone et al. (1984) extended the mirror-reading paradigm to HD patients, a double dissociation between recognition memory and skill learning emerged. Although alcoholic Korsakoff patients performed as described by Cohen and Squire (1980), the HD patients were significantly impaired in the acquisition of the visuomotor skill despite normal recognition of the words employed on the test. On the basis of these findings, Martone et al. (1984) suggested that the learning of motor skills and the storage of factual (i.e., data-based) materials might depend on the integrity of the basal ganglia (especially the caudate nucleus) and limbic-diencephalic regions, respectively.

In addition to comparisons between amnesic and HD patients, recent investigations from our laboratory have also focused upon the performance of patients with Alzheimer's disease on episodic (Tulving, 1983), semantic (Tulving, 1983), and implicit (Graf & Schacter, 1985; Schacter, 1987) memory tasks. The findings, which will be reviewed in this chapter, have not only demonstrated the heuristic value of these taxonomic concepts but also provided clues as to their neuroanatomical substrates. The relevance for Cummings and Benson's (1984) proposed distinction between "cortical" and "subcortical" dementia will also be discussed.

Tulving (1983) has defined episodic memories as those dependent on temporal and/or spatial cues for their retrieval. For instance, attempts to recall the previous day's breakfast meal or a specific encounter with a colleague requires the use of temporal and spatial contextual cues and, therefore, would represent retrieval from episodic memory. Most of the traditional verbal learning techniques (e.g., paired-associate learning, list learning) employed by experimental psychologists are categorized as episodic memory tasks. In comparison with episodic memories, semantic memories are totally independent of contextual cues for their retrieval. Various numerical (e.g., the number of feet in a yard), historical (e.g., the name of the first President of the United States and geographical (e.g., the capital of California), facts serve as examples of semantic memories. Although it is possible for new information to enter either episodic or semantic memory directly, memories which are initially episodic in nature may become context-free and part of an individual's semantic fund of knowledge after much repetition and overlearning.

Implicit memory refers to a class of diverse memory tasks which, unlike traditional tests of recall and recognition, do not require the explicit, conscious recollection of previous experiences (Schacter, 1987), and are usually preserved in severely amnesic patients (Squire, 1987). Classical conditioning, lexical and semantic priming, motor skill learning, and perceptual learning have all been considered forms of implicit memory. In all of these cases, individuals' performances are facilitated "unconsciously" by the prior exposure of stimulus material (Kihlstrom, 1987). It should be stressed that the distinction between explicit and implicit memory is intended to be purely descriptive, and it remains to be determined how valid this dichotomy will be when applied to the entire spectrum of learning and memory phenomena. Also, whether various types of implicit memory are mediated by a single or different neurological entities has not been adequately addressed.

The Alzheimer patients who participated in our recent studies were diagnosed using the clinical criteria developed by the National Institute on Neurological and Communicative Disorders and Stroke and the Alzheimer's Disease and Related Disorders Association (McKhann et al., 1984). All patients scored at or above 104 out of a possible 144 points on the Dementia Rating Scale (DRS), a mental status examination which assesses a broad spectrum of cognitive functions (Mattis, 1976). In addition, the patients averaged 7 to 10 errors out of a possible 33 errors on Fuld's (1978) adaptation of the Information–Memory–Concentration Test (Blessed, Tomlinson, & Roth, 1968), and they earned 21 to 24 correct responses out of a possible 30 on the Mini-Mental State examination (Folstein, Folstein, & McHugh, 1975).

The HD patients were similar to those described by Butters (1984). They have a genetically transmitted disorder resulting in a progressive atrophy of the basal ganglia, especially the caudate nucleus. The most common behavioral symptoms included choreiform movements, a progressive dementia, and in most cases marked personality changes (e.g., depression, increased irritability). Although the first onset of symptomatology is difficult to determine, almost all of the patients used in these investigations initially evidenced choreiform movements in the third, fourth, or fifth decades of life. These HD patients had a mean age of 46 years and had been diagnosed 3 months to 19 years prior to testing. Although some of the HD patients had moderate choreiform movements (i.e., many had only mild chorea), none was considered in the terminal stages of the disease.

Most of the amnesic patients in these studies were alcoholics with Korsakoff's syndrome. They were male veterans with a mean age of 58 years. They all had 20- to 30-year histories of alcohol addiction accompanied by malnutrition prior to the onset of their Wernicke–Korsakoff syndrome. At the time of testing, all of the Korsakoff patients were residing in a Veterans Administration facility or nursing home. They had severe anterograde and retrograde amnesias, as measured by the Wechsler Memory Scale and on the basis of clinical assessment, but their general intellectual functioning, as measured by the Wechsler Adult Intelligence Scale, was within normal limits. Although it is generally assumed that these patients' severe amnesia is related to hemorrhagic lesions in the medial diencephalon (Victor, Adams, & Collins, 1971), there is some evidence that alcoholic Korsakoff patients, like patients with DAT, may also have a significant loss of neurons in various structures of the basal forebrain (Arendt, Bigl, Arendt, & Tennstedt, 1983).

## EPISODIC AND SEMANTIC MEMORY

The dichotomy between *episodic* and *semantic* memory has been used to differentiate the impairments of amnesic and demented patients (Martin & Fedio, 1983; Weingartner, Grafman, Boutelle, Kaye, & Martin, 1983). Although both amnesic and demented patients are impaired in the acquisition and recall of materials associated with particular temporal and/or spatial contexts (i.e., episodic memory), only demented patients are severely impaired in recalling general knowledge such as rules of grammar and multiplication tables (i.e., semantic memory). In one study, Weingartner and his colleagues (1983) compared the performances of alcoholic Korsakoff patients with those of patients with progressive dementias (presumably Alzheimer's disease) on both episodic (e.g., verbal list learning) and semantic (e.g., sentence completion, verbal fluency) memory tasks. As anticipated, both the Korsakoff and demented patients were severely impaired in the acquisition of word lists and the immediate recall of short passages, whereas only the demented patients evidenced severe deficits in the completion of highly structured sentences and on a letter fluency task. Other studies utilizing verbal fluency tasks to assess semantic memory have reported significant impairments even during the early stages of Alzheimer's and Huntington's diseases (Butters, Sax, Montgomery, & Tarlow, 1978; Ober, Dronkers, Koss, Delis, & Friedland, 1986; Rosen, 1980).

In addition to demonstrating the existence of episodic and/or semantic memory problems in amnesic and demented patients, some investigations have focused on the processess underlying these cognitive deficiencies. Although alcoholic Korsakoff patients encounter more difficulty with episodic than with semantic memory tasks, their performances on both are marked by several indices of increased sensitivity to proactive interference. For example, AK patients are highly prone to prior-item (list, passage) intrusions on short-term memory tasks (Butters & Cermak, 1980), verbal paired-associate learning (Winocur & Weiskrantz, 1976), recall of short passages (Butters, Wolfe, Granholm, & Martone, 1986), and on verbal fluency tests (Butters et al., 1986). In comparison with AK patients, HD patients appear to be severely impaired on both episodic and semantic memory tasks due to a general retrieval problem. On list-learning tests and tasks involving memory of prose passages, HD patients perform as poorly as do Korsakoff patients when recall measures are employed, but the HD patients are superior to amnesic patients if recognition tests are introduced (Butters et al., 1986; Butters, Wolfe, Martone, Granholm, & Cermak, 1985). On letter fluency tasks, HD patients generate fewer correct responses (as well as perseverative errors) than do AK patients. This double dissociation between HD and Korsakoff patients on verbal recognition and verbal fluency tests has been cited as evidence that HD patients are impaired in the initiation of systematic strategies for searching both episodic and semantic memory (Butters et al., 1986). More specifically, as the retrieval demands are reduced (e.g., the use of recognition rather than recall memory tests) or increased (e.g., letter fluency test), the performances of HD patients change dramatically in comparison with those of amnesic subjects.

Butters and his colleagues (Butters, Granholm, Salmon, Grant, & Wolfe, 1987) have extended these analyses of episodic and semantic memory to patients with dementia of the Alzheimer type (DAT). The performances of DAT, HD, and alcoholic Korsakoff patients were compared with those of young and elderly intact control subjects on memory for passages (i.e., episodic memory) and two (letter, category) verbal fluency tasks (i.e., semantic memory). Based on previous findings (Butters et al., 1986; Butters et al., 1985), it was anticipated that the quantitative and qualitative features of the AK and HD patients' responses would again reflect the roles of an increased sensitivity to proactive interference (AK patients) and a general retrieval deficit (HD patients). Since patients with DAT also commit numerous perseveration and intrusion errors on episodic (Butters, Albert, Sax, Miliotis, & Sterste, 1983; Fuld, 1983) and semantic (Ober et al., 1986) memory tasks, some similarities in the memory deficiencies of the AK and Alzheimer patients were anticipated. However, in view of Alzheimer patients' aphasic difficulties, they were expected to demonstrate a distinctive pattern of problems on the letter and category fluency tasks. If searching for exemplars of an abstract concept (i.e., animals) requires that the hierarchic organization of semantic knowledge be relatively intact (Martin, 1987), Alzheimer patients should be more impaired on category than on letter fluency tasks, especially in the very early stages of the disease.

A total of 60 subjects participated in Butters et al.'s (1987) study: 12 HD patients; 13 patients with DAT; nine AK patients; 13 young normal controls age-matched to the HD patients; and 13 old (i.e., elderly) normal controls age-matched to the patients with DAT. The three patient groups were matched in terms of overall degree of dementia as assessed with the DRS. Such matching for general cognitive loss helps reduce the confounding of differences due to disease entity (e.g., HD vs. DAT) with those due to severity of dementia (e.g., mild vs. severe dementia). As might be expected, only the Alzheimer patients showed a moderate degree of aphasia (i.e., dysnomia).

The episodic memory task involved the recall of four thematically neutral stories similar in format and length to the Logical Memory Passages of the Wechsler Memory Scale. Following the presentation of each story, the subjects were asked to count backwards from 100 by 3's for 30 seconds, and then were asked to recall as much of the story as they could remember. All stories were scored according to a verbatim scale which gave one point credit for each verbatim informational unit (maximum of 23 units per story) recalled by the subject. In addition to the items correctly recalled, the examiner recorded prior-story intrusion errors (i.e., a correctly recalled item from one story which is recalled as part of a subsequent story) and extra-story intrusion errors (i.e., ideas recalled by the subject which were never presented in any story).

The evaluation of semantic memory was comprised of two parts: a letter fluency task (FAS) developed by Benton and his colleagues (Benton, 1968; Borkowski, Benton, & Spreen, 1967), and a category fluency task. On the letter fluency task, the subjects were read the letters "F," "A," and "S" sequentially and asked to produce "as many *different* words as they could think of" that began with the given letter. For each of the three letters, the subjects were allowed 60 seconds to generate words orally. On the category fluency task, the subjects were allowed 60 seconds to produce "as many different *animals* as they could think of." The subjects' responses on the two fluency tasks were categorized into four types: (1) correct responses; (2) perseveration errors (i.e., the repetition of a correct word within a given trial); (3) intrusion errors (i.e., responses which did not conform with the criteria established for the given letter or animal category); and (4) variation errors (i.e., words repeated within a given trial with a different or added suffix).

On the episodic memory task (i.e., memory for passages), all three patient groups were found to be severely impaired in comparison with their age-matched controls in the number of phrases they correctly recalled. The major differences among the three patient groups became apparent when the numbers of prior-story and extra-story intrusion errors were examined. Both the AK patients and the patients with DAT made more intrusion errors than did their age-matched controls and the HD patients. When the performances of the patient groups were

evaluated in terms of proportions (%) of total responses, the differences among
the three patient groups were even more striking. Although the HD patients did
not recall many phrases from the four stories, what little they did recall was
usually correct (78%). In contrast, fewer than 50% of the impaired recall of the
AK and Alzheimer patients was correct; most of their recall represented some
combination of prior- and extra-story intrusion errors.

The results for the fluency tasks revealed four major differences among the
patient groups: (a) The HD patients were severely impaired on both letter and
category fluency tasks. Of the three patient groups, the HD patients produced the
fewest number of correct words on both tests. (b) The AK patients showed a
mild-to-moderate impairment on both fluency tests, and like the HD patients, the
severity of their fluency problem was not related to the linguistic constraints
(i.e., letter vs. category fluency) of the semantic memory task. (c) The performance of the Alzheimer patients was directly related to the linguistic demands of
the two fluency tasks. On the letter fluency test, the patients with DAT generated
almost as many correct words as did their age-matched controls and actually
produced more correct words than did the HD and AK patients. However, on the
category fluency task, the performance of the patients with DAT was severely
impaired. They generated significantly fewer correct animal names than did their
elderly age-matched controls, and their performance was indistinguishable from
that of the severely impaired HD patients. (d) On the letter fluency task, both the
DAT and AK patients made significantly more perseveration errors than did the
HD patients and the two groups of control subjects.

These findings indicate that patients with DAT have a pattern of deficits on
episodic and semantic memory tasks which differentiates them from other dementing (e.g., HD) and amnesic (e.g., AK) disorders. When asked to recall
short passages, the patients with DAT remembered few correct facts and made
numerous prior-story and extra-story intrusion errors. The ubiquitousness of
these intrusions exemplifies the Alzheimer patients' increased sensitivity to
proactive interference and confirms other reports that intrusion errors are an
important characteristic of these patients' episodic memory disorder (Fuld, 1983;
Fuld, Katzman, Davies, & Terry, 1982).

On the two fluency tasks (i.e., semantic memory) the Alzheimer patients
were adversely affected by their aphasic disorder as well as by their increased
sensitivity to interference. Although the patients with DAT generated nearly as
many correct responses as did the intact elderly controls on the letter fluency
task, they emitted significantly more perseveration errors. Of even greater import
for the Alzheimer patients' problems with semantic memory was the difference
in their performances on the category and letter fluency tests. They were severely
impaired in producing names of animals but encountered few problems on the
letter fluency task. That is, their deficits in semantic memory were most apparent
when they had to search for exemplars of an abstract category (i.e., animals). If,
as Martin and Fedio (1983) and Ober et al. (1986) have suggested, the Alzheimer

patients' language problems involve a reduction in the number of exemplars comprising an abstract category, scores on the category fluency task should be a highly sensitive measure of deficiencies in semantic memory. Since the letter fluency task can be performed using phonemic cues to search a very extensive set of appropriate exemplars, impairments on this task may not be apparent until the disease has progressed beyond its earliest stages.

The HD patients' performances on the story recall and fluency tasks indicate that their episodic and semantic memory disorders involve processes different from those of Alzheimer patients. The HD patients were impaired on story recall and fluency measures, but their pattern of deficits and errors does not suggest a special role for proactive interference and general language dysfunctions. The HD patients produced relatively few intrusion and perseveration errors in comparison with Alzheimer patients, and yet were severely impaired on *both* letter and category fluency tests. Although Butters et al.'s (1987) study was not designed to evaluate the hypothesis that HD patients' episodic and semantic memory disorders reflect a general retrieval deficit (Butters, 1984; Butters et al., 1986; Caine, Hunt, Weingartner, & Ebert, 1978), the findings are certainly consistent with this notion. Patients who encounter unusual difficulty in retrieving successfully stored information should be impaired on virtually all fluency tasks regardless of their linguistic demands.

The alcoholics with Korsakoff's syndrome performed as anticipated on the episodic memory task. They recalled few verbatim items from the stories and made numerous prior- and extra-story intrusion errors. The prior-story intrusions serve as another indicator of the Korsakoff patients' well-known increased sensitivity to proactive interference (Butters & Cermak, 1980), whereas the extrastory intrusions may be a remnant of these patients' tendency to confabulate during the acute phase of the disorder. The Korsakoff patients' propensity for perseverative intrusion errors was also evident on one of the semantic memory tasks (i.e., letter fluency), where they often repeated correct words (e.g., *field, found, factory, field*) during the 60-second test period. Apparently, whether episodic or semantic memory is being assessed, those memories dominating a Korsakoff patient's response hierarchy at a given moment will be repeatedly emitted and remain unmonitored by any inhibitory feedback.

The parallels in the performances of the Korsakoff and Alzheimer patients are deserving of some mention. As Butters (1985) reported in a preliminary comparison of these patients' story recall and letter fluency, both Alzheimer and Korsakoff patients are prone to perseveration and intrusion errors. Although such error tendencies are not necessarily indicative of a specific brain dysfunction or etiology (Shindler, Caplan, & Hier, 1984), one recent neuropathological report provides some basis for considering a common neurochemical factor in these two disorders. Arendt and his colleagues (1983) have reported that the number of neurons in basal forebrain structures was reduced by 70% and 47% in the brains of Alzheimer and Korsakoff patients, respectively. Examination of the brains of

HD patients revealed a significant loss of neurons in the globus pallidus, but not in the basal forebrain. Given that the basal forebrain is the source of cholinergic input to the hippocampus and frontal association cortex, one might speculate that the common error patterns of Alzheimer and AK patients might reflect a similar underlying cholinergic deficiency. Although this suggestion is certainly worthy of further neurochemical and neuropathological investigation, the differences between Alzheimer and AK patients in terms of aphasic and dyspraxic symptoms must not be overlooked. The lack of aphasia and severe constructional apraxia in alcoholic Korsakoff patients may be due to differences in the extent of basal forebrain damage or may be indications that the noted similarities in the two disorders are coincidental.

Another recent study (Granholm & Butters, 1988) provides further support for some common underlying deficits in Korsakoff and Alzheimer patients. Using an encoding specificity paradigm (Tulving & Thomson, 1973), Cermak, Uhly, and Reale (1980) found that Korsakoff patients were so impaired in their encoding of the semantic relationships between two words that they could not use the product of such encoding to facilitate retrieval. The encoding specificity hypothesis, as developed from verbal memory studies with normal subjects (Thomson & Tulving, 1970), predicts that words present at both encoding and retrieval, whether strong or weak associates, should be the most effective retrieval cues. However, unlike intact subjects, AK patients consistently benefited more from strong associates than from weak associates of the to-be-remembered (TBR) word, regardless of which associate was present during encoding (Cermak et al., 1980). Granholm and Butters (1988), using the same stimuli and design employed by Cermak et al. (1980), examined the associative encoding and retrieval abilities of Alzheimer and HD patients. If, as Martin, Brouwers, Cox, and Fedio (1985) have suggested, Alzheimer patients have a limited ability to perform adequate semantic encoding during presentation, they should demonstrate a pattern of performance similar to that of the AK patients. Since HD patients' memory deficits primarily involve retrieval problems (Butters et al., 1986), it was anticipated that these patients should evidence a pattern of performance on the encoding specificity task similar to that of intact controls.

Forty subjects participated in this study: 10 HD patients; 10 patients with DAT; 10 middle-aged normal controls (i.e., age-matched to the HD patients); and 10 elderly normal controls (i.e., age-matched to the patients with DAT). Since the HD and DAT patient groups did not differ in terms of their DRS scores, they appeared to be matched in terms of overall severity of dementia.

The materials and design employed in this study are described in detail elsewhere (Cermak et al., 1980; Granholm & Butters, 1988). Briefly, 60 word triads were constructed, consisting of a to-be-remembered (TBR) word plus a strong and weak associate of the TBR word (e.g., TBR word = DAY; strong associate = night; weak associate = sun). The 60 TBR words were then divided into five lists of 12 words each, and printed on index cards in uppercase letters.

Four encoding/retrieval conditions and a free-recall condition were created by varying the types of cues (i.e., strong: S; weak: W; or no cues: 0) that were available at presentation and recall. The five experimental conditions were designated by the following abbreviated terms: 0–0, S–S, W–W, W–S, and S–W. For example, condition 0–0 was a standard free-recall condition with no associates present at either presentation or recall. In the S–S condition, each TBR word was accompanied by a strong cue at presentation (e.g., DAY – night), and the subjects were cued with the same strong associate at recall. In condition W–S, each TBR word was accompanied by a weak associate (e.g., DAY – sun) at presentation, and subjects were cued with an appropriate strongly associated (but not previously presented) word (e.g., night) at recall, and so on.

Subjects were presented a list of 12 word pairs, each consisting of a capitalized TBR word and, in the four encoding/retrieval conditions, an associated word printed in lowercase letters and enclosed in parentheses above the TBR word. First, the subject was shown a sample card and told to read aloud and memorize each capitalized word and also to pay attention to the related word as a possible aid in recalling the capitalized one at a later time. Following the presentation of this practice card, each of the 12 word pairs was presented individually for three seconds. After a second presentation of the 12 word pairs, the subject was given a sheet of paper containing a typed column of 12 cue words with a space beside each for the appropriate TBR words. The subject was instructed that each word on the list was a cue or aid to recalling one of the capitalized words that he or she had read aloud. The subject was told to write the words remembered in the space next to the cue that helped him or her. Words remembered without the help of a cue were to be written separately on the page. In the 0–0 condition subjects were shown no cues at recall; rather, they were handed a sheet containing 12 blank spaces and asked to recall as many of the TBR words as possible. A maximum of 5 minutes was allowed for each recall test. The same procedures were followed for each of the five experimental conditions. Subjects were allowed a 2–3 minute rest period between lists.

In addition to the number of words correctly recalled, the number of omission errors, prior-list intrusion errors (i.e., words recalled which were present as either TBR words or cues on a previous trial), and extralist intrusion errors (i.e., words recalled by the subject which were not presented as TBR words or cues in any other list) were also recorded.

Figure 1 shows the total number of correctly recalled words for the four subject groups in the free-recall condition and each of the four encoding/retrieval conditions. Both the HD and Alzheimer patients were impaired relative to their age-matched controls in total words recalled. Although the two patient groups demonstrated similar overall levels of recall performance, they displayed different patterns of performance across the five experimental conditions. For all four subject groups, recall performance was best in the S–S condition (i.e., strong associates presented both at encoding and retrieval) and was worst in the S–W

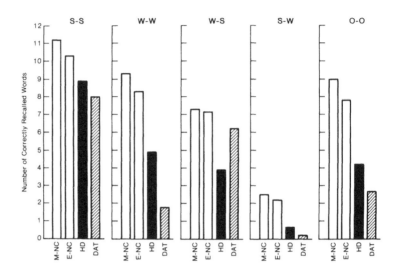

*FIGURE 1* Total number of correctly recalled words in each of the five conditions for the middle-aged normal control (M-NC) subjects, elderly normal control (E-NC) subjects, Huntington's disease (HD) patients, and patients with dementia of the Alzheimer type (DAT). Adapted from Granholm and Butters (1988).

condition. The HD group, like the two control groups, also demonstrated a similar level of recall on the three remaining conditions (i.e., W–W, W–S, 0–0). In contrast, the DAT group performed significantly better in the W–S condition than in the W–W and 0–0 conditions. These different patterns of performance were still apparent when proportion scores (percentage of total correct responses) were used to correct for group differences in the total number of words recalled (Figure 2).

Analyses of prior-list intrusions, extralist intrusions, and omission errors also revealed different patterns of performance between the HD and DAT groups. Specifically, the Alzheimer patients made a larger proportion (i.e., percentage of total errors) of extralist intrusions than did the HD patients, while the HD patients produced a larger proportion of omission errors.

The findings of this encoding specificity study are consistent with our previous demonstrations that the semantic memory impairments of DAT and HD patients involve different underlying processes. Although both patient groups evidenced poor recall overall, they were clearly distinguished by their ability to utilize strong and weak cues for retrieving TBR words. As anticipated by their general difficulty with initiating systematic retrieval processes (Butters, 1984; Butters et al., 1986; Caine et al., 1978) the HD patients demonstrated the same pattern of performance with the various combinations of weak and strong cues at encoding and retrieval as did the two intact control groups. The HD patients and

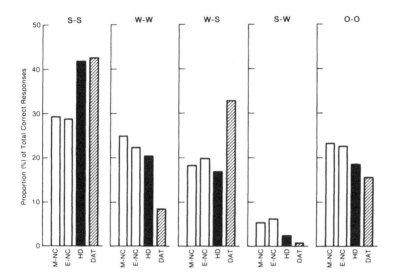

*FIGURE 2*    Recall performance in each of the five conditions is presented as a proportion of total correctly recalled words for the middle-aged normal control (M-NC) subjects, elderly normal control (E-NC) subjects, Huntington's disease (HD) patients, and patients with dementia of the Alzheimer type (DAT). Adapted from Granholm and Butters (1988).

control subjects were generally most successful recalling words when the strength of the cues was identical during encoding and retrieval, and were least successful when the cue words differed during presentation and recall. It appears, then, that both the HD patients and control subjects successfully encoded the relationships between the cue and TBR words and subsequently were able to use the cue word to facilitate retrieval. The HD patients' overall impaired performance probably demonstrates their inability to initiate efficient retrieval strategies despite relatively intact encoding.

The Alzheimer patients' pattern of performance with the various combinations of strong and weak cues indicated that they either did not encode the relationships between cue and TBR words or were unable to utilize the product of encoding at the time of cued recall. In comparison with the HD patients, the Alzheimer patients were severely deficient in recall when the same weak associate was shown at both encoding and retrieval. Also, the Alzheimer patients performed relatively well whenever a strong cue was present at recall, regardless of whether a strong or weak cue was present at encoding. These results suggest that the encoding of specific relationships between associates and TBR words was not responsible for the Alzheimer patients' success in retrieval with strong cues. Instead of relying upon semantic encoding the patients with DAT appear to have simply generated their most dominant associations to the cue words during recall testing. Such an associative strategy would account for the huge discrepancies in the DAT patients' performance when strong and weak associates were available during recall. Free associating to a strong associate is obviously much more likely to result in the chance production of the TBR word. The other subject groups, relying upon the product of their encoding as a retrieval cue, were hindered whenever the same associate was not present at both encoding and retrieval.

The results of the error analyses are also consistent with this interpretation of the Alzheimer patients' performance. Any tendency to free associate to retrieval cues should result not only in an increased probability of recalling TBR words when strong associates are present but also in a marked increment in extralist intrusion errors regardless of cue conditions. Since HD patients and intact control subjects did rely primarily upon the product of the encoding during stimulus presentation, they should not have been prone to generating such extralist intrusions.

The Alzheimer patients' pattern of performance on this task, though different from that of the HD patients, was strikingly similar to the pattern reported by Cermak et al. (1980) for alcoholic Korsakoff patients. Both DAT and AK patients recalled significantly more words in the W–S condition than in the W–W condition, and neither groups performance differed significantly from that of control subjects in the W–S condition. These results suggest that Alzheimer and Korsakoff patients are both impaired in their ability to utilize semantic information present at encoding to facilitate recall performance. Again, whether such similarities in cognitive mechanisms truly reflect some common neurological dysfunction (e.g., loss of cells in the basal forebrain) can only be determined by future neuropathological investigations.

Finally, the findings of our recent investigations (Butters et al., 1987; Granholm & Butters, 1988) not only support the notion that episodic and semantic memory are disturbed in the dementias, but also demonstrate that the processes underlying failures in episodic and semantic memory systems may vary from one form of dementia to another. Patients with HD perform poorly on both episodic and semantic memory tasks because of their inability to initiate suitable retrieval strategies, whereas the deficits of patients with DAT on these same memory tasks reflect linguistic aberrations, an increased sensitivity to proactive interference, and reduced semantic encoding ability. It appears then that the notion that all dementias may be characterized as a loss of both episodic and semantic memory seems too simplistic and likely blurs many important distinctions among various degenerative diseases of the central nervous system.

## IMPLICIT MEMORY

In addition to the differences between HD and Alzheimer patients on explicit tests of episodic and semantic memory, there is now some evidence that these patient groups may be dissociated by their performance on implicit memory tests as well. Martone and her colleagues (1984) found that HD patients were impaired in their ability to acquire a visuomotor skill (i.e., reading mirror-reversed words), whereas Eslinger and Damasio (1986) have reported that Alzheimer patients could acquire in a normal fashion the motor skills underlying a pursuit rotor task. Together, these results suggest that the neostriatum (damaged in HD but preserved in the early stages of DAT) may be critically involved in the acquisition of visuomotor skills. That is, in addition to the well-known motor dysfunctions (e.g., chorea, bradykinesia, tremor, rigidity) associated with basal ganglia lesions, patients with various forms of the so-called "subcortical" dementias (Cummings & Benson, 1984) may be deficient in forming the motor programs and links so vital to the acquisition of motor skills.

To assess this hypothesis, Heindel, Butters, and Salmon (1988) compared the ability of HD and Alzheimer patients to learn a pursuit rotor task. This classical test of skill learning has a major methodological advantage over mirror reading in that patients' initial level of performance may be equated readily by adjusting the speed of rotation of the disk. Since HD patients' initial level of performance on a mirror-reading task is much slower than that of intact controls and even other neurological groups (Martone et al., 1984), ceiling and floor effects may cloud any interpretation of significant group differences in rate of learning.

A total of 44 patients participated in Heindel et al.'s (1988) study: 10 HD patients; 10 patients with DAT; four amnesic patients of mixed etiologies; and 20 intact control subjects. As in our other studies (Butters et al., 1987; Granholm & Butters, 1988), the three patient groups were matched for overall degree of dementia with the DRS. The small group of amnesic patients was included to confirm previous findings of spared motor learning in amnesia (Cermak, Lewis, Butters, & Goodglass, 1973; Corkin, 1968).

Subjects were asked to maintain contact between a stylus held in their preferred hand and a small metallic disk (2 cm in diameter) on a rotating turntable (25 cm in diameter). The turntable could be adjusted to rotate at 15, 30, 45, or 60 rotations per min (rpm) for a given 20-sec trial. All subjects were tested over three sessions of eight trials each, with each session separated by approximately 30 min of other psychometric testing. Within each test session, subjects were also allowed a 1-min rest interval between the fourth and fifth trials, thereby creating six blocks of four trials each. The total time on target was recorded for each 20-sec trial.

For each subject the first test session was preceded by a block of practice trials to determine the speed of rotation (i.e., 15, 30, 45, 60 rpm) of the turntable. On each successive practice trial the speed of the turntable was increased. The turntable was then set for the remainder of the subject's testing to that speed associated with a score (i.e., time on target) closest to 5 sec (i.e., contact maintained 25% of time). In this manner, the initial level of performance on the pursuit rotor task was equated for the four subject groups.

The results showed that three of the four groups evidenced systematic skill learning over the six blocks of testing. Specifically, the Alzheimer and amnesic

patients and normal control subjects all improved their performance to approximately 52% time on target on Block 6, whereas the HD patients maintained
contact between the stylus and the disk for only 36% of the time on this last test
block. When difference scores (Block 6 – Block 1) were calculated to measure
the amount of skill acquisition, the HD patients demonstrated significantly less
learning than did the other three groups. As anticipated, the amnesic and
Alzheimer patients did not differ from the intact control subjects on any measure
of skill acquisition.

Like previous findings, the results of Heindel et al.'s (1988) study support
the notion that the basal ganglia (especially the neostriatum) are involved in the
acquisition of motor skills. Since the four subject groups were matched for initial
level of performance on the pursuit rotor task, the impairment of the HD patients
cannot be attributed to ceiling or floor effects. Furthermore, the HD patients with
the least amount of functional disability were found to be as impaired on this task
as were those with the greatest disability, indicating that pursuit rotor learning in
HD does not appear to be directly related to primary motor deficits. It should also
be noted that the matching of the three patient groups in terms of overall level of
dementia with the DRS reduces the possibility that the differences in the learning
of the motor skill might reflect differences in degree of overall cognitive loss
(i.e., dementia).

The proposed linkage between motor skill learning and the basal ganglia is
consistent with current understanding of the organization of the motor system.
The neostriatum along with the other subcortical components of the ex-
trapyramidal motor system (i.e., the pallidum, substantia nigra, and subthalamic
nucleus) appears to influence voluntary motor behavior in an indirect way
through thalamocortical projections to the pyramidal system. In addition, basal
ganglia dysfunction has been associated more with an impairment in self-
inititated movements than simply with the direct control of movement per se
(Evarts & Wise, 1984). Given the massive topographical projection from most of
the neocortex to the neostriatum (Kemp & Powell, 1970), the neostriatum may
play a role in converting general strategies for motor action formed by the
association cortex into purposeful motor behavior (Brooks, 1986; Groves, 1983).

Given the HD patients' impairment in acquiring visuomotor skills, the
question arises concerning the general role of the basal ganglia in implicit
memory. Are the basal ganglia critically involved in all forms of implicit
memory, or are different forms of implicit memory mediated by their own
distinct neural systems? An investigation of verbal priming in amnesic and
demented patients (Shimamura, Salmon, Squire, & Butters, 1987) supports the
latter hypothesis. Priming, another form of implicit memory, has been defined as
the temporary (and unconscious) facilitation of performance via prior exposure to
stimuli. Shimamura et al., using a lexical priming paradigm in which subjects
were asked to complete three-letter word stems with the first words that came to
mind, found that AK patients, HD patients, and normal controls all demonstrated
a similar tendency to complete these stems with previously presented stimuli.

Alzheimer patients, however, were found to be severely impaired in their lexical priming ability. These results suggest that this form of implicit memory is not dependent on the integrity of the basal ganglia, but rather is mediated by a neural system that is selectively disrupted in DAT.

Since patients with DAT show marked pathology in temporal, parietal, and frontal association cortices along with a relative sparing of the primary sensory areas (Brun, 1983), their impaired priming ability may be related to damage to those neocortical association regions which store the lexical representations of semantic memory. This notion that Alzheimer patients are deficient in activating pre-existing representations stored in semantic memory is also consistent with the difficulty Alzheimer patients have on explicit tests of semantic memory such as category fluency (Butters et al., 1987; Martin, 1987; Martin & Fedio, 1983; Ober et al., 1986). In both instances, the Alzheimer patients' impairment may be related to a breakdown in the hierarchic organization of their semantic knowledge.

To explore further these possible ties between patients' priming and semantic memory deficits, Salmon, Shimamura, Butters, and Smith (1988) administered a semantic priming task to Alzheimer, HD, and intact control subjects. Subjects were asked to judge categorically or functionally related word pairs (e.g., BIRD–ROBIN, NEEDLE–THREAD) and later to say the first word that comes to mind (i.e., "free associate") when presented with the first word (e.g., BIRD, NEEDLE) of a pair. Semantic priming, as well as an intact organization of semantic memory, are indicated by the subjects' tendency to produce the second word of the related word pairs. Nine patients with DAT, 10 HD patients, 9 elderly control subjects, and 10 middle-aged control subjects participated in this study. The Alzheimer and HD patients were again matched for overall level of dementia with the DRS.

Forty-eight *functional* word pairs were created by pairing 24 stimulus words with both a "strong" associate and a "moderate" associate. The two words in each of these functional pairs were semantically related either by common function (e.g., NEEDLE–THREAD), by tendency to occur in the same context (e.g., DOCTOR–NURSE), or by part–whole relationships (e.g., HAND–FINGER). Forty-eight *categorical* pairs (e.g., BIRD –ROBIN) were also created by pairing 24 different stimulus words with both a "strong" and "moderate" exemplar. Six additional words pairs, three categorical and three functional, were designated as filler pairs, and used to control for primacy and recency effects. Another six word pairs with no apparent semantic association were created. These unrelated pairs were used to control for the possibility that subjects might respond with target words during the free association task, not because an existing semantic association had been primed, but simply because the two words had been presented together.

The test was administered in three identical blocks, which were composed of a rating task and a free-association task. Subjects were presented pairs of words one pair at a time, and were asked to rate how closely the two words were related on a five-point scale. Each group of 12 word pairs (4 categorical, 4 functional, 2 unrelated, 2 filler) was presented to each subject twice in succession, in the same order. Of the categorical and functional pairs, half of each type were strong associates, the other half moderate associates. Filler pairs were always presented first and last in each group of 12 pairs.

Immediately following the second presentation of word pairs in each block, the free-association task was presented. The examiner never mentioned that this task was related to the previous rating task. Subjects were told that single words would be presented visually and they were to say "the first word that came to mind" in response to each stimulus word. Stimuli for the free-association task included the first words of the categorical, functional, and unrelated pairs presented during the rating task. In addition, eight distractors (four strong associates and four moderate associates) were presented; they were members of categorical and functional stimulus pairs which had not been presented to the subjects at any time. Distractors were included as a measure of the probability of a correct response due simply to chance. The same procedures were followed for the remaining two blocks.

Figure 3 shows the percentage of previously presented words produced on the semantic priming task by each group. Since the production of previously presented words from unrelated word pairs was extremely rare and isolated, subjects in all four groups apparently treated the task as one of free association

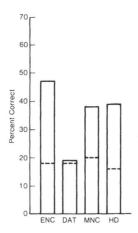

*FIGURE 3* The percentage of previously presented words correctly produced in the free association task by patients with dementia of the Alzheimer type (DAT), patients with Huntington's disease (HD), elderly normal control subjects (ENC), and middle-aged normal control subjects (MNC). The baseline guessing rate of each group is indicated by the broken line. Adapted from Salmon et al. (1988).

rather than adopting a conscious recall strategy. The HD patients demonstrated normal semantic priming in this task, and performed significantly better than did the Alzheimer patients. The DAT group was significantly impaired compared with their control group, and was the only group that did not prime above baseline guessing rates. The priming performance of the four groups was further subdivided into categorical vs. functional items (Fig. 4) as well as strongly vs. moderately associated items. In all four cases, the Alzheimer, but not the HD patients, were severely impaired in their semantic priming ability.

The results of this study support the idea that Alzheimer patients experience a breakdown in the associative structure of their semantic memory. The categorical and functional cues may have failed to activate traces of previously presented stimuli due to the dissolution of the semantic network governing verbal materials. For example, the cue "BIRD" may not have evoked an unconscious activation of the categorical associate "ROBIN" because the association between the two words has been greatly weakened. Such a disruption of the organization of semantic memory would also account for the Alzheimer patients' previously noted impairment on a lexical priming task (Shimamura et al., 1987). That is, the association in semantic memory between a word stem such as "MOT" and the word "MOTEL" may be sufficiently disrupted to negate the facilitating effect of the word's presentation.

This interpretation of the semantic priming results allows for the integration of the Alzheimer patients' performance on explicit and implicit semantic mem-

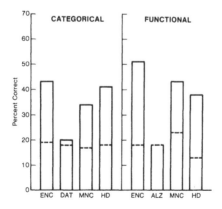

FIGURE 4   The percentage of previously presented words correctly produced in response to categorically or functionally related semantic associates in the free-association task by patients with dementia of the Alzheimer type (DAT), patients with Huntington's disease (HD), elderly normal control subjects (ENC), and middle-aged normal control subjects (MNC). The baseline guessing rate of each group is indicated by the broken line. Adapted from Salmon et al. (1988).

ory tasks. Like deficits in semantic priming, deficiencies in the effortful retrieval of specific exemplars of an abstract category may also reflect significant changes in the structure and organization of semantic memory. As Martin and Fedio (1983) have noted, using a supermarket fluency task, the number of specific exemplars associated with a given category is greatly reduced in DAT. Alzheimer patients can often name many of the general categories of items found in a supermarket (e.g., meats, vegetables, fruits) but may be unable to produce specific examples (e.g., veal, beef, tomatoes, lettuce, apples) of these categories.

The intact semantic priming of HD patients supports the conclusion drawn from the lexical priming study (Shimamura et al., 1987) that the integrity of the basal ganglia is not critical for the activation of stored representations in semantic memory. These results, in conjunction with those from the skill learning studies (Eslinger & Damasio, 1986; Heindel et al., 1988; Martone et al., 1984), suggest that different forms of implicit memory do depend on different anatomical substrates. Specifically, the HD patients' impairments on pursuit rotor and mirror-reading tests are consistent with a critical role of the basal ganglia in skill learning, whereas the Alzheimer patients' deficiencies on lexical and semantic priming tasks may be attributable to the cortical neuropathology reported in DAT (Terry & Katzman, 1983).

The double dissociation between the HD and Alzheimer patients on implicit memory tasks has relevance for Cummings and Benson's (1984) distinction between cortical and subcortical dementias. Patients with subcortical dementias (e.g., HD) usually have much less dysphasia and dyspraxia than do patients with cortical dementias (e.g., Alzheimer's disease) but are also much slower to initiate and complete most cognitive, as well as motor, processes than are patients with cortical degenerative diseases. The present results suggest that patients with cortical and subcortical dementias can also be differentiated by their performance on different implicit memory tasks. Patients with cortical dementias may have a preserved capacity to acquire and retain motor skills, but may be severely impaired on other tests of implicit memory which depend on the intactness of the association cortex in the dominant hemisphere. In contrast, patients with some forms of subcortical dementia may appear very limited in their ability to learn motor skills despite their normal performance on implicit memory tasks mediated by verbal processes (e.g., lexical priming).

In a recently completed study, Heindel, Salmon, Shults, Walicke, and Butters (1989) evaluated whether this double dissociation between the two implicit memory tasks and the DAT and HD patients would generalize to patients with idiopathic Parkinson's disease (PD). Although not included in James Parkinson's (1817) original description of the disorder, dementia has consistently been found to occur more frequently in PD than would be expected in a general population of the same age (Brown & Marsden, 1984; Lieberman et al., 1979). Although there is now general agreement that dementia can be an integral feature of the disease, considerable disagreement still exists concerning the underlying nature of the dementia. Since the primary lesion in PD appears to be a loss of cells in the substantia nigra pars compacta, several investigators (Albert, 1978; Huber, Shuttleworth, Paulson, Bellchambers, & Clapp, 1986; Mayeux, Stern, Rosen, & Benson, 1981) have stressed the common features (e.g., preserved language) of the dementias of PD, HD, and other subcortical dementias. However, others (Alvord et al., 1974; Boller, Mizutani, Roessmann, & Gambetti, 1980) have noted that the dementing form of PD shares many neuropathological features with DAT and may be the result of the superimposition of Alzheimer-type changes upon primary subcortical pathology. In view of these uncertainties about the etiology and neurological basis of the dementia of PD, the performances of demented PD patients on priming and motor skill learning tasks seem of some importance.

Heindel and his colleagues (1989) administered to demented and non-demented PD patients two of the implicit memory tasks (pursuit rotor learning, stem-completion priming) found to differentiate DAT from HD patients. If the dementia of PD is similar to that of DAT, impaired performance on lexical priming, combined with intact motor skill learning would be expected. Conversely, if demented PD patients manifest deficient skill learning combined with normal lexical priming, their cognitive impairments should appear similar to those of HD patients.

A total of 68 subjects participated in this study: 16 patients with DAT; 13 HD patients; 8 demented PD patients; 9 nondemented PD patients; 12 elderly control subjects; and 10 middle-aged control subjects. The demented PD patients all obtained DRS scores that were at least two standard deviations below the mean of the elderly control subjects (i.e., fewer than 134). The nondemented PD group, in contrast, did not differ significantly on the DRS from either control group. All PD patients were rated from 0 (absence of symptom) to 4 (greatest severity) on each of the three classic parkinsonian symptoms; i.e., tremor, rigidity, and bradykinesia. Ten of the HD patients were also rated with a five-point scale for the severity of their choreiform movements.

The lexical priming paradigm used in this study was adapted from that used by Shimamura et al. (1987). Briefly, subjects were shown 10 words (e.g., MOTEL, ABSTAIN) one at a time and were asked to rate how much they liked each word on a five-point scale. Three additional filler words were placed at the beginning of the list and two at the end in order to reduce primacy and recency effects, respectively. After the subjects completed this initial rating of the entire set of 10 words, the examiner requested that they perform a second rating of the same words presented in the same order. Following the two presentation trials, subjects were shown 20 three-letter word stems (e.g., MOT, ABS) and were asked to complete each stem with the first word that came to mind. Ten of the stems could be completed using study words, and the other 10 stems were used to assess baseline guessing rates. The entire stem-completion study/test procedure was then repeated in exactly the same manner using a different list of 10 words. In this way, stem completion was assessed twice, using two different lists of 10 words.

The procedure for the pursuit rotor task was identical to that used in the previously described study by Heindel et al. (1988).

As can be seen in Figure 5, all six subject groups began the pursuit rotor task at about the same level of performance (i.e., 25% time on target). Despite these similar initial levels, the HD and demented PD groups both demonstrated significantly less learning over the six test blocks than did their control groups (Figure 6). The HD and demented PD groups, though not differing significantly from each other, also demonstrated significantly less motor learning than did both the DAT and nondemented PD groups. In contrast, the Alzheimer and nondemented PD patients did not differ from their controls in the amount they learned on this task.

The motor learning ability of the HD patients was found to be significantly correlated with their scores on the DRS, but not with the severity of their choreiform movements. Similarly, the performance of the PD patients (demented and nondemented combined) was significantly correlated with DRS, but not with the severity of their tremor, rigidity, or bradykinesia. Thus, motor learning in

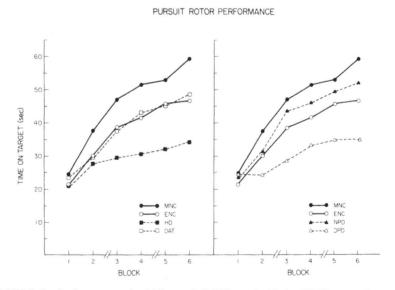

PURSUIT ROTOR PERFORMANCE

**FIGURE 5** Performance of middle-aged (MNC) and elderly (ENC) normal control subjects, Huntington's disease (HD) patients, patients with dementia of the Alzheimer type (DAT), and demented (DPD) and nondemented (NPD) Parkinson's disease patients on the pursuit rotor task. Adapted from Heindel et al. (1989).

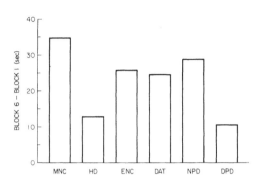

*FIGURE 6* Difference in performance between the last and first test blocks on the pursuit rotor task for middle-aged (MNC) and elderly (ENC) normal control subjects, Huntington's disease (HD) patients, patients with dementia of the Alzheimer type (DAT), and demented (DPD) and nondemented (NPD) Parkinson's disease patients. Adapted from Heindel et al. (1989).

both HD and PD patients appears to be related more to the severity of their dementia than to the severity of their motor dysfunction.

The results of the lexical priming task are shown in Figure 7. Baseline guessing rates (dotted lines) did not differ across the groups, indicating that the subject groups were very similar in their ability to perform the basic stem-completion task. Although the HD and nondemented PD groups demonstrated normal priming ability, the DAT and demented PD groups were both severely impaired relative to their control groups. Furthermore, the DAT and demented PD groups were both impaired in their priming ability compared with the HD and nondemented PD groups, but did not differ significantly from each other.

Besides providing a replication of the previously reported dissociations between HD and DAT patients on the two implicit memory tasks (Heindel et al., 1988; Shimamura et al., 1987), these findings suggest that demented PD patients may not fit neatly into Cummings and Benson's (1984) "cortical-subcortical" taxonomy of dementia. The impaired performances of the demented PD patients on both pursuit rotor and lexical priming tasks indicate that these patients share some common features with *both* HD and DAT patients. The demented PD patients' deficiencies in acquiring motor skills may be due to their basal ganglia dysfunction, whereas their lack of lexical priming may have its origins in neuropathological changes in cortical association areas. It appears likely then that previous attempts to define the dementia of PD may have been hampered by the failure to recognize the coexistence of both "cortical" and "subcortical" features within the same disease.

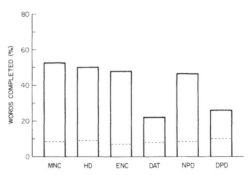

FIGURE 7   The percentage of word stems completed with previously presented words on the lexical priming task by middle-aged (MNC) and elderly (ENC) normal control subjects, Huntington's disease (HD) patients, patients with dementia of the Alzheimer type (DAT), and demented (DPD) and nondemented (NPD) Parkinson's disease patients. Adapted from Heindel et al. (1989).

## CONCLUSIONS

The neuropsychological studies reviewed in this chapter are consistent with the notion that patients with dementias of different etiologies can be differentiated from each other and from patients with amnesic conditions. Although both patients with DAT and HD patients are impaired on episodic and semantic memory tasks, they seem to fail for quite distinct reasons. The HD patients' capacity to store new verbal information seems relatively preserved, but these patients appear extremely deficient in initiating systematic retrieval strategies when asked to recall information from either episodic or semantic memory. In contrast, patients with DAT encounter unusual difficulty in consolidating new information, and their attempts to recall information from semantic memory are often hindered by their dysphasia. The deleterious effects of proactive interference are also more apparent in the episodic and semantic memory deficits of Alzheimer than of HD patients.

Investigations focusing upon the learning of motor skills and other types of implicit memory usually preserved in amnesic patients suggest additional dissociations between cortical and subcortical dementias. Although HD patients appear severely impaired in their attempts to acquire motor skills, they perform normally on stem-completion priming tasks. The opposite relationship is seen in patients with DAT. Alzheimer patients acquire and retain motor skills with the same facility as intact controls and amnesic patients, but they evidence little tendency to complete three-letter stems with words previously exposed to them.

These findings suggest that the learning of motor skills and stem-completion priming depend on different neuroanatomical systems and also lend support to the previously proposed distinction between cortical and subcortical dementias. The impaired performances of demented PD patients on both tests of implicit memory suggest the presence of both cortical and subcortical dysfunctions in this disorder.

From a clinical perspective, it is important to stress again that the present findings emanate from the application of concepts borrowed from cognitive psychology and from careful analyses of the processes underlying the patients' achievements and deficits. These demonstrations of the utility of experimental concepts with pathological populations also provide the constructs themselves with a form of validity and legitimacy unavailable through studies limited to normal subjects. In our view, the mutual benefits that have been described represent an ideal model for the interaction between experimental and clinical approaches to neuropsychology. Certainly, such interactions between clinical and experimental phenomena lie at the core of Luria's neuropsychology and are essential to the success of any process-achievement analyses.

## ACKNOWLEDGMENTS

The research reported in this manuscript was supported by funds from the Medical Research Service of the Veterans Administration, by NIAAA grant AA–00187 to Boston University, and by NIA grants AG-05131 and AG-08204 to the University of California at San Diego.

## REFERENCES

Albert, M. L., (1978). Subcortical dementia. In R. Katzman, R. D. Terry, & K. L. Bick (Eds.), *Alzheimer's disease: Senile dementia and related disorders* (pp. 173–180). New York: Raven Press.

Albert, M. S., & Kaplan, E. (1980). Organic implications of neuropsychological deficits in the elderly. In L. Poon, J. Fozard, L. Cermak, D. Arenberg, & L. Thompson (Eds.), *New directions in memory and aging* (pp. 403–432). Hillsdale, NJ: Lawrence Erlbaum Associates.

Alvord, E. C., Forno, L. S., Kusske, J. A., Kaufman, R. J., Rhodes, J. S., & Goetowski, C. R. (1974). The pathology of parkinsonism: A comparison of degeneration in cerebral cortex and brainstem. In F. McDowell & A. Barbeau (Eds.), *Advances in neurology, Vol. 5: Second Canadian-American conference on Parkinson's disease* (pp. 175–193). New York: Raven Press.

Arendt, T., Bigl, V., Arendt, A., & Tennstedt, A. (1983). Loss of neurons in the nucleus basalis of Meynert in Alzheimer's disease. *Acta Neuropathologica, 61,* 101–108.

Benton, A. L. (1968). Differential behavioral effects in frontal lobe disease. *Neuropsychologia, 6,* 53–60.

Blessed, G., Tomlinson, B. E., & Roth, M. (1968). The association between quantitative measures of dementia and of senile change in the cerebral grey matter of elderly subjects. *British Journal of Psychiatry, 114,* 797–811.

Boller, F., Mizutani, T., Roessmann, U., & Gambetti, P. (1980), Parkinson disease, dementia, and Alzheimer disease: Clinicopathological correlations. *Annals of Neurology, 7,* 329-335.

Borkowski, J. G., Benton A. L., & Spreen, O. (1967). Word fluency and brain damage. *Neuropsychologia, 5,* 135–140.

Brooks, V. B. (1986). *The neural basis of motor control.* New York: Oxford University Press.

Brown, R. G., & Marsden, C. D. (1984). How common is dementia in Parkinson's disease? *Lancet, 2,* 1262–1265.

Brun, A. (1983). An overview of light and electron microscopic changes. In B. Reisberg (Ed.), *Alzheimer's disease* (pp. 37–47). New York: Free Press.

Butters, N. (1984). The clinical aspects of memory disorders: Contributions from experimental studies of amnesia and dementia. *Journal of Clinical Neuropsychology, 6,* 17–36.

Butters, N. (1985). Alcoholic Korsakoff's syndrome: Some unresolved issues concerning etiology, neuropathology and cognitive deficits. *Journal of Clinical and Experimental Neuropsychology, 7,* 181–210.

Butters, N., Albert, M. S., Sax, D. S., Miliotis, P., & Sterste, A. (1983). The effect of verbal elaborators on the pictorial memory of brain-damaged patients. *Neuropsychologia, 21,* 307–323.

Butters, N., & Cermak, L. S. (1980). *Alcoholic Korsakoff's syndrome: An information-processing approach to amnesia.* New York: Academic Press.

Butters, N., Granholm, E., Salmon, D. P., Grant, I., & Wolfe, J. (1987). Episodic and semantic memory: A comparison of amnesic and demented patients. *Journal of Clinical and Experimental Neuropsychology, 9,* 479–497.

Butters, N., Sax, D. S., Montgomery, K., & Tarlow, S. (1978). Comparison of the neuropsychological deficits associated with early and advanced Huntington's disease. *Archives of Neurology, 35,* 585–589.

Butters, N., Wolfe, J., Granholm, E., & Martone, M. (1986). An assessment of verbal recall, recognition and fluency abilities in patients with Huntington's disease. *Cortex, 22,* 11–32.

Butters, N., Wolfe, J., Martone, M., Granholm, E., & Cermak, L. S. (1985). Memory disorders associated with Huntington's disease: Verbal recall, verbal recognition and procedural memory. *Neuropsychologia, 6,* 729–744.

Caine, E., Hunt, R., Weingartner, H., & Ebert, M. (1978). Huntington's dementia: Clinical and neuropsychological features. *Archives of General Psychiatry, 35,* 377–384.

Cermak, L. S., Lewis, R., Butters, N., & Goodglass, H. (1973). Role of verbal mediation in performance of motor tasks by Korsakoff patients. *Perceptual and Motor Skills, 37,* 259–262.

Cermak, L. S., Uhly, B., & Reale, L. (1980). Encoding specificity in the alcoholic Korsakoff patient. *Brain and Language, 11,* 119–127.

Cohen, N. J., & Squire, L. R. (1980). Preserved learning and retention of pattern analyzing skills in amnesia: Dissociation of knowing how and knowing that. *Science, 210,* 207–210.

Corkin, S. (1968). Acquisition of motor skill after bilateral medial temporal-lobe excision. *Neuropsychologia, 6,* 255–265.

Cummings, J. L., & Benson, D. F. (1984). Subcortical dementia: Review of an emerging concept. *Archives of Neurology, 41,* 874–879.

Eslinger, P. J., & Damasio, A. R. (1986). Preserved motor learning in Alzheimer's disease: Implications for anatomy and behavior. *Journal of Neuroscience, 6,* 3006–3009.

Evarts, E. V., & Wise, S. P. (1984). Basal ganglia outputs and motor control. In D. Evered & M. O'Connor (Eds.), *Functions of the basal ganglia: Ciba foundation symposium 107* (pp. 83–102). London: Pitman Press.

Folstein, M. F., Folstein, S. E., & McHugh, P. R. (1975). "Mini-Mental State": A practical method for grading the cognitive state of patients for the clinician. *Journal of Psychiatric Research, 12,* 189–198.

Fuld, P. (1978). Psychological testing in the differential diagnosis of the dementias. In R. Katzman, R. D. Terry, & K. L. Bick (Eds.), *Alzheimer's disease: Senile dementia and related disorders* (pp. 185–193). New York: Raven Press.

Fuld, P. A.(1983). Word intrusion as a diagnostic sign in Alzheimer's disease. *Geriatric Medicine Today, 2,* 33–41

Fuld, P. A., Katzman, R., Davies, P., & Terry, R. D. (1982). Intrusions as a sign of Alzheimer's dementia: Chemical and pathological verification. *Annals of Neurology, 11,* 155–159.

Graf, P., & Schacter, D. L. (1985). Implicit and explicit memory for new associations in normal and amnesic subjects. *Journal of Experimental Psychology. Learning, Memory, and Cognition, 11,* 501–518.

Granholm, E., & Butters, N. (1988). Associative encoding and retrieval in Alzheimer's and Huntington's disease. *Brain and Cognition, 7,* 335–347.

Groves, P. M. (1983). A theory of the functional organization of the neostriatum and the neostriatal control of voluntary movement. *Brain Research Reviews, 5,* 109–132.

Heindel, W. C., Butters, N., & Salmon, D. P. (1988). Impaired learning of a motor skill in patients with Huntington's disease. *Behavioral Neuroscience, 102,* 141–147.

Heindel, W. C., Salmon, D. P., Shults, C. W., Walicke, P. A., & Butters, N. (1989). Neuropsychological evidence for multiple implicit memory systems: A comparison of Alzheimer's, Huntington's, and Parkinson's disease patients. *Journal of Neuroscience, 9,* 582–587.

Huber, S. J., Shuttleworth, E. C., Paulson, G. W., Bellchambers, M. J. G., & Clapp, L. E. (1986). Cortical vs subcortical dementia: Neuropsychological differences. *Archives of Neurology, 43,* 392–394.

Kemp, J. M., & Powell, T. P. S. (1970). The cortico-striate projection in the monkey. *Brain, 93*, 525–546.

Kihlstrom, J. F. (1987). The cognitive unconscious. *Science, 237*, 1445–1452.

Lieberman, A., Dziatolowski, M., Kupersmith, M., Serby, M., Goodgold, A., Korein, J., & Goldstein, M. (1979). Dementia in Parkinson disease. *Annals of Neurology, 6*, 355–359.

Luria, A. R. (1966a). *Higher cortical functions in man.* New York: Basic Books.

Luria, A. R. (1966b). *Human brain and psychological processes.* New York: Harper & Row.

Luria, A. R. (1976). *The neuropsychology of memory.* Washington, DC: V. W. Winston.

Martin, A. (1987). Representation of semantic and spatial knowledge in Alzheimer's patients: Implications for models of preserved learning in amnesia. *Journal of Clinical and Experimental Neuropsychology, 9*, 191–224.

Martin, A., Brouwers, P., Cox, C., & Fedio, P. (1985). On the nature of the verbal memory deficit in Alzheimer's disease. *Brain and Language, 25*, 323–341.

Martin, A., & Fedio, P. (1983). Word production and comprehension in Alzheimer's disease: The breakdown of semantic knowledge. *Brain and Language, 19*, 124–141.

Martone, M., Butters, N., Payne, M., Becker, J., & Sax, D. S. (1984). Dissociations between skill learning and verbal recognition in amnesia and dementia. *Archives of Neurology, 41*, 965–970.

Mattis, S. (1976). Mental status examination for organic mental syndrome in the elderly patient. In L. Bellack & T. B. Karasu (Eds.), *Geriatric Psychiatry* (pp. 77–121). New York: Grune & Stratton.

Mayeux, R., Stern, Y., Rosen, J., & Benson, D. F. (1981). Subcortical dementia: A recognizable clinical entity. *Annals of Neurology, 10*, 100–101.

McKhann, G., Drachman, D., Folstein., M., Katzman, R., Price, D., & Stadlan, E. M. (1984). Clinical diagnosis of Alzheimer's disease: Report of the NINCDS-ADRDA Work Group under the auspices of Department of Health and Human Services Task Force on Alzheimer's Disease. *Neurology, 34*, 939–944.

Milberg, W., Hebben, N., & Kaplan, E. (1986). The Boston process approach to neuropsychological assessment. In I. Grant & K. Adams (Eds.), *Neuropsychological assessment of neuropsychiatric disorders* (pp. 65–86). New York: Oxford University Press.

Ober, B. A., Dronkers, N. F., Koss, E., Delis, D. C., & Freidland, R. P. (1986). Retrieval from semantic memory in Alzheimer-type dementia. *Journal of Clinical and Experimental Neuropsychology, 8*, 75–92.

Parkinson, J. (1817). *An essay on the shaking palsy.* London: Sherwood, Neely, & Jones.

Rosen, W. G. (1980). Verbal fluency in aging and dementia. *Journal of Clinical Neuropsychology, 2*, 135–146.

Salmon, D. P., Shimamura, A. P., Butters, N., & Smith, S. (1988). Lexical and semantic priming deficits in patients with Alzheimer's disease. *Journal of Clinical and Experimental Neuropsychology, 10*, 477–494.

Schacter, D. L. (1987). Implicit memory: History and current status. *Journal of Experimental Psychology. Learning, Memory, and Cognition, 13,* 501–517.

Shimamura, A. P., Salmon, D. P., Squire, L. R., & Butters, N. (1987). Memory dysfunction and word priming in dementia and amnesia. *Behavioral Neuroscience, 101,* 347–351.

Shindler, A. G., Caplan, L. R., & Hier, D. B. (1984). Intrusions and perseverations. *Brain and Language, 23,* 148–158.

Squire. L. R. (1987). *Memory and brain.* New York: Oxford University Press.

Terry, R. D., & Katzman, R. (1983). Senile dementia of the Alzheimer type. *Annals of Neurology, 14,* 497–506.

Thomson, D. M., & Tulving, E. (1970). Associative encoding and retrieval: Weak and strong cues. *Journal of Experimental Psychology, 86,* 255–262.

Tulving, E. (1983). *Elements of episodic memory.* New York: Oxford University Press.

Tulving, E., & Thomson, D. M. (1973). Encoding specificity and retrieval processes in episodic memory. *Psychological Review, 80,* 352–373.

Victor, M., Adams, R. D., & Collins, G. H. (1971). *The Wernicke–Korsakoff syndrome.* Philadelphia: F. A. Davis.

Weingartner, H., Grafman, J., Boutelle, W., Kaye, W., & Martin, P. (1983). Forms of memory failure. *Science, 21,* 380–382.

Winocur, G., & Weiskrantz, L. (1976). An investigation of paired-associate learning in amnesic patients. *Neuropsychologia, 14,* 97–110.

# 6

# A Reinterpretation of Memorative Functions of the Limbic System[1]

*Paul D. MacLean*

*National Institute of Mental Health*

The word "memorative" in the title of this chapter has a double connotation—applying to memory and also meaning commemorative. The word, therefore, answers a dual purpose for my contribution to a volume commemorating the life and work of Alexandr Romanovich Luria.

In this chapter a main focus of attention is on a condition that has been traditionally referred to as a loss of recent memory. But this would seem to be a mistaken characterization because it is not possible to lose what is not possessed. Hence it is necessary to substitute another expression. Clinically, the term amnesia, the Greek word for forgetfulness, refers to a memory loss, but also means a *lack* of memory. Clinicians recognize two main forms of amnesia— anterograde and retrograde amnesia. Anterograde amnesia pertains to a person's inability to recall ongoing experiences *subsequent to* some disease, trauma, or other affliction, whereas a retrograde amnesia applies to a failure to remember experiences throughout a particular period (or periods) *prior to* such an

[1]In evolution, the forebrain of advanced mammals has developed as a triune structure, comprising three neural assemblies that, anatomically and chemically, reflect an ancestral relationship to reptiles, early mammals, and late mammals. The paleomammalian brain represents an inheritance from early mammals, consisting of cortical and subcortical structures now known as the limbic system (for recent review, see MacLean, 1985). In this article the limbic system will be understood as comprising the cortex of the great limbic lobe of Broca and structures of the brainstem with which it has primary connections. It is made up of three main cortico-subcortical subdivisions. The cortical areas of the two phylogenetically older subdivisions are primarily innervated by telencephalic nuclei located, respectively, in the amygdala and septum. The cingulate cortex of the third subdivision receives its afferents primarily from the anterior thalamic nuclei, as well as from parts of the medial dorsal nucleus and certain intralaminar nuclei. In addition to reciprocal connections with the nuclear groups just mentioned, parts of the limbic cortex project to the olfactostriatum and several hypothalamic nuclei, including the mammillary bodies that are one focus of the present article.

affliction. The term affliction covers a wide range of conditions, such as a blow to the head, carbon monoxide poisoning, a viral encephalitis, an epileptic seizure.

Depending on the nature of the affliction, the duration of a retrograde amnesia may involve periods of minutes, hours, days, months, or years. Without documentation it may be impossible to conclude whether or not a retrograde amnesia is actually a failure to recall something that was once remembered or whether the memory deficit is attributable to a pre-existing anterograde amnesia that made impossible the acquisition of memories. When, as may be the case in anterograde amnesia, there is an inability to recall information derived via all the sensory systems, the condition is referred to as a global amnesia.

For present purposes, it is necessary to take into account another kind of memory variously characterized as "immediate" or "short-term," usually implying a fleeting memory.

Anterograde amnesia is of primary interest here because it is a condition that has led to the recognition of cerebral structures accounting for the memory of ongoing experiences that, in turn, is requisite for learning. Hence, it has proved to be a matter of utmost significance and unweaning interest that destruction of certain parts of the limbic system may result in a profound anterograde amnesia. The following account deals successively with (1) The history of clinical findings relevant to anterograde amnesia; (2) Attempts of animal experimentation to duplicate the clinical picture; (3) Insights provided by the analysis of the amnesia of epileptic automatisms; and (4) The results of anatomical and electrophysiological studies on intero- and exteroceptive inputs to the limbic cortex. The analysis of the assorted material leads to the proposal that the limbic integration of information derived from intero- and exteroceptive systems is a prerequisite for a sense of self-identity and a memory of self-involved experience.

## ANTEROGRADE AMNESIA: BACKGROUND

A chronological account of the revelation of brain structures involved in anterograde amnesia requires one to deal successively with the mammillary bodies, hippocampal formation, and medial dorsal nucleus of the thalamus.

In a textbook on diseases of the brain, Wernicke in 1881 described a condition that he called "polio-encephalitis superior hemorrhagica," characterized by diplopia, ataxia, delirium, and mental confusion. Six years later, Korsakoff (1887) published a report of cases of alcoholism in which in addition to a multiple neuritis there was a mental disorder most strikingly manifested by a disturbance of "recent memory." He later referred to it as a "psychic disorder in conjunction with multiple neuritis" (1889; see Victor & Yakovlev, 1955). The condition subsequently became known as Korsakoff's psychosis. In cases showing both the memory deficit and the other neurological signs, the condition is referred to as the Wernicke–Korsakoff syndrome. Many, if not all, of the symptoms have been ascribed to a deficiency of thiamine (vitamin $B_1$) (Jolliffe, Colbert, & Joffe 1936; Phillips, Victor, Adams, & Davidson, 1952). The pathology is characterized by a noninflammatory type of reaction primarily affecting the vasculature of certain structures of the diencephalon and lower brainstem. The ocular paralysis of Wernicke's encephalopathy is attributable to disease of parts of the nuclei of the third and sixth nerves, while the ataxic condition can be ascribed to loss of Purkinje cells in the vermis and uvula of the cerebellum (Victor, Adams, & Collins, 1971). The structures believed to be involved in the memory deficit will be dealt with after giving a clinical picture of the amnestic syndrome, beginning with a description in Korsakoff's own words (see Victor and Yakovlev, 1955):

> The disorder of memory manifests itself in an extraordinarily peculiar amnesia, in which the memory of recent events, those which just happened, is chiefly disturbed, whereas the remote past is remembered fairly well. . . . At first, during conversation with such a patient, it is difficult to note the presence of psychic disorder; the patient gives the impression of a person in complete possession of his faculties; he reasons about everything perfectly well, draws correct deductions from given premises, makes witty remarks, plays chess or a game of cards; in a word, comports himself as a mentally sound person. (pp. 397–398)

Yet later, Korsakoff continues, one discovers that the patient "remembers absolutely nothing of what goes on around him." In conversation the same thing may be repeated "twenty times." "Patients of this type," he points out, "may read the same page over and over again sometimes for hours, because they are absolutely unable to remember what they have read."

This last statement recalls the description of the behavior of a monkey which, after bilateral temporal lobectomy may pick up and examine a nail "a hundred times" as though it had never been seen before (Klüver & Bucy, 1939). Clinically, what may be the most surprising contrast is that the patient's apparently normal social comportment and intellectual functioning are interlarded with glaring memory lapses. This is illustrated by the conversation of a man who had been in the navy to whom I offered a ride as he seemed to be rushing for shelter from an approaching thunderstorm. He was so polite and well spoken that I might have left him at his destination without having been aware of his mental derangement, had not the tower of the naval hospital kept coming in and out of view as we drove along the highway. Every time his eye caught the tower of the hospital, he would repeat, almost word for word, an experience that he had had there many years before.

Based on a study of 245 patients, Victor, et al. (1971) found that *retrograde* amnesia occurs in conjunction with *anterograde* amnesia in individuals suffering from Korsakoff's psychosis. They point out that the retrograde amnesia is "variable in extent and degree," but usually extends back several years prior to the present illness. They cite one extreme case, that of a 40-year-old woman who could remember nothing since leaving Ireland at the age of 19. In most cases, the retrograde amnesia is not complete and, comparable to a partly destroyed videotape randomly spliced together, the patients recount remembered periods as though they had occurred successively. Such ill-remembered past experiences may contribute to the clinical impression that patients with Korsakoff's psychosis are inclined to confabulation.

Victor (1981, p. 10) observes that in patients who recover from Korsakoff's psychosis, the anterograde and retrograde amnesia "always recover together." It seems quite probable that when there appears to be a permanent gap in memory for a period prior to the onset of the present illness, there may have been a pre-existing anterograde amnesia.

In anticipating the account of animal experimentation, it is to be emphasized that "the capacity for immediate recall or so-called short-term memory" is unimpaired, as evident by the patient's ability to repeat a series of six to nine numbers (Victor, 1981, p. 10)

## Clinico-pathological Correlations

In 1896, in an article illustrating the peripheral nerve findings in alcoholic polyneuritis, Hans Gudden (1896) (not to be confused with Bernard von Gudden) also described partial to extensive degeneration in the medial mammillary nucleus in three of the four cases (sections not available in fourth case). Some 30 years later, Gamper (1928), an Austrian neurologist, called attention to these observations when reporting findings on nine men and six women with Korsakoff's psychosis. Since lesions of the mammillary bodies were the "constant" finding in all of his cases, Gamper regarded damage of this structure as a crucial factor accounting for the psychological changes characteristic of Korsakoff's psychosis. He referred to current views that the mammillary bodies constituted a nodal structure in the cerebral regulation of autonomic function.

Since then, there have been repeated reports of the high incidence of lesions of the mammillary bodies in Korsakoff's psychosis. In two of the most extensive case studies, however, the conclusions of the respective authors were in disagreement regarding the significance of the mammillary lesions. In 1956, Malamud and Skillikorn described the cerebral pathology in 70 institutionalized cases of Korsakoff's disease in which the memory deficit was documented. Their finding of the presence of disease of the mammillary bodies in 67 of the cases (95.7%) was a clear indication to them that Gamper was correct in his conclusions that damage to these structures was primarily responsible for the manifestations of Korsakoff's disease. The periventricular and periaqueductal gray matter was variously involved in all 70 cases. Contrary to the case study next to be mentioned, the medial dorsal nucleus of the thalamus was involved in only 37 cases (52.8%), while the pulvinar was damaged in three (4.2%).

In their monograph on the Wernicke–Korsakoff syndrome, Victor, Adams, and Collins (1971) report the cerebral pathology in 62 cases. They found that the mammillary bodies were grossly involved in 46 of the cases (74%). The lesions were almost always symmetrical in distribution and occupied the central part of the medial nuclei. Hemorrhages were present in 10% of the cases. The walls of the third ventricle were grossly involved in 24% of the cases. It should be emphasized that a zone 0.5 to 1.0 mm in width immediately next to the ependyma was always spared. Parts of the thalamus were available for examination in 45 cases. Material from 43 cases revealed disease of the medial dorsal nucleus in 38 (88.4%). The medial pulvinar was examined in 20 cases and showed involvement in 17 (85%). Of the thalamic structures in general, the authors noted that "the degree of cell loss was always greatest in the medial dorsal nucleus and medial pulvinar" (p. 112). Of interest in the light of recent findings on frontal lobe and thalamic connections, there might also be extensive cell loss in the anterior and lateral dorsal nuclei and in the submedius, medial ventral, and parataenial nuclei. There was loss of myelinated fibers in the ventral anterior and medial dorsal nuclei and in the medial pulvinar.

In discussing clinico-pathological correlations, Victor et al. (1971) point out that with respect to the memory defect, analysis showed a high degree of correlation with disease of the mammillary bodies, the medial dorsal nucleus, and the medial part of the pulvinar. In regard to the question as to which structures are crucial, they emphasized that five patients in their series who had shown no memory defect were found to have disease of the mammillary bodies and that in none of them could it be described as "minimal." Significantly, in all five the medial dorsal nucleus was "free of disease." There were an additional five cases in which there had been a serious defect in memory and in which the medial dorsal nucleus "was virtually the only thalamic nucleus affected." On the basis of these findings the authors concluded that "the mammillary bodies may be significantly affected in the absence of a memory defect" (p. 132), whereas there was strong evidence that disease of the medial dorsal nucleus may be the critical factor.

As opposed to cases of Korsakoff's psychosis with its multiple lesions, Delay and Brion (1954) have reported a case in which there was anterograde amnesia and in which the postmortem findings revealed a hamartoma that resulted in an almost exclusive destruction of the mammillary bodies. Other evidence, next to be considered, indicates that the mammillary bodies, regardless of the nature of their specific functions, lie within a circuit of structures that are requisite for the retention and recall of ongoing experiences.

## Hippocampal Formation

Bechterew (1900), the renowned Russian physiologist and neurologist, is credited with being the first to call attention to the involvement of the hippocampal formation in memorative functions. As briefly described in an abstract, the author presented before the Moscow Society the case of a 60-year-old patient with alcoholic polyneuritis and a psychosis who, for 20 years, suffered from a memory disturbance. Examination of the brain revealed bilateral softening of the uncinate gyrus and hippocampus.

In 1951, Conrad and Ule described a case of Korsakoff's psychosis with bilateral lesions of the hippocampal formation that were ascribed to a toxoplasma infection. There was transneuronal degeneration of the mammillary bodies. In discussing these findings, Ule (1951) referred to a case described by Grünthal in 1947 in which a bilateral destruction of the hippocampus subsequent to insulin coma was associated with advanced intellectual and emotional deterioration. In 1952, Glees and Griffith described a case in which there was bilateral destruction of the hippocampus in a patient in whom there had been a longstanding loss of memory. Although the fornix is said to have had only about 25% of "the normal population" of fibers, the mammillary bodies presented a normal appearance. In the light of these findings, the authors suggested that the hippocampal formation is "essential for recent memory."

The possible role of the hippocampal formation in memorative functions began to attract wider interest in 1958 when Penfield and Milner reported two cases of severe anterograde amnesia following unilateral extirpation of a large part of the hippocampal formation for the treatment of psychomotor epilepsy. It was believed that the memory impairment in these two cases resulted from bilateral hippocampal damage because, after partial destruction of the hippocampal formation in the dominant hemisphere, there remained a "more or less completely destructive" lesion of the right hippocampal zone (p. 488). The outcome in the case of these two patients was regarded as remarkable because the memory loss "appeared in isolation from any disturbance of reasoning, attention, or concentration" (p. 496). The first patient was a glove cutter and the second a civil engineer. The surgery did not produce any significant alteration in the IQ, as witnessed by the engineer's postoperative score of 125, as opposed to a former score of 120. The outstanding finding in each case was the inability to retain the memory of any ongoing experience for longer than 5 minutes, particularly if there occurred any interruption. Extensive psychological testing revealed that "the difficulty with recent memory was a general one, affecting both verbal and nonverbal material. There was no corresponding loss of attention, concentration, or reasoning ability" (p. 493). As was noted in regard to Korsakoff's psychosis, there was in these two patients a retrograde amnesia, extending over the preceding 4 years for the glover and for the preceding 2 months for the civil engineer.

In 1951, when visiting the Montreal Neurological Institute, I saw the civil engineer (patient P. B.) about 2 months after his operation. At that time he was totally dependent on a little notebook which he carried in his hand for finding his way around and keeping appointments. His keeping it in his hand served as a continual tactile and visual reminder of why it was there to refer to. Tasks to which he had been long accustomed were performed, so to speak, automatically. He had, for example, been in the habit of following the weather and recording the daily temperature and barometric pressure. He continued to carry out this routine following surgery. In this respect, it is of interest to mention that prior to surgery he would sometimes have epileptic automatisms during which he would observe and record the temperature and barometric pressure, having no memory of it afterwards.

In response to a question about his capacity to experience emotion, he said to me that generally things did not bother him so much because he so quickly forgot them.

Support for the inference that the memory deficit in the two cases under consideration was owing to disease and malfunction of the remaining hippocampus was obtained when P. B. died 15 years later. It is said that the pathological examination by Dr. Gordon Mathieson disclosed that the "right hippocampus was atrophic, the extent of destruction actually exceeding that on the left caused by the surgical removal" (Milner, Corkin, & Teuber, 1968, p. 231).

The most extensively studied case of a patient subjected to a bilateral surgical ablation of the medial temporal region is that of a man who has become widely known in the literature as H. M. On September 1, 1953, H. M. underwent a "bilateral medial temporal-lobe resection" by the late William B. Scoville, who explained that "this frankly experimental operation" was undertaken with the hope that it would remedy the patient's incapacitation by major and minor seizures uncontrolled by various forms of maximal medication (Scoville & Milner, 1957). The patient was a 29-year-old motor winder with a history of epilepsy since the age of 16. The bilateral medial temporal lobe resection is said to have extended posteriorly for a distance of 8 cm from the tips of the temporal lobes and that the temporal horns constituted the lateral edges of the resection. Although it is more than risky to assume that the extent of the ablations agrees with the operative description, the patient's symptomatology will be briefly described because he has now been followed for 30 years and has become better known than any other case of this kind. After operation, the patient "could no longer recognize the hospital staff nor find his way to the bathroom, and he seemed to recall nothing of the day-to-day events of his hospital life" (p. 14). There was also a partial retrograde amnesia extending back 3 years prior to surgery, as dated by his failure to remember the death of a favorite uncle 3 years earlier. Conforming with the description given above by Korsakoff, he would "read the same magazines over and over again without finding their contents familiar" (p. 14). A half an hour after luncheon, he could not remember a single item of food that he had eaten. "Yet," it is said, "to a casual observer this man seems like a relatively normal individual, since his understanding and reasoning are undiminished" (p. 14).

In 1968, Milner, Corkin, and Teuber described the condition of this same patient 14 years after his surgery. Throughout that period he continued to have a "profound amnesia for most ongoing events." H. M., they explained, "still fails to recognize people who are close neighbors or family friends" (p. 216) with whom he became acquainted subsequent to his operation. He had not lost any of his social graces, and kept himself neat. "It is characteristic," the authors state, "that he cannot give us any description of his place of work, the nature of his job, or the route along which he is driven each day. . . ." (p. 217). Yet he was able to draw an accurate floor plan of the place in which he lived, and he seemed familiar with the neighborhood within, but not beyond, three blocks from home base. He would describe his condition as like that of "waking from a dream," apparently because of a failure to remember what went on before. H. M. had been given a wide assortment of tests, all of which were indicative of a memory disability rather than one of intelligence and perception. For example, on an alternate form of the Wechsler memory scale, he achieved only a quotient of 64, which is "grossly abnormal" and in striking contrast to his full-scale IQ of 118. He proved superior to controls on Mooney's facial perception task, but showed marked impairment in the delayed matching of photographed faces. Given a shortened version of a visual or tactual maze, he proved capable of some learning and partial retention.

Some other notable items are the authors' observations that H. M. rarely mentions being hungry; does not report physical pain such as headache or stomach ache; and lacks sexual interest. They do not refer to his subjective response to feelings associated with urination and defecation. Speaking of his "emotional tone," they state that it is instructive that a feeling of uneasiness associated with the vague knowledge of his mother's illness, appeared to fade away rapidly.

In addition to these and other case reports of anterograde amnesia with bilateral lesions of the hippocampus, there is some evidence that unilateral destruction of the hippocampus, together with atrophy of the fornix and anterograde transneuronal degeneration, may contribute to the same kind of impairment (Schenk, 1959). For example, Torch, Hirano, and Solomon (1977) have since described a case of impairment of "recent and short-term memory" in which severe unilateral atrophy of the fornix, mammillary body, mammillothalamic tract, and anterior thalamic nucleus followed an infarction of the posterior hippocampal and fusiform gyrus. Boudin, Brion, Pépin, and Barbizet (1968) have cited cases, including one of their own, in which asymmetrical lesions of the limbic system are associated with a Korsakoff-type deficit in memorization. In their own case there was an occipitotemporal softening on the left side, including the posterior hippocampus and fornix, while on the right side there was a softening of the anterior cingulate gyrus and other structures fed by the right anterior cerebral artery.

Finally, mention should be made of two cases in which large parts of the limbic lobe were destroyed by a viral infection and in which, in addition to cognitive and emotional deficits, there was a severe anterograde amnesia (Friedman & Allen, 1969; Gascon & Gilles, 1973). The case described by Friedman and Allen, for example, was that of a 50-year-old automobile mechanic who survived 11 years following the onset of his symptoms. The "amnestic syndrome was characterized by complete loss of memory for the period of the acute illness and total impairment of recording of new memoranda. Instantaneous retention of sequential perceptions . . . was intact, but nothing could be retained from one minute to the next" (p. 680). Consequently, although he retained the ability to spot a mechanical difficulty in a car and to use tools correctly, he could no longer carry out repairs.

In view of the experimental work to be described and the question of the role of the amygdala in memorative functions, mention should be made of a case of anterograde amnesia following bilateral infarction of the hippocampal formation, in which it is specifically stated that the amygdaloid complex was "normal" (DeJong, Itabashi, & Olson, 1969).

## THE AMNESTIC SYNDROME IN ANIMALS

Since the recognition that the limbic structures of the temporal lobe are implicated in memorative functions, numerous experiments have been performed on rats, cats, dogs, and monkeys in an attempt to define the nature of the deficit and to identify specific structures involved. As a generality, it may be said that the results of such experimentation are difficult to evaluate because of (1) The variation in the location of the brain lesions; (2) The failure in most cases to provide *volumetric* measurements of the amount of particular brain structures destroyed; and (3) Lack of expert neuropathological analysis of the nature and extent of changes in surrounding tissue as a result of surgical probing and interference with the arterial blood supply and venous drainage. One might also regret the lack of information regarding the pre- and postoperative bioelectrical activity of the brain in the region of the surgery, as well as elsewhere. For example, the discrepancies in the findings of some experiments might be attributable to discharges occurring in injured brain tissue. It should be noted, however, that the placement of electrodes themselves may result in damage that will give rise to an irritable focus. The implantation of an electrode in the hippocampus, for example, may occlude a small vessel, with nerve cell death and gliosis leading to a discharging focus (personal observations). The numerous hippocampal ablation studies that have been performed on rats present special difficulties in their interpretation, not only because of the great variation in the location and size of the lesions, but also because of the uneven experience of the workers performing the surgery and assessing the anatomical extent of the lesions.

Apart from such considerations, the experimental work on animals has been generally frustrating for investigators because of the failure to produce the kind of amnestic deficit observed clinically in patients with lesions of the hippocampus and neighboring structures. In the research on nonprimates it is noteworthy for comparative purposes to call attention to experiments such as those conducted by Olton and coworkers (Olton, 1978). They use a radial arm maze that they believe provides a test of spatial memory. In a maze with bait at the end of the arms, a fasted rat will usually obtain the bait in one arm and then go on to another. Rats with hippocampal lesions, however, may repeatedly enter an arm in which they had already obtained the bait. They are reminiscent of the Korsakoff patient who will keep rereading the same page, or the Klüver–Bucy monkey that keeps examining the same object as though it had not been seen before. Since reviews by Isaacson (1982) and others (e.g., Douglas, 1967; Weiskrantz & Warrington, 1975) have dealt with the outcome of hippocampal experimentation on nonprimate animals, the following account will deal with the results of experiments on monkeys.

## Tests Used for Experiments on Monkeys

The tests usually employed in work with primates are (1) the delayed response test, (2) the delayed alternation test, and (3) the delayed matching-from-sample tests. The delayed response test involves baiting one of two cups to the right and left of a monkey enclosed in a Wisconsin-type apparatus. One of the cups is baited in a random manner and then an opaque screen is lowered between the monkey and the cups for a period usually ranging from 5 to 10 sec. A correct response requires that the monkey go directly to the baited cup and uncover it to obtain food. A variation of this test is to bait alternately the right- and left-hand cups. Interestingly, this delayed alternation test has proved to be a more difficult task for the monkey than the delayed response test. (Correll & Scoville, 1967; Orbach, Milner, & Rasmussen, 1960).

Tests involving *delayed matching-from-sample* or *nonmatching-to-sample* have been advocated as preferable methods for assessing deficits in retention. In such tests, a left–right orientation can be minimized. A delayed matching-from-sample test, for example, may simply involve the presentation of a red or green light as the cue which, after a delay of 5 sec., the monkey is required to indicate the matching color upon the simultaneous appearance of green and red lights. The color to be matched is randomly presented as is the position of the two lights. The delayed nonmatching-to-sample test will be described when the reason is explained for its introduction in recent experimentation.

Since tests involving repeated trials lead to a "learning set" (namely, the animal's learning an approach to the test that facilitates its accomplishment), advantage may be taken of this factor for assessing retention of memory. Once an animal has reached criterion in the performance of a test, one can, after a lapse of several days or weeks, administer the test again and obtain a measure of how many trials it requires for the animal again to reach criterion. Rapid relearning is indicative of retention of the learning set. In this way, one obtains a measure of an animal's long-term retention before and after surgery.

All of the tests that have been described thus far involve the use of vision. Consequently, it is necessary after brain surgery to confirm that a deficit in performing a test is not owing to a loss of vision. For this purpose, animals are trained in a task in which they must visually differentiate between two objects.

In tests of memorization, it is also important to show whether or not the loss is attributable to other sensory deficits. For this purpose, one has access to tests involving retention of information conveyed via auditory, somesthetic, and other channels.

## Combined Amygdala and Hippocampal Ablations

In 1960, Orbach et al. reported the first extensive study in monkeys in which an attempt was made to duplicate the kind of memory deficit attributed to damage of the hippocampal formation in human beings. Eleven of their macaques survived lesions of various medial temporal structures. In seven subjects the amygdala, hippocampus, and hippocampal gyrus were aspirated via a frontal approach. In addition there was one animal with an amygdalectomy and transection of the fornix; a ninth with an amygdalectomy; a tenth with the hippocampus aspirated via a posterior approach; and an 11th subject with a partial bilateral lesion of the amygdala and hippocampus. For comparison, there were two animals with ablations of the inferior temporal cortex; one with a transection of the olfactory tracts; two with electrolytic lesions of the cingulate gyrus; and two with electrolytic lesions of the pulvinar.

As tests of "short-term memory," the investigators used the delayed response and delayed alternation tests. For assessing long-term retention, they administered tests of visual and tactile discrimination. Finally, they observed the effects of distraction on the performance of tests involving short-term and long-term retention.

The main findings were these: None of the monkeys with extensive removals of the amygdala and hippocampus showed savings in relearning the delayed alternation test. The delayed response test had not been administered prior to surgery. Following surgery, the animals with extensive medial temporal lesions learned to perform both the delayed response and delayed alternation tests with a 5-sec. delay as readily as the controls. The introduction of a distraction during trials did not interfere with their performance. The seven monkeys with extensive medial temporal lesions showed impaired retention, as well as retardation in relearning the visual discrimination problem. A similar impairment in a tactile, size-discrimination problem indicated that the retention and relearning deficits were not modality specific.

*Comment.* It is evident that the deficits observed in this study seemed to correspond only in part to those that have been described in connection with hippocampal destruction in human beings. The results would indicate that medial temporal ablations involving a large part of the hippocampus and the amygdala affected long-term memory, but had no apparent effect on the so-called "short-term memory."

## *Delayed Matching-from-sample Tests*

Lawicka and Konorski (1959), were among those who called into question the use of the delayed response and delayed alternation tests for assessing impairment of "short-term memory." It was pointed out that animals might bridge the delay by maintaining orientation with respect to one baited cup or the other. Drachman and Ommaya (1964) used a delayed matching-from-sample test that was designed to avoid this objection. First, they trained eight macaque monkeys in a matching-from-sample test and then in a delayed matching-from-sample test, using an apparatus in which the use of display of white, green, and red lights avoided spatial cues. After reaching criterion, the subjects were tested again 7 to 10 weeks later so as to obtain a measure of their retention. Five monkeys were subjected to surgery, and three served as controls. There were three monkeys in which the amygdala and the greater part of the body of the hippocampus were aspirated. In matching-from-sample, these three subjects required more trials to attain criterion than in the preoperative assessment, but there were "considerable savings." In the delayed matching-from-sample (5-sec. delay), these same three animals required more trials to relearn this task than did two monkeys with small medial temporal ablations and the three unoperated animals. However, they were as readily trained to delay for 12 sec. as the two animals with small lesions. It was also shown that the introduction of a distraction did not interfere with performance in the delayed matching-from-sample test.

In the early 1960s, Correll and Scoville had also been investigating the effects of medial temporal lesions on memory and learning. In one study utilizing the delayed matching-from-sample test (1965), they compared the performance of 13 rhesus monkeys—4 that had amygdala-hippocampal ablations; 4 with amygdala-uncal ablations; 3 with combined hippocampus and hippocampal gyrus ablations; and 2 that were sham-operated. The preoperative retention scores showed "a high degree of stability in performance." Postoperatively, however, the animals with extensive bilateral amygdala and hippocampal ablations showed a statistically significant deficit in both the matching-from-sample and the delayed matching-from-sample tests with delays of 5 sec. The authors concluded, however, that the deficit was attributable to the conditional structure of the problem rather than to a "rapid decay of the memory trace."

*Comment.* In each of the studies involving delayed matching-from-sample, the investigators were in agreement that the ability to bridge a delay is not impaired after extensive bilateral temporal lesions. Drachman and Ommaya (1964) concluded that the "loss of pre-operative retention and impairment of acquisition are the important factors" that explain the retarded reacquisition of delayed matching-from-sample (p. 423). According to their interpretation, the "studies of short-term memory in human beings and animals are in reality testing different properties" (p. 412). Since the terms "short-term" or "immediate" now tend to be used clinically for evanescent memory, the term "recent," in Korsakoff's sense, would more appropriately refer to what the authors had in mind. In other words, they were referring to anterograde amnesia in which there is a failure to acquire and store memories of ongoing experiences, whereas the animal experiments seem to involve the testing of short-term (immediate) retention, of which a patient with anterograde amnesia is capable.

## Delayed Nonmatching-to-sample

Mishkin (1978, 1982) contends that none of the tests heretofore used on animals is comparable to those used in assessing human amnesia. Consequently, he has employed a test of the kind that appeared to be effective in disclosing the memory impairment of the patient H. M. who has been described. Referred to as the delayed nonmatching-to-sample test, it involves a one-trial object recognition for which the animal receives a peanut. A monkey is tested in a Wisconsin general testing apparatus in which it is required to show that a new object just presented is not the same as the one to which it had been exposed 10 sec. before. Since no object is seen more than twice, the experimenter draws upon a collection of 300 dissimilar objects. The new object presented in each test becomes the familiar item of the next test. The procedure thus "exploits" the monkey's natural tendency to focus upon the novel object. After reaching criterion of 90 correct choices in 100 trials, monkeys are tested with longer delays between the presentation of the sample and nonmatching objects.

Mishkin (1978, 1982) undertook to learn whether or not this test would distinguish monkeys with bilateral ablations of the amygdala and the greater part of the hippocampus from subjects that had been submitted either to an amygdalectomy or hippocampectomy (including much of the fusiform-hippocampal gyrus). There were three animals in each group, as well as three controls. Two weeks following surgery, the operated animals were retrained to criterion and then tested under conditions in which the delay was increased from 10 to 30 to 60 to 120 sec. All of the monkeys achieved criterion, except those with the combined lesions in which the average score was 60% correct, "or just above chance."

Mishkin interpreted the results of this study as demonstrating that combined ablation of the amygdala and hippocampus resulted in a loss of memory comparable to that seen in patients. It was proposed that the amygdala and hippocampus have overlapping projections to the diencephalon that allow one structure to compensate for the loss of the other.

On the basis of experiments conducted by Horel (1978), however, there was the question of whether or not Mishkin's findings were owing to an interruption of the "temporal stem" that corresponds to the white matter above the lateral ventricle and which contains connections going to and from the neocortex of the temporal lobe. Accordingly, Zola–Morgan, Squire, and Mishkin (1982) carried out a study in which they compared the effects of transecting the temporal stem, as opposed to a bilateral removal of the amygdala and hippocampus by an approach that left the stem intact. The performance of the delayed nonmatching-to-sample test of the animals with the temporal stem lesions was essentially no different from that of the controls, whereas the results with respect to the combined amygdala-hippocampal ablations were practically the same as in the previous study.

*Medial Thalamic Lesions.*    As was noted under clinical findings, lesions of the medial dorsal nucleus of the thalamus may be responsible for the anterograde amnesia of Korsakoff's psychosis. In proposing an explanation for the apparent deficit resulting from combined amygdala and hippocampal lesions, Mishkin (1978, 1982) noted that the amygdala projects to the medial part of the medial dorsal nucleus whereas the hippocampal formation projects to the anterior group. With Aggleton (1983), it was found that lesions of the medial thalamus involving both the anterior group and the medial dorsal nucleus resulted in the same kind of impairment in the delayed nonmatching-to-sample test as that following combined amygdala and hippocampal ablations.

*Role of Different Sensory Modalities.*    Using a test comparable with the delayed nonmatching-to-sample, Murray and Mishkin (1983) found that monkeys with combined amygdala and hippocampal lesions also showed a memory deficit when performance required tactile recognition. They inferred from these findings that combined amygdala-hippocampal ablations probably resulted in a global type of amnesia. These observations recall those of Stepien, Cordeau, and Rasmussen (1960). Using Konorski's tests involving compound stimuli, they compared the effects of various medial temporal lesions on the ability of green monkeys to bridge a delay when required to indicate whether or not one of two sounds (clicks at 5 sec. and at 20 sec.) or intermittent photic stimuli (also at 5 sec. and at 20 sec.) were presented. Although anatomical confirmation was not available, it was said that combined amygdala and hippocampal ablations impaired performance in both tests. Posterior inferior temporal ablations interfered only with the visual test, whereas ablation of the cortex rostral to the primary auditory area interfered only with the auditory test. In testing these same animals 2 years later, Cordeau and Mahut (1964) concluded that the deficits resulting from medial temporal ablations were transitory.

*Unresolved Role of Hippocampus.*    Based on the studies that have been reviewed, there is evidence that combined ablations of the amygdala and hippocampus result in some impairment of retention of past experience, as well as the registration and recall of ongoing experience. But there remain opposing views as to whether or not hippocampal ablations alone impair memorative functions. Kimble and Pribram (1963) conducted experiments on monkeys that led them to conclude that hippocampal lesions interfere with the sequential performance of a task, rather than "short-term" memory per se. Waxler and Rosvold (1970) called into question the current view that impairment of delayed alternation was "an inevitable consequence of removing the hippocampus." In a study involving eight monkeys with hippocampal lesions and eight controls they found that failure in performing the delayed alternation test might or might not occur regardless of the size or locus of hippocampal destruction. It was their impression that the test itself presented the inherent difficulty of requiring the animal to withhold responding to the just-baited cup, and that some monkeys were able to bridge the delay by learning to orient in a manner not evident to the experimenter. The authors, however, failed to take into account the possibility that an irritative focus near the site of hippocampal destruction may have in some cases resulted in hippocampal discharges or cerebral dysrhythmias that might have had a disrupting effect on performance.

Recently, Mahut, Zola–Morgan, and Moss (1982) reported their findings that ablations primarily involving the hippocampus and adjacent hippocampal-fusiform gyrus significantly interfere with nonspatial, "short-term" memory. They used the delayed nonmatching-to-sample test, as well as a test involving recollection of a list of objects. A "concurrent discrimination task" was also employed.

In seeking an explanation of the discrepant findings on the hippocampus, Squire and Zola–Morgan (1983) reviewed the descriptions of the postmortem examination of the brain in 20 different studies. In those cases in which there was a frontotemporal approach, they thought it likely that the amygdala and the greater part of the hippocampus back to the level of the lateral geniculate body had been ablated. In the cases, however, in which there had been a caudal approach to the hippocampus, it seemed probable, as Orbach et al. (1960) had found, that a considerable segment of the hippocampus proximal to the amygdala was left intact. They attributed this situation to the operator's caution against not extending the ablation rostrally into the amygdala. It was estimated that in many cases 20% to 30% of the body of the hippocampus toward the amygdala might be left intact.

## The Mammillary Bodies

As was noted, Victor et al. (1971) were inclined to believe that disease of the mammillary bodies does not contribute significantly to the amnestic syndrome of Korsakoff's psychosis. Goldberg (1984) has suggested that the mammillary bodies are linked in one of two circuits that must be damaged "in order to produce massive amnesia." There are only a few experimental studies that bear on this question. Thus far, it has not been possible to induce lesions of the mammillary bodies in monkeys (e.g., Witt & Goldman–Rakic, 1983) by giving diets deficient in thiamine, and damage of these structures is only an irregular occurrence in carnivores subjected to thiamine deficiency (Jubb, Saunders, & Coates, 1956). In a study on squirrel monkeys, Ploog and MacLean (1963) found that electrocoagulations of the mammillary bodies did not interfere with a conditioned avoidance test in which a short delay was introduced between the conditional stimulus and the called-for response. Dahl, Ingram, and Knott (1962) obtained essentially the same results in experiments on cats.

## A Comparison of Experimental and Clinical Findings

As was illustrated, verbal ability and verbal communication may be intact in cases in which lesions of parts of the limbic system are associated with an anterograde type of amnesia. The same applies to forms of reasoning and perception that are dependent on verbal ability. Therefore, it would appear that discrepancies between clinical and experimental findings cannot necessarily be ascribed to unbridgeable differences·between animals and human beings because of verbal factors.

A major difficulty in comparing the experimental and clinical findings on memorative functions arises in part because of differing interpretations with respect to what is designated as recent memory. As was noted, Drachman and Ommaya (1964) put their finger on one source of the problem by their emphasis on the distinction between an evanescent retention of an experience, as opposed to the registration and storage of an experience that makes it possible for it to be recalled at a later time. The capability of monkeys with medial temporal ablations to bridge a short delay in delayed-response tests would correspond to the patient with a Korsakoff deficit ability to recall temporarily a list of items, followed by an evanescence of this memory. The delayed nonmatching-to-sample test used by Mishkin (1978, 1982) was calculated to show whether or not animals with medial temporal lesions were able to recall a novel object after much longer delays than routinely used with delayed response tests. It will be recalled that monkeys with combined amygdala and hippocampal lesions tested at just above chance level with 2-minute delays. This type of test, however, still seems to leave in doubt whether or not an animal with such lesions is capable of meaningful assimilation of new forms of experiences into its day-to-day existence. Perhaps situations might be devised in a quasinatural environment with one or more conspecifics or unlike species that would more adequately demonstrate whether or not an experimental subject had the capacity to register, store, and recall ongoing experiences.

## SIMILARITY TO THE AMNESIA OF ICTAL AUTOMATISMS

Subsequent to the initial aura, patients with psychomotor epilepsy (complex partial seizures) may engage in simple or complex automatisms for which they have no memory. Clinically, there appears to be general agreement that such patients have a complete absence of recall of anything that happens after the onset of the automatism. In this respect, it is to be noted that interviews of patients under sodium amytal sedation have failed to elicit any evidence of awareness during the automatism (Stevens, Glaser, & MacLean, 1955). Yet patients may be capable of performing such complex sequential acts as driving a train, delivering a baby, and playing an organ. Performances of this kind would be indicative of competent neocortical function. The preservation of cognitive functions for dealing with new situations is remarkably illustrated by Jackson's case Z, the young physician who was able during an automatism to continue examining a patient, make a diagnosis, and write an appropriate prescription (Jackson, 1888). Years later a postmortem examination revealed in Z's brain a small cystic lesion near the junction of the left hippocampus and amygdala (Jackson & Colman, 1898).

Since patients are unable to recall anything that happens after the onset of an automatism, the memory lapse would compare to an anterograde type of amnesia. Starting with the onset of the automatism, there appears to be an interference with cerebral processes that account for the registration, storage, and recall of ongoing experience. At the same time, it is evident that because of the preservation of motor skills and verbal capacities that have been illustrated, neocortical functions must be relatively intact. Experimentally, it has been observed that

during propagating hippocampal seizures sensory stimulation may evoke potentials in the neocortex like those recorded under normal conditions (Flynn,
MacLean, & Kim, 1961).

Since it has been shown clinically and experimentally that seizures induced
in the limbic cortex by electrical stimulation propagate preferentially in the
limbic system, it has been inferred that such propagation may result in a
"functional ablation" of the involved structures (MacLean, Flanigan, Flynn,
Kim, & Stevens, 1955/1956). An inference of this kind is partly based on
neurosurgical observations that seizures induced in the region of Broca's area,
for example, may result in a postictal paresis of speech for several minutes, or
that seizures induced in the medial occipital region may be followed by a
bilateral hemianopsia lasting many minutes. Because of the regularity with
which automatisms and the associated amnesia occur with afterdischarges initiated by electrical stimulation in the medial temporal region, Feindel and Penfield
(1954) were inclined to regard the amygdala and the hippocampal formation as
requisite for the registration of memories.

*Ingredients of a Sense of Individuality.*    What might be unique about the
role of these structures in memory? This leads to the question of what accounts
for a feeling of individuality—a sense of self—that is basic to a consideration of
neural mechanisms of memory. Without a sense of individuality there is, so to
speak, no place to deposit a memory. Philosophical and other writings have
skirted the issue of what it is that accounts for a feeling of individuality, as well
as the uniqueness of being an individual. Through introspection it becomes
evident that the condition that psychologically most clearly distinguishes us as
individuals is our twofold source of information from the internal private world
and the external public world. Signals to the brain from the world within are
entirely private, being self-contained, whereas those from the outside world can
be publicly shared and lend themselves to a comparison among individuals
(MacLean, 1969).

Where in the forebrain might one look for structures strategically located for
effecting a fusion of internally and externally derived experience? Although the
neocortex, together with its related subcortical structures, must obviously exert
control over respiration and other somatovisceral functions, it serves primarily to
promote the organism's orientation and survival with respect to the external
environment. The evolution of the neocortex goes hand in hand with the elaboration of the visual, auditory, and somatic systems, which more than any other of
the "sensory" systems, provide a refined differentiation and discrimination of
happenings in the external environment. Interestingly, the signals to which these
systems are receptive are the only ones that lend themselves to electronic
amplification and radiotransmission (MacLean, 1972). Smells, tastes, and in-
teroceptions have no such avenue for communication.

Until relatively recent times the cortex of the great limbic lobe of Broca was regarded as part of the rhinecenphalon, depending primarily on information received from the olfactory apparatus and the "oral senses." The phenomenology of psychomotor epilepsy would indicate otherwise: Symptoms experienced during the aura may be of the kind associated with any one of the intero- and exteroceptive systems. Hence, we undertook experimentation to clarify the nature of inputs to the limbic cortex.

## ELECTROPHYSIOLOGICAL AND ANATOMICAL DATA

In our own work on the question just referred to we used squirrel monkeys for the electrophysiological and anatomical studies now to be summarized.

### *Microelectrode Findings*

Altogether in experiments employing closed-system, microelectrode exploration in awake sitting squirrel monkeys, we have tested the responsiveness of 14,000 nerve units to various forms of stimulation. About 40% of the units were located in limbic structures. In brief summary, we found that photic stimulation evoked unit responses in the posterior parahippocampal gyrus and retrosplenial cingulate cortex (MacLean, Yokota, & Kinnard, 1968). Units responding specifically to gustatory, somatic, and auditory stimulation were located in the insular cortex overlying the claustrum (Sudakov, MacLean, Reeves, & Marino, 1971). It was well known that olfactory stimulation evoked responses in the piriform area. With intracellular recording in awake sitting monkeys we found that stimulation of the olfactory bulb elicited excitatory postsynaptic potentials (EPSPs), but not unit discharges, in entorhinal and hippocampal neurones (Yokota, Reeves, & MacLean, 1970).

In the supracallosal cingulate cortex nearly 20% of the units were responsive to vagal volleys (Bachman, Hallowitz, & MacLean, 1977). Stimulation of other sensory systems was ineffective. Vagal volleys also activated units in the limen insulae, amygdala, and hippocampus (Radna & MacLean, 1981). In the hippocampus 24% of the recorded units were responsive and were located in all its cytoarchitectural areas. Triple shocks applied to the vagus every 4 sec. entrained respiration, and in the hippocampus, amygdala, and limen insulae a small percentage (6%) of the units discharged with a periodicity commensurate with the respiratory rhythm.

The septum is regarded as one source of interoceptive inputs to the hippocampus. Significantly, as will be discussed, septal volleys elicited EPSPs that reached threshold for unit discharge (Yokata et al., 1970).

*Anatomical Findings*

In the rat, cat, and monkey, the use of autoradiography and the horseradish peroxidase methods has shown that both the vagal and gustatory components of the solitary nucleus project to the parabrachial region, which in turn projects to certain parts of the forebrain, including the amygdala (Loewy and Burton, 1978; Mehler, 1980; McBride and Sutin, 1976; Norgren, 1976; Ricardo & Koh, 1978).

In regard to visual inputs, we traced in the monkey degeneration from the lateral geniculate body leading via Meyer's loop to the posterior parahippocampal gyrus and retrosplenial cortex (MacLean & Creswell, 1970). In infraprimates the use of new anatomical techniques not only supports such findings (Akopyan, 1982), but also has provided evidence of direct connections from the retina to the anterior dorsal nucleus (Conrad & Stumpf, 1975), which in turn projects to the retrosplenial cortex (Itaya, Van Hoesen, & Jenq, 1981). Visual information may also reach this area via connections from the lateral dorsal nucleus which receives an innervation from the superior colliculus and pretectal nuclei (Akopyan, 1982; Robertson, Kaitz, & Robards, 1980).

There is also anatomical evidence of direct subcortical gustatory, auditory, and somatic pathways to the insular cortex overlying the claustrum (see Sudakov et al., 1971, for refs.). In addition to direct olfactory connections to the hippocampal rudiment, there are pathways to the hippocampus via the piriform and entorhinal cortex (see Heimer, 1978).

## CONCLUDING DISCUSSION

Since the hippocampal formation receives connections from all the limbic areas innervated by extero- and interoceptive systems, it is in a position to achieve a synthesis of internally and externally derived information and, in turn, to influence the activity of the hypothalamus and other structures involved in somatovisceral functions variously called upon in self-preservation, procreation, and family-related behavior. In addition to its direct projections to the mammillary bodies and anterior thalamic nuclei, its connections with the amygdala and septum provide it the capacity to exert an extensive influence on the medial dorsal nucleus (MD), which, as was noted, is one of the structures primarily implicated in Korsakoff's disease. Relevant to the matter of internal inputs, we found that 27% of 367 units tested in MD were responsive to vagal stimulation (Hallowitz & Maclean, 1977). Luria and coworkers observed that frontal lobe lesions interfered with the vegetative components of the orienting response (see Luria & Homskaya, 1964.)

Based on our microelectrode findings and other considerations, we originally proposed the following hypothesis in regard to how the differential effects of intero- and exteroceptive systems on hippocampal pyramids might be conducive to memory and learning: Impulses conducted by interoceptive inputs are highly effective in producing neuronal discharge because of their excitatory effects near the cell bodies, whereas impulses of external origin induce only partial depolarization because excitation occurs primarily at the distal part of the apical dendrites (see Figs. 9 and 10, MacLean, 1972). In terms of classical conditioning, interoceptive impulses transmitted by the septum would be comparable to unconditional stimuli, since they are capable by themselves of inducing unit discharge, whereas olfactory and other exteroceptive impulses conducted by the perforant pathway would compare to conditional stimuli, being incapable, when at first acting alone, of bringing about a discharge (Gergen & Maclean, 1964; Maclean, 1969).

A study on cats in which we observed the effects of propagated hippocampal seizures on conditioned visceral and viscerosomatic responses is relevant to this hypothesis (Flynn et al., 1961; MacLean et al., 1955/1956). For this study, we used classical *trace* conditioning in which the conditional stimulus was the sound of a buzzer followed 15 sec. later by an unconditional stimulus consisting of a shock to the foreleg. Under these conditions, cardiac and respiratory changes are regularly elicited after about 40 trials. The animal, however, never develops an anticipated leg response. The visceral and viscerosomatic responses are characterized by cardiac slowing and accelerated shallow respiration. During the electrically induced hippocampal afterdischarges there is an elimination of the autonomic responses if the seizure propagates to the opposite side. The neocortical activity appears unaffected, and evoked auditory responses are unaltered. Moreover, if single muscle units are recorded in the foreleg during the propagated afterdischarge, there is no change in the rate of their discharge.

Subsequently, Flynn and Wasman (1960), attempted to show whether or not the cat was capable of *learning* during hippocampal seizures. For this purpose they used a classical conditioning method in which the termination of a conditional stimulus (the sound of a buzzer) coincided with a shock to the foreleg. Under these conditions, they observed an anticipatory leg response. The outcome in this experiment is perhaps relevant to evidence that patients with a Korsakoff memory deficit appear to manifest some degree of learning when performing a simple maze test involving the use of a stylus (Milner et al., 1968). Such a test might be regarded as comparing to the experimental situation in the cat where there is an *overlap* of the conditional and unconditional stimuli.

According to what has been proposed, either a temporary "functional ablation" during an attack of psychomotor epilepsy or bilateral disease or destruction of the hippocampal formation would interfere with the integration of internal and external experience and thereby tend to eliminate a sense of self. During the aura of psychomotor epilepsy, and prior to the automatism, some patients may have exaggerated feelings of self-awareness or, on the contrary, there may be feelings of bodily detachment and depersonalization which Jackson characterized as "mental diplopia" (Jackson & Stewart, 1899). In the light of what was said about extrapersonal information derived by the neocortex, it is of interest to recall Penfield's patient who, during the aura, experienced "mental diplopia," having the feeling as though she were two persons, with one watching the other. When asked with which person she seemed identified, she replied, "I felt as though I were the one watching" (Penfield & Perot, 1963).

This last observation recalls the clinical condition known as paramnesia, in which a patient may ascribe a personal experience to someone else. Talland (1965) reported such a disturbance of self-reference in a patient who developed a Korsakoff type of memory deficit following an acute attack of "inclusion body encephalitis." When the patient described what he remembered about his brother's fatal automobile accident, Talland reminded him that this was a good example of the preservation of his memory prior to his present illness. To that the patient countered, "But was it not *you* who has just told me about [it]?" (p. 69). It further reflects on this patient's disruption of self-reference that his family were in the habit of holding up a mirror to him so that he could observe and identify himself. Talland suggests that in this case, as has also been observed in Korsakoff patients with an alcoholic etiology, there were deficits in olfactory and gustatory discrimination and that this may have contributed to his inability to maintain a feeling of self-reference. Patients with a Korsakoff type of memory disturbance secondary to strokes or other disease may also have problems with self-reference. For example, when asked if they have a need to go to the bathroom, they may reply, "*You* have to go."

To sum up, it is proposed that the anterograde type of amnesia associated with ictal automatisms results from an interference with the integration of internal and external experience by a bilateral propagation of a seizure discharge that leads to a "functional ablation" of the hippocampal formation. It is suggested that a like failure of integration would occur in cases of anterograde amnesia in which there is an actual destruction of hippocampal tissue. Squire (1986) has recently reported a case of a severe 5-year anterograde amnesia secondary to an anoxic episode. At autopsy the major finding was a disappearance of the pyramidal cells of CA1 throughout the hippocampus. One might contend that a "clasp" of internal and external experience is as essential for memory as the antigen-antibody union in the anamnestic immune reaction. With no self-reference to the internal world there is, so to speak, no place to deposit the recollection of an experience.[2]

---

[2]Space precludes the consideration of another significant limbic factor in memory. There is a saying that "something does not exist until you give it a name." The study of the affective nature of the auras in psychomotor epilepsy suggests that there may be an essential precondition and that something does not exist unless it is imbued by an affective feeling, no matter how slight.

## FINAL COMMENT

In his clinical studies, Luria gave emphasis to concepts of "system" localization of functions. According to these concepts, he said, "each mode of psychological activity is a functional system based upon a complex interaction of jointly functioning parts of the brain. . . ." (Luria, 1973, p. 3). In discussing the disturbance of vegetative components of the orienting reflex observed in cases of frontal lobe lesions, he and Homskaya (1964) commented that damage to a "whole self-regulatory system" involved in the system-selective organization of behavior resulted not only in deterioration of the highest forms of attention, but also in the "most complicated control of memory processes." Luria adhered to a faith that *precise* experiments might open up wholly new vistas in such problem areas of neuropsychology.

## ACKNOWLEDGMENT

I am grateful to Judith Osler Newman for her typing and reading the manuscript.

## REFERENCES

Aggleton, J. P., & Mishkin, M. (1983). Memory impairments following restricted medial thalamic lesions in monkeys. *Exp. Brain Res., 52,* 199–209.

Akopyan, E. V. (1982). Visual thalamic afferents to field 29 of the rat limbic cortex. *Neurophysiology* [Russia], *14,* 135–139.

Bachman, D. S., Hallowitz, R. A., & MacLean, P. D. (1977). Effects of vagal volleys and serotonin on units of cingulate cortex in monkeys. *Brain Res., 130,* 253–269.

Bechterew, W., von (1900). Demonstration eines Gehirns mit Zerstörung der vorderen und inneren Theile der Hirnrinde beider Schlafenlappen. *Neurol. Zentbl. 19,* 990–991.

Boudin, G., Brion, S., Pepin, B., & Barbizet, J. (1968). Syndrome de Korsakoff d'étiologie artériopathique, par lésion bilatérale, asymétrique du système limbique. *Rev. Neurol. (Paris), 119,* 341–348.

Conrad, C. D., & Stumpf, W. E. (1975). Direct visual input to the limbic system: Crossed retinal projections to the nucleus anterodorsalis thalami in the tree shrew. *Exp. Brain Res., 23,* 141–149.

Conrad, K., & Ule, G. (1951). Ein Fall von Korsakow-psychose mit anatomischen Befund und Klinischen Betrachtungen *Dtsch Z. Nervenheilk. 165,* 430–445.

Cordeau, J. P., & Mahut, H. (1964). Some long-term effects of temporal lobe resections on auditory and visual discrimination in monkeys. *Brain, 87,* 177–190.

Correll, R. E., & Scoville, W. B. (1965). Performance on delayed match following lesions of medial temporal lobe structures. *J. Comp. Physiol. Psych., 60,* 360–367.

Correll, R. E., & Scoville, W. B. (1967). Significance of delay in the performance of monkeys with medial temporal lobe resections. *Exp. Brain Res., 4,* 85–96.

Dahl, D., Ingram, W. R., & Knott, J. R. (1962). Diencephalic lesions and avoidance learning in cats. *Arch. Neurol., 7,* 314–319.

DeJong, R. N., Itabashi, H. H., & Olson, J. R. (1969). Memory loss due to hippocampal lesions. Report of a case. *Arch. Neurol., 20,* 339–348.

Delay, J., & Brion, S. (1954). Syndrome de Korsakoff et corps mamillaires. *L'Encéphale, 43,* 193–200.

Douglas, R. J. (1967). The hippocampus and behavior. *Psychol. Bull., 67,* 416–442.

Drachman, D. A., & Ommaya, A. K. (1964). Memory and the hippocampal complex. *Arch. Neurol., 10,* 411–425.

Feindel, W., & Penfield, W. (1954). Localization of discharge in temporal lobe automatism. *Arch. Neurol. Psych., 72,* 605–630.

Flynn, J. P., MacLean, P. D., & Kim, C. (1961). Effects of hippocampal afterdischarges on conditioned responses. In D. E. Sheer (Ed.), *Electrical stimulation of the brain.* Austin: University of Texas Press, pp. 380–386.

Flynn, J. P., & Wasman, M. (1960). Learning and cortically evoked movement during propagated hippocampal afterdischarges. *Science, 131,* 1607–1608.

Friedman, H. M., & Allen, N. (1969). Chronic effects of complete limbic lobe destruction in man. *Neurology, 19,* 679–690.

Gamper, E. (1928). Zur Frage der Polioencephalitis haemorrhagica der chronischen Alkoholiker. Anatomische Befunde beim Alkoholischen Korsakow und ihre Beziehungen zum klinischen Bild. *Dtsch. Z. Nervenheilk., 102,* 122–129.

Gascon, G. G., & Gilles, F. (1973). Limbic dementia. *J. Neurol. Neurosurg. Psychiat., 36,* 421–430.

Gergen, J. A., & MacLean, P. D. (1964). The limbic system: Photic activation of limbic cortical areas in the squirrel monkey. *Ann. N.Y. Acad. Sci., 117,* 69–87.

Glees, P., & Griffith, H. B. (1952). Bilateral destruction of the hippocampus (Cornu Ammonis) in a case of dementia. *Mschr. Psychiat. Neurol., 123,* 193–204.

Goldberg, E. (1984). Papez circuit revisited: Two systems instead of one? In L. R. Squire & N. Butters (Eds.), *Neuropsychology of memory.* New York: Guilford Press, pp. 183–193.

Grünthal, E. (1947). Über das klinische Bild nach umschriebenem beiderseitigen Ausfall der Ammonshornrinde. *Mschr. Psychiat. Neurol., 113,* 1–16.

Gudden, H. (1896). Klinische und anatomische Beitrage zur Kenntniss der multiplen Alkoholneuritis nebst Bemerkungen über die Regenerationsvorgange im peripheren Nervensystem. *Arch. f. Psych., 28,* 643–741.

Hallowitz, R. A., & MacLean, P. D. (1977). Effects of vagal volleys on units of intralaminar and juxtalaminar thalamic nuclei in monkeys. *Brain Res., 130,* 271–286.

Heimer, L. (1978). The olfactory cortex and the ventral striatum. In K. E. Livingston & O. Hornykiewicz (Eds.), *Limbic mechanisms.* New York: Plenum Press. pp. 95–187.

Horel, J. A. (1978). The neuroanatomy of amnesia. A critique of the hippocampal memory hypothesis. *Brain, 101,* 403–445.

Isaacson, R. L. (1982). *The limbic system.* New York: Plenum Press, 2nd ed.

Itaya, S. K., Van Hoesen, G. W., & Jenq, C.-B. (1981). Direct retinal input to the limbic system of the rat. *Brain Res., 226,* 33–42.

Jackson, J. H. (1888). On a particular variety of epilepsy ("intellectual aura"), one case with symptoms of organic brain disease. *Brain, 11,* 179–207.

Jackson, J. H., & Colman, W. S. (1898). Case of epilepsy with tasting movements and "dreamy state"—very small patch of softening in the left uncinate gyrus. *Brain, 21,* 580–590.

Jackson, J. H., & Stewart, P. (1899). Epileptic attacks with a warning of a crude sensation of smell and with the intellectual aura (dreamy state) in a patient who had symptoms pointing to gross organic disease of the right temporosphenoidal lobe. *Brain, 22,* 534–549.

Jolliffe, N., Colbert, C. N., & Joffe, P. M. (1936). Observations on etiologic relationship of vitamin B ($B_1$) to polyneuritis in alcohol addict. *Am. J. Med. Sci., 191,* 515–526.

Jubb, K. V., Saunders, L. Z., & Coates, H. V. (1956). Thiamine deficiency encephalopathy in cats. *J. Comp. Path., 66,* 217–227.

Kimble, D. P., & Pribram, K. H. (1963). Hippocampectomy and behavior sequences. *Science, 139,* 824–825.

Klüver, H., & Bucy, P. C. (1939). Preliminary analysis of functions of the temporal lobes in monkeys. *Arch. Neurol. Psychiat. (Chicago), 42,* 979–1000.

Korsakoff, S. S. (1887). Disturbance of psychic function in alcoholic paralysis and its relation to the disturbance of the psychic sphere in multiple neuritis of non-alcoholic origin. *Vestnik Psichiatrii, 4,* fascicle 2.

Korsakoff, S. S. (1889). Psychosis Polyneuritica s. Cerebropathia Psychica Toxaemica. *Medizinskoje Obozrenije, 31*(13).

Lawicka, W., & Konorski, J. (1959). Physiological mechanism of delayed reactions. III. The effects of prefrontal ablations on delayed reactions in dogs. *Acta. Biol. Exp. (Warsz), 19,* 221–231.

Loewy, A. D., & Burton, H. (1978). Nuclei of the solitary tract: Efferent projections to the lower brain stem and spinal cord of the cat. *J. Comp. Neurol., 181,* 421–450.

Luria, A. R. (1973). The frontal lobe and the regulation of behavior. In K. H. Pribram & A. R. Luria (Eds.), *Psychophysiology of the frontal lobes.* New York: Academic Press, pp. 3–26.

Luria, A. R., & Homskaya, E. D. (1964). Disturbance in the regulative role of speech with frontal lobe lesions. In J. M. Warren & K. Akert (Eds.), *The frontal granular cortex and behavior.* New York: McGraw–Hill, pp. 353–371.

MacLean, P. D. (1969). The internal-external bonds of the memory process. *J. Nerv. Ment. Dis., 149,* 40–47.

MacLean, P. D. (1972). Implications of microelectrode findings on exteroceptive inputs to the limbic cortex. In C. H. Hockman (Ed.), *Limbic system mechanisms and autonomic function.* Springfield, IL: Charles C. Thomas, pp. 115–136.

MacLean, P. D. (1985). Brain evolution relating to family, play and the separation call. *Archives of General Psychiatry, 42,* 405–417.

MacLean, P. D., & G. Creswell (1970). Anatomical connections of visual system with limbic cortex of monkey. *J. Comp. Neurol., 138,* 265–278.

MacLean, P. D., Flanigan, S., Flynn, J. P., Kim, C., & Stevens, J. R. (1955/1956). Hippocampal function: tentative correlations of conditioning, EEG, drug, and radioautographic studies. *Yale J. Biol. Med., 28,* 380–395.

MacLean, P. D., Yokota, T., & Kinnard, M. D. (1968). Photically sustained on-responses of units in posterior hippocampal gyrus of awake monkey. *J. Neurophysiol., 31,* 870–883.

McBride, R. L., & Sutin, J. (1976). Projections of the locus coeruleus and adjacent pontine tegmentum in the cat. *J. Comp. Neurol., 165,* 265–284.

Mahut, H., Zola–Morgan, S., & Moss, M. (1982). Hippocampal resections impair associative learning and recognition memory in the monkey. *J. Neuroscience, 2,* 1214–1229.

Malamud, N., & Skillikorn, S. A. (1956). Relationship between the Wernicke and the Korsakoff syndrome. *Arch. Neurol. Psychiat. (Chic.), 76,* 585–596.

Mehler, W. R. (1980). Subcortical afferent connections of the amygdala in the monkey. *J. Comp. Neurol, 190,* 733–762.

Milner, B., Corkin, S., & Teuber, H.–L. (1968). Further analysis of the hippocampal amnesic syndrome: 14-year follow-up study of H. M. *Neuropsychologia, 6,* 215–234.

Mishkin, M. (1978). Memory in monkeys severely impaired by combined but not by separate removal of amygdala and hippocampus. *Nature, 273,* 297–298.

Mishkin, M. (1982). A memory system in the monkey. *Phil. Trans. R. Soc. Lond. B., 298,* 85–95.

Murray, E. A., & Mishkin, M. (1983). Severe tactual memory deficits in monkeys after combined removal of the amygdala and hippocampus. *Brain Res., 270,* 340–344.

Norgren, R. (1976). Taste pathways to hypothalamus and amygdala. *J. Comp. Neurol., 166,* 17–30.

Olton, D. S. (1978). The function of septo-hippocampal connections in spatially organized behaviour. In K. Elliott & J. Whelan (Eds.), *Functions of the septo-hippocampal system.* Amsterdam: Elsevier, pp. 327–349.

Orbach, J., Milner, B., & Rasmussen, T. (1960). Learning and retention in monkeys after amygdala-hippocampus resection. *Arch. Neurol., 3,* 230–251.

Penfield, W., & Milner, B. (1958). Memory deficit produced by bilateral lesions in the hippocampal zone. *Arch. Neurol. Psych., 79,* 475–497.

Penfield, W., & Perot, P. (1963). The brain's record of auditory and visual experience. A final summary and discussion. *Brain, 86,* 596–696.

Phillips, G. B., Victor, M., Adams, R. D., & Davidson, C. S. (1952). A study of the nutritional defect in Wernicke's syndrome: The effect of a purified diet, thiamine, and other vitamins on the clinical manifestations. *J. Clin. Invest., 31*, 859–871.

Ploog, D. W., & MacLean, P. D. (1963). On functions of the mammillary bodies in the squirrel monkey. *Exp. Neurol., 7*, 76–85.

Radna, R. J., & MacLean, P. D. (1981). Vagal elicitation of respiratory-type and other unit responses in basal limbic structures of squirrel monkeys. *Brain Res., 213*, 45–61.

Ricardo, J. A., & Koh, E. T. (1978). Anatomical evidence of direct projections from the nucleus of the solitary tract to the hypothalamus, amygdala, and other forebrain structures in the rat. *Brain Res., 153*, 1–26.

Robertson, R. T., Kaitz, S. S., & Robards, M. J. (1980). A subcortical pathway links sensory and limbic systems of the forebrain. *Neurosci. Letters, 17*, 161–165.

Schenk, V. W. D. (1959). Unilateral atrophy of the fornix. In A. Biemond et al. (Eds.), *Recent neurological research*. Amsterdam: Elsevier, pp. 168–179.

Scoville, W. B., & Milner, B. (1957). Loss of recent memory after bilateral hippocampal lesions. *J. Neurol. Neurosurg. Psychiat., 20*, 11–21.

Squire, L. R. (1986). Mechanisms of memory. *Science, 232*, 1612–1919.

Squire, L. R., & Zola–Morgan, S. (1983). The neurology of memory: The case for correspondence between the findings for human and nonhuman primate. In *The physiological basis of memory*. New York: Academic Press, pp. 199–268.

Stepien, L. S., Cordeau, J. P., & Rasmussen, T. (1960). The effect of temporal lobe and hippocampal lesions on auditory and visual recent memory in monkeys. *Brain, 83(part 3)*, 470–489.

Stevens, J. R., Glaser, G. H., & MacLean, P. D. (1955). The influence of sodium amytal on the recollection of seizure states. *Trans. Am. Neurol. Assoc., 79*, 40–45.

Sudakov, K., MacLean, P. D., Reeves, A. G., & Marino, R. (1971). Unit study of exteroceptive inputs to claustrocortex in awake, sitting, squirrel monkey. *Brain Res., 28*, 19–34.

Talland, G. A. (1965). An amnesic patient's disavowal of his own recall performance and its attribution to the interviewer. *Psychiat. Neurol., 149*, 67–76.

Torch, W. C., Hirano, A., & Solomon, S. (1977). Anterograde transneuronal degeneration in the limbic system: Clinical-anatomic correlation. *Neurology, 27*, 1157–1163.

Ule, G. (1951). Korsakow-Psychose nach doppelseitiger Ammonshornzerstörung mit transneuronaler Degeneration der Corpora mamillaria. *Dtsch. Z. Nervenheilk, 165*, 446–456.

Victor, M. (1981). Diseases of the nervous system due to nutritional deficiency. In J. Spittell, Jr. (Ed.), *Clinical Medicine*. Philadelphia: Harper & Row, pp. 1–30.

Victor, M., Adams, R. D., & Collins, G. H. (1971). The Wernicke–Korsakoff Syndrome. A Clinical and Pathological Study of 245 Patients, 82 with Post-Mortem Examinations. Philadelphia: F. A. David.

Victor, M., & Yakovlev, P. I. (1955). S. S. Korsakoff's psychic disorder in conjunction with peripheral neuritis. A translation of Korsakoff's original article with brief comments on the author and his contribution to clinical medicine. *Neurology, 5*(6), 394–406.

Waxler, M., & Rosvold, H. E. (1970). Delayed alternation in monkeys after removal of the hippocampus. *Neuropsychologia, 8*, 137–146.

Weiskrantz, L., & Warrington, E. K. (1975). The problem of the amnesic syndrome in man and animals. In R. L. Isaacson & K. H. Pribram, (Eds.), *The hippocampus.* New York: Plenum, Vol. 2, pp. 411–428.

Wernicke, C. (1881). *Lehrbuch der Gehirnkrankheiten fur Artze und Studierende.* Kassel: Theodor Fischer, Vol 2, pp. 229–242.

Witt, E. D., & Goldman-Rakic, P. S. (1983). Intermittent thiamine deficiency in the rhesus monkey. I. Progression of neurological signs and neuroanatomical lesions. *Ann. Neurol. 13*, 376–395.

Yokota, T., Reeves, A. G., & MacLean, P. D. (1970). Differential effects of septal and olfactory volleys on intracellular responses of hippocampal neurons in awake, sitting monkeys. *J. Neurophysiol., 33*, 96–107.

Zola-Morgan, S., Squire, L. R., & Mishkin, M. (1982). The neuroanatomy of amnesia: Amygdala-hippocampus versus temporal stem. *Science, 218*, 1337–1339.

# 7

# Hemispheric Interaction and Decisional Dominance

*Edoardo Bisiach*

*Institute di Clinica Neurologica dell'Università di Milano*

> Somewhere along the line–and it is not easy to determine just when and by whom—the hypothesis of cerebral dominance took origin. The term is an unsatisfactory one, for it suggests a suzerainty of the cerebral hemispheres over some other unnamed structure of the brain. What is no doubt implied, though not explicitly stated, is a relative preponderancy of one half of the cerebrum over the other. (Critchley, 1972)

Critchley's words indicate the mild annoyance with which the worn-out concept of cerebral dominance may nowadays be received. Although a faithful reconstruction would indeed be laborious, we may trace the root of this concept back to Jackson's (1874) principle of hemispheric leadership and view its further development as a partial distortion of this principle.

In his writings, Hughlings Jackson explicitly exonerates himself of any attempt to imply a misconceived segregation of brain activities. His idea of a leading side is a dynamic one and refers to the migration of the primary stages of an activity to the locus where suitable brain structures can be found for the *execution of that activity*. Moreover, the leadership is not absolute but apportioned: the left hemisphere is held by Jackson to lead the "voluntary" expression of language, to the "automatic" inception of which the right hemisphere contributes; the reverse applies, in his view, to the "revival of images."

In the fervent years of rising neuropsychology, however, the apparent implication of left-hemisphere pathology in a series of conspicuous behavioral disorders besides dysphasia was sufficient to cloud the role of the right hemisphere in highest nervous functions. In 1926, Henschen, stressing the slight share of the right hemisphere in a series of mental functions, wondered whether it was a regressing organ or, to the contrary, an organ capable of training and "reserved for future higher development and possibly for new facilities." Such a striking departure from Jackson's views shows, among other things, how neglectful those years were of the important role played by the right hemisphere in the representation of egocentric space. Attestations to this role, in fact, had already appeared in literature at the close of the last century, culminating in Zingerle's 1913 article on dyschiria and in Babinski's 1914 and 1918 addresses concerning anosognosia for left hemiplegia.

A crisis in the notion of the absolute left-hemisphere dominance in the coordinated activity of the two halves of the brain was determined, however, by the ascent of experimental neuropsychology in the years following World War II. In his 1962 book on *The Higher Cortical Functions in Man,* Luria hinted at the incipient revision of this issue, which, in his view, still needed to be brought into sharper focus. This was prompted by the amazing wealth of contributions which followed Brenda Milner's pioneering work of the late 1950s (1954, 1958) on hemispheric functional asymmetries. The old concept of hemispheric dominance gave way to the idea of specific competences, relative to functions conceived along lines such as those suggested by Luria, that is as interlaced, multi-component paths of neural activity involving modules common to different paths. This conception predicts interhemispheric shifts of activity closely related not only to the nature of the stimuli but also to the program of the task in which they are involved.

The concept of hemisphere-specific processing competence, however, does not seem to exhaust all of the implications of terms such as "cerebral dominance" or "leadership." In spite of the fact that the two hemispheres are widely connected through commissures into a larger system and have some complementary competences, they may seem to constitute the machinery of two distinct minds. The question therefore arises as to their respective participation in decisional acts relative to processes which either hemisphere might be competent to initiate and carry on. The possibility of interhemispheric conflicts is indeed suggested by phenomena such as diagonistic dyspraxia (Akelaitis, Risteen, Herren, & Van Wagenen, 1942) observed in split-brain patients. The notion of interhemispheric rivalry, however, has also been applied to the intact brain (e.g., Critchley, 1972). Thus the problem of cerebral dominance, considered as *decisional dominance,* independent of specific functional competences, has still to be faced on at least one front. It might well turn out to be a pseudoproblem, an illusion due to a penchant, difficult to eradicate from our mind, toward anthropomorphic explanations, or due to ignorance of the full extent of the repercussions of a massive interconnection such as that provided by the corpus callosum. Pending resolution it remains a problem worth pursuing.

Investigations more or less explicitly directed toward a solution of the problem of (strictly conceived) cerebral dominance are scanty and their results do not fully corroborate one another. This stands in striking contrast to the host of investigations which have been, and are, generating data relative to hemispheric functional competences. Whether this is due to widespread lack of interest in this issue or to the unquestionable difficulty in finding adequate experimental paradigms to address it, is unclear. The next sections give an overview of these sparse efforts.

## COMPARATIVE CHRONOMETRY

Robert Efron (1963a) investigated temporal comparisons between stimuli delivered to symmetrical points of the sensory surface. Suprathreshold electric shocks to the left and right index fingers were given to nine right-handers. Light spots subtending a visual angle of three degrees were flashed to the nasal side of each retina (26 degrees lateral to the fixation point and 17 degrees above the horizontal midline) in 11 right-handers. The mean results showed that verbal judgments of simultaneity were given when the left distal stimulus preceded the right by 3.32 msec. for shocks ($p < .005$) and 3.81 msec. for lights ($p < .005$). The site of the comparison thus appeared to be located in the left hemisphere, and the delay due to transfer of information relative to the left stimulus from the right to the left hemisphere. The same pattern of results was obtained in an experiment in which no overt verbal response was required, but the subjects themselves adjusted a delay circuit so that the two lights were experienced as being simultaneous. This ruled out an explanation grounded on the lateralization of speech. By surveying the literature, Efron found a few similar results which had not, however, been examined in terms of hemispheric functional asymmetries. Of special interest is the fact that further experiments conducted on a right-hander allowed Efron (1963a, pp. 274–276) to suggest that a left-hemisphere mechanism was involved in cross-modality temporal comparisons even when *both* stimuli were initially addressed to the right hemisphere. Efron also found (1963b) that if stimulus intensity was decreased, the delay of the presumed interhemispheric transfer increased proportionately.

Defending his position against a hypothesis that explained his data as due to slower transmission along the pathways directed to the right hemisphere, Efron quoted investigations which had failed to find latency differences between left and right cortical evoked potentials due to contralateral somatosensory or visual stimulation.

## CONFLICTING BILATERAL STIMULATION

Efron and Yund (1974) gave five right-handers pairs of dichotic chords, the first of which was obtained by stimulating the left ear with a 1900-Hz and the right with a 1500-Hz tone or vice versa; in the second chord, which followed after a 1-sec. interval, the combination ear-tone was reversed. The subject had to report verbally whether he heard a high-low or a low-high sequence. The sound pressure level was varied in one ear from 80 to 30 dB, in steps of 10 dB, while the sound pressure level in the opposite ear was kept constant at 80 dB. The results were amazing: Whereas in all subjects a difference of 10 dB between the two ears caused the acoustic image to shift toward the ear which received the louder stimulation, pitch judgments were consistently given on the basis of the sequences heard by one ear, even when the source of the stimulation was experienced by the other, until very marked differences in sound pressure level between the two ears were reached. The right ear was dominant in four subjects and the left ear in one, whose right-handedness, however, was questionable. Nonetheless, after having subjected a population of 70 subjects to an identical test, Yund and Efron (1975) found that 31% were right-ear dominant, 33% left-ear dominant, and 36% showed no significant ear dominance. No correlation between ear dominance thus assessed and handedness or ear dominance for speech sounds was found (Efron 1974). It is worth noting that when the difference in sound pressure level between the two ears was such that a transition began between reporting the sequences heard by one ear only and those heard by the opposite ear only, the subjects were sometimes aware of a contradictory double percept which they described in one of three ways: (a) "I hear both sequences and don't know which to report," (b) "In one respect I feel compelled to report that the sequence is high-low but some other part of my mind tells me that the sequence is low-high," or (c) "I *hear* one sequence, perhaps the low-high, but I want to say the other one (high-low)" (Efron & Yund, 1974, p. 255).

A similar attempt at generating a state of conflict between the two hemispheres, the resolution of which might uncover the locus where the decision was taken, was later made by my coworkers and myself (Basso, Bisiach, & Capitani, 1977). Horizontally elongated gray rectangles of three graded shades were tachistoscopically presented across the fixation point to 58 right-handers. The stimuli appeared on four different backgrounds: full white, full black, white in the left half, and black in the right, and vice versa. After each exposition the subject was given a multiple-choice display on which five horizontal gray stripes were juxtaposed, from the lightest (top) to the darkest (bottom), the three in the middle being identical to those tachistoscopically projected. Our subjects made the expected wrong choice whenever the gray rectangle was surrounded by a uniform white or black background, but, somewhat to our surprise, all of them were remarkably accurate on trials with chimerical backgrounds. This showed that, wherever it may be located in the brain, the mechanism responsible for the decision weighed the conflicting information initially available to each hemisphere with the impartiality needed to pass Solomonian judgments. It is worth mentioning that our subjects were unaware of the presence of nonuniform backgrounds.

## STIMULATION IN SPLIT-BRAIN PATIENTS

Levy, Trevarthen, and Sperry (1972) gave commissurotomized patients tachistoscopic stimuli constructed by juxtaposing the left half of a face to the right half of a different face. The subjects had to recognize the stimuli in a multiple-choice display containing all the full faces from which the stimuli had been prepared. A correct choice was made on the basis of the *left* half of the stimulus in 89% of responses given by the *left* hand and in 75% of responses given by the *right* hand (the error rate being 1% and 5%, respectively). Switching to a condition in which verbal identifications were required (in the form of names which the patients had previously learned with "unusual difficulty . . . succeeding eventually only by assigning some verbal label to a distinctive feature of each face"), correct responses were given on the basis of the *right* half of the stimulus in 49% of trials and of the *left* half in 30% of trials (the error rate having increased in 15%). In either condition the patients showed no awareness of the chimerical nature of the stimuli, although in exceptional instances a double correct pointing seemed to reflect the conflict between two concurrent percepts. Similar results were obtained with random shapes, pictures of familiar objects, and groups of geometrical shapes.

A further study by Levy and Trevarthen (1976) showed that the interhemispheric switching of control in split-brain patients did not merely depend on whether the required response involved overt speech or not. In this experiment, chimerical configurations of common objects had to be matched to one of several drawings, exposed to free vision, on the basis of two different criteria: (a) visual similarity (such as that existing between a pair of open scissors and crossed fork and spoon) and (b) conceptual relatedness (such as that existing between scissors and spools of thread or between crossed fork and spoon on one side and a cake on the other). If the instructions were ambiguous about the criterion that the subject had to adopt, choices for visual similarity were made by the right hemisphere (on the basis of the left halves of chimerical stimuli), whereas choices for conceptual relatedness were made by the left hemisphere (on the basis of the right halves). If instructions were such as to force criterion (a) on some trials and criterion (b) on other trials, the results were not uniform. In fact, on some observations, change of instruction determined a shift both in strategy and in locus of control, so that command was assumed by the hemisphere which was more competent in the required strategy. On other observations, however, there was a dissociation, either in the sense that changing strategy was not accompanied a by shift of hemispheric control or that only the latter occurred, while the strategy—despite the instructions—remained unchanged.

These data are important since they show that *in patients with telencephalic commissurotomy* the locus of command may switch beforehand from one hemisphere to the other, depending on factors which are not exclusively related to hemisphere-specific processing competences. Moreover, they show that the expression of hemispheric dominance is not merely due to a "speed contest between the two halves of the brain." As to the precise nature of the factors determining which of the two hemispheres will be in charge in a given task, we are still far from having a satisfactory answer. All we may infer, so far, is that the pivot of what Levy and Trevarthen called "metacontrol of hemispheric functions" appears to be located in subcortical structures unaffected by surgical disconnection.

## UNILATERAL HEMISPHERIC DAMAGE

Similarity judgments between multivariate stimuli, by apparently implying an *optional* performance, might in principle reflect the coexistence of alternative cognitive rules, of which one may, for a variety of reasons, be dominant. Therefore, unlike tasks implying *optimal* performance (and, consequently, a more constrained and fixed chain of processing steps firmly bound to specific hemispheric competences), investigation of optional performance tasks in patients with unilateral hemisphere damage might uncover different neural strategies and a relative hierarchy for choice order as well as the side of the brain by which this order is imposed.

We explored this issue (Bisiach & Capitani, 1976) by asking patients with lesions confined to either hemisphere to classify a series of rectangles, in which shape and area were orthogonally manipulated, as more similar to one or the other of two standards (Figure 1). The results are depicted in Figure 2, in which the inclination of the vectors representative of various groups of subjects is a measure of the relative weight given to area (A) and shape (S) in the judgments of similarity. A vector lying on the abscissa would correspond to judgments made exclusively on the basis of shape, whereas a vector lying on the ordinate would reflect judgments made on the basis of area alone (see the original paper for further details). Figure 2 shows that in control subjects (C) and in right brain-damaged patients with and without visual field defects on confrontation perimetry (R+ and R–, respectively) choices were virtually made on the basis of shape alone. No significant differences existed between these groups. By contrast, the two stimulus variables were equally weighed in the choices made by both groups of left brain-damaged patients (L+ and L–), which did not differ from each other, whereas their performance was significantly different from that of the other three groups.

Since, independently of their location, lesions of the left hemisphere seemed to "release a processing mechanism which is apparently more adherent to the overall physical characteristics of the stimuli" (and the results, therefore, could not be interpreted as being due to failures in hemisphere-specific processing of either feature), they were seen as uncovering a subordinate—right-hemisphere

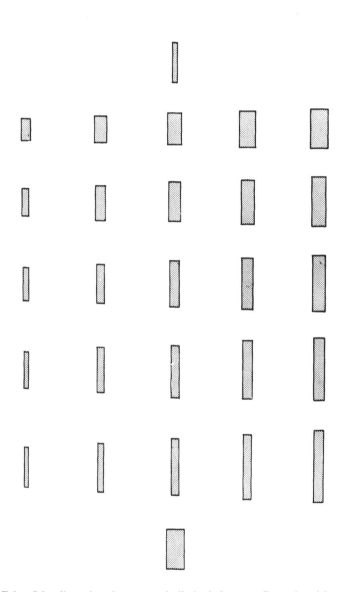

**FIGURE 1.** Stimuli employed to assess similarity judgments. Reproduced from Bisiach and Capitani (1976).

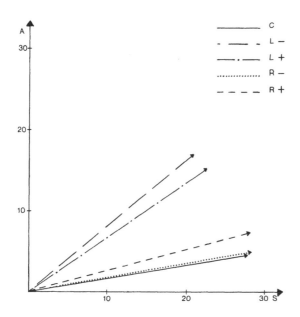

**FIGURE 2.** Similarity judgments given by brain-damaged and control subjects. See text for explanation. Reproduced from Bisiach and Capitani (1976).

idiosyncratic—cognitive style, which in the intact brain is inhibited by a dominant alternative tied to left-hemisphere functioning. In the original paper we hinted at the possibility that these findings could fit the concept of cerebral dominance *stricto sensu,* that is orthogonal to the partition of specific technical competences between the two hemispheres and conceivably justified by the necessity of imposing any order on the chaos that might possibly arise from competing processes occurring in parallel in two connected systems, each of which is to a considerable extent the replica of the other. Such a conclusion, however, would appear to be totally unwarranted. Indeed, if we assume that under environmental pressures the nervous system has evolved in such a way as to privilege shape detection, the assumption of optionality relative to similarity judgments appears to be fallacious. Any argument concerning the location of the mechanism involved in these judgments would seem therefore to relapse once again into the question of hemispheric competencies.

## LATERALIZATION OF THE DECISION STAGE

In a further attempt at disentangling a decision stage from processing stages likely to be dependent on specific hemispheric resources, we asked 32 right-handers to perform a go/no-go task in which they had to react with either hand to single dots tachistoscopically projected to a fixed point in either visual hemifield and to abstain from responding to two dots simultaneously appearing, one to the left, and one to the right of the fixation point (Bisiach, Mini, Sterzi, & Vallar, 1982; Vallar, Bisiach, & Sterzi, 1984). A previous investigation (Bisiach, Capitani, & Tansini, 1979) had failed to find left-right differences in the detection of this type of stimuli.

The results of a preliminary experiment with simple RTs to single lateralized dots are shown in Figure 3a. Whereas field and hand effects were not significant,

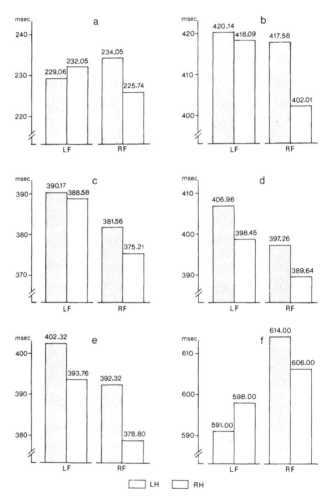

**FIGURE 3.** Mean RTs recorded in normal subjects on various tasks (see text) involving presentation of stimuli in the left (LF) or right (RF) visual field and left-hand (LH) or right-hand (RH) responses.

their interaction was ($p < .001$). Faster ipsilateral responses were in fact quite expected and in agreement with the literature quoted in our article; they are generally interpreted as being due to shorter neural pathways and to spatial S–R compatibility. Choice RTs are shown in Figure 3b. Here, a significant field effect ($p < .001$) and a significant hand $\times$ field interaction ($p < .005$) were found.

Choice RTs of this group of subjects are consistent with a model in which the decision is taken by a mechanism permanently located in the left hemisphere. We compared this mechanism with an *exclusive*-OR logic gate giving an output (*go* response) if and *only* if only one of the two inputs accepted by the mechanism was positive. This requires the additional assumption of a warm-up phase— initiated by either input—longer than the time taken by left-field stimuli to be transferred to the left hemisphere. Without this assumption, the right-field stimulus of the no-go pattern, arriving at the gate before the left, would cause it to give an output also in the no-go condition. This model predicts shorter RTs to right-field stimuli and shorter right-hand reactions when the right visual field is stimulated.

On the contrary, the hypothesis of an itinerant decision mechanism, switching to the left or to the right, according to the side of visual input or to the side of the responding hand, is untenable. In fact, assuming that left-field stimuli activate a right-hemispheric decision stage, left-hand reactions to such stimuli ought to be faster than right-hand reactions, as in simple RTs; this prediction is not confirmed by our results. Conversely, assuming that pretuning of the left hand for responding preactivates a right-hemispheric decision stage would imply faster reactions of this hand to left-field stimuli, as in simple RTs, which again is in contrast to the results.

In order to ascertain whether the decision stage may shift to the right hemisphere if the left one is engaged in a concurrent task, the experiment was replicated in a different group of 20 right-handers in two different conditions: The first identical to the original, the second differing in that stimuli were given while the subject was engaged in counting backwards aloud by three, starting with a number which changed from trial to trial (Vallar, Bisiach, Cerizza, & Rusconi, 1988).

Figure 3c shows the results of the exact replica of the original *go-no go* experiment. The general profile is similar to that of Figure 3b. Whereas the field effect was significant ($p < .007$), the hand effect did not reach significance. In contrast to the early experiment, no significant hand $\times$ field interaction was found. Figure 3d shows RTs recorded in the condition in which the concurrent task was added. Again, the outline of the results remains roughly unchanged. The field effect was fairly significant ($p < .01$) whereas the hand effect only approached significance ($p < .053$); their interaction was not significant. These results suggest that although the concurrent task engaging the left hemisphere caused a slight overall increase in choice RTs—hinting at the involvement of a common processing resource—the decision stage remained anchored to this hemisphere. In order to test further the security of this anchoring, our last step was to determine whether the locus of the decision mechanism would remain the same even in a condition in which all information needed for the decision was first available to one hemisphere.

A new group of 20 right-handers participated in an experiment which differed from the original in that no-go stimuli were pairs of dots appearing one above the other either in the left or in the right visual field. The RTs of this experiment are shown in Figure 3e, from the inspection of which it is evident that the pattern of results remains substantially unchanged. The field effect was even more clear-cut ($p < .0001$); the hand effect was also significant ($p < .05$); their interaction was not significant. Thus, the decision stage appears to remain in the left hemisphere even when all information required for the choice is primarily addressed to the right hemisphere.

The question arises as to what happens when choices are required for complex stimuli for which interhemispheric processing asymmetries are known to exist. Rizzolatti, Umiltà and Berlucchi (1971) investigated hemispheric competence in the perception of human faces by asking 12 right-handers to react as fast as possible with the forefinger of either hand to either of two faces (go stimuli) tachistoscopically presented in either visual hemifield. The subjects had to refrain from any reaction on trials in which one of two other faces (no-go stimuli) was presented. Figure 3f has been drawn from the results obtained in this experiment to simplify comparison with our results. Rizzolatti et al. found a significant left-field superiority ($p < .005$), whereas the hand effect and the field × hand interaction were not significant. However, except for the skewness due to the increase of RTs to right-field stimuli, the profile of their results is unquestionably more similar to that obtained in our experiment with simple RTs (Figure 3a) than to those we obtained in experiments with choice RTs to poorly structured stimuli (Figures 3b–e). This profile is predicted by a model in which the decision to respond is taken by the hemisphere which first receives the stimulus, no matter how efficient this hemisphere is in processing such stimuli.[1]

## CONCLUSIONS

In retrospect, experiments such as those of Efron and Yung, Yund and Efron, and Basso et al. do not allow one to draw firm inferences about the location of a decision stage. These results merely show the proportion in which

---

[1]Rizzolatti et al. employed the same experimental paradigm with letters as stimuli. A right-field superiority ($p < .005$) was found. Left-field RTs were 448 and 452 msec for the left and the right hand respectively; right-field RTs were 432 and 431 msec for the left and the right hand, respectively.

information initially available to each hemisphere merges in a unitary percept on the basis of which a response is given. The variable privilege given to one channel over the other, found in Yund and Efron's subjects, does not necessarily imply that the decision concerning the response is taken by a mechanism located in the hemisphere to which the major sensory component is initially conveyed. The remarkable equilibrium of the two channels found in the subjects who participated in our experiment with gray stimuli on chimerical backgrounds suggests that the degree of informational exchange between the two halves of the brain may be such as to mask any presumed lateralization of the decision mechanism.

Shifts in similarity judgments after unilateral brain damage, as we have seen, are also equivocal since they may simply reflect the recruitment of hemisphere-specific competencies applied to the most adaptive end. The appearance of a different criterion for similarity judgments after left-hemisphere lesion does not necessarily imply that in the intact brain a decision must be made between two conflicting criteria: one of them could, in fact, have been pre-selected due to its ecological advantage.

Although we cannot fully generalize from data obtained in commissurotomized patients to normal brain function, the observations made by Levy et al. (1972) and by Levy and Trevarthen (1976) are most enlightening. They have provided unequivocal evidence of lateralized decision mechanisms, the dominance of which may shift independently of hemispheric competence in processing sensory information. This undermines the concept of dominance as a fixed, general supremacy of one hemisphere over the other and reveals a much more articulated hemispheric interaction.

What remains to be settled, is the principle which determines the migration of the decision stage and the mechanisms by which this migration is realized. Apparently, a clue to the former must be sought not only in the features of the stimuli involved in certain decisional processes but also in those aspects of the program according to which sensory information is processed in different tasks.[2] What does determine left dominance in tasks such as those requiring judgments of simultaneity, investigated by Efron (1975), or choice reactions to lateralized visual stimuli, investigated by my colleagues and myself? In both cases, the structure of the stimuli was not such as to favor hemisphere-specific processing mechanisms. The kind of response (verbal vs. nonverbal) was found to be immaterial in Efron's experiments and no verbal response was required in ours. Verbal instructions, on the other hand, cannot be suspected of being determi-

---

[2]Mention should be made of an important point concerning conclusions drawn from some of the reviewed experiments. The results of these experiments have been published as group statistics, leaving aside the question of possible individual differences. This procedure may be dangerous, since it averages patterns of behavior which might be highly variant. Future research should consider carefully this point.

nants of left dominance in these tasks, since they are also used in experiments measuring simple RTs (see Figure 3a), or choice RTs in which no permanent location of the decision stage in one hemisphere has been found (Figure 3f).

This is all the more evident if one considers that in Rizzolatti et al.'s (1971) experiment verbal instructions were presumably more complex than in Efron's experiments.

A possibility to be considered is that, independent of the way in which the instructions are given, the complexity of the algorithm inherent in some tasks may be such as to require a propositional mediation afforded by the left hemisphere. I am not suggesting, of course, that inner speech must recite, as it were, the algorithm at each trial. This would be incompatible with RTs as short as those found in our choice tasks as well as with the results shown in Figure 3d, where a mediation by inner speech would have presumably been severely disrupted by the concurrent task. However represented in the brain, the rule that responses must obey in these tasks should be available for rapid access and read-out and should be relatively unimpeded by a concurrent task as cognitively demanding as the one we employed in our experiment. It could be suggested that the unnaturalness of the principle distinguishing go and no-go conditions in our choice tasks (Figures 3b–e) requires some kind of explicit propositional rule which is not necessary in the tasks studied by Rizzolatti et al., involving the recognition of human faces; consequently, a stable left-hemisphere dominance results in the former tasks not in the latter. This interpretation, however, hardly applies to simultaneity judgments. The algorithm, here, is quite simple and the task demands a minimum of memory; instead, a very careful comparison of two elementary sensations on a temporal dimension is required.

In order to formulate an adequate hypothesis, one must find out what the decisions relative to simultaneity judgments and choice responses to poorly structured visual stimuli have in common, but that they do not share with the decisions involved in the detection of suprathreshold stimuli (simple RTs) and in choice reactions to faces.

One might submit that the former, but not the latter, require a more "analytical" set and therefore are more congenial to the left hemisphere. This suggestion finds a somewhat weak support in the rather dubious (cf. Bradshaw & Nettleton, (1981) "analytical-holistic" dichotomy of hemispheric competences.

Alternatively, one might suggest that simultaneity judgments and highly artificial choice responses to unstructured, meaningless stimuli require more deliberate control, whereas simple detection of suprathreshold stimuli and choice reactions to natural stimuli, such as faces, are likely to be carried out more automatically. As a consequence, the former would be more strictly dependent on the left hemisphere, whereas the whole control over the latter would be taken by the hemisphere which first received the sensory input. This interpretation, which might (somewhat tendentiously) appeal to Jacksonian doctrine, could find some support in the well-known dissociation between automatic activities—

correctly carried out—and voluntary activities (severely impaired) in cases of apraxia due to left-hemisphere lesions. A similar dissociation was present in a patient observed in our department after a left occipitotemporal stroke, who complained of loss of visual imagery: He was perfectly able to carry out routine activities of any kind unless he tried to represent explicitly to himself the sequence of the visuomotor events occurring in these activities (Basso, Bisiach, & Luzzatti, 1980).

A mentalistic vocabulary might be avoided by rephrasing this "voluntary-automatic" distinction in terms of sequential vs. parallel cognitive processes. Whereas the latter are likely to occur in both hemispheres in nearly the same way, the former might be peculiar to the left hemisphere as a form of nonverbal thought originating from an introjection of speech in accordance with the theory of the regulatory function of inner speech developed by Vygotsky and Luria.


## ACKNOWLEDGEMENTS

It was a fair October evening when I entered Frunze street the first time. Enclosed between the old buildings on each side, the sudden darkness made a sharp contrast to the brightness of the red star lit on the top of the Kremlin tower I had just left behind. Two elderly women were seated on the threshold of N. 13 and I had to interrupt their chat to ask the way to Professor Luria's flat. They stared at me. Then at each other; blankly. As I renewed my request mentioning the first name and patronymic of my host, they brightened at once and be-nevolently showed me a door on the opposite side of the small court. A few moments later, I was comfortably seated in an armchair, next to a massive desk overcrowded with papers and objects of all kinds. There I spent some hours enjoying the lively conversation of the tall, smiling, white-haired man to whom I had been asked to pay merely a courtesy visit, far from imagining myself on the verge of a totally unforeseen course of events.

At the end of the evening, Alexandr Romanovich suddenly turned to address me in Russian. Once apparently satisfied that I could somehow manage to follow him, he succinctly declared that the motives that had taken me to Moscow were not so compelling after all, that I had better forget them and train in neuropsychology (starting next morning), that I should therefore refrain from speaking or reading any language except Russian for the next six months and that he himself would take care of all documents required to free myself from the engagements required by the grant which brought me to Moscow. On the following day I started my training under the direction of the best man I ever met. As for the treasure of his advice, the pleasantness of his friendship and my debt of gratitude to him, I will never be able to express all that adequately.

## REFERENCES

Akelaitis, A. J., Risteen, W. A., Herren, R. Y., & Van Wagenen W. P. (1942). Studies on the corpus callosum III. A contribution to the study of dyspraxia following partial and complete section of the corpus callosum. *Archives of Neurology and Psychiatry 47*, 971–1007.

Babinski, M. J. (1914). Contribution à 'étude des troubles mentaux dans l'hémiplégie organique cérébrale (Anosognosie). *Revue Neurologique 27*, 845–848.

Babinski, M. J. (1918). Anosognosie. *Revue Neurologique 31*, 365–367.

Basso, A., Bisiach, E., & Capitani, E. (1977). Decision in ambiguity: Hemispheric dominance or interaction? *Cortex 13*, 96–99.

Basso, A., Bisiach, E., & Luzzatti, C. (1980). Loss of visual imagery: A case study. *Neuropsychologia 18*, 435–442.

Bisiach, E., & Capitani, E. (1976). Cerebral dominance and visual similarity judgments. *Cortex, 12*, 347–355.

Bisiach, E., Capitani, E., & Tansini, E. (1979). Detection from left and right hemifields on single and double simultaneous stimulation. *Perceptual and Motor Skills, 48*, 960.

Bisiach, E., Mini, M., Sterzi, R., & Vallar, G. (1982). Hemispheric lateralization of the decisional stage in choice reaction times to visual unstructured stimuli. *Cortex, 18*, 191–198.

Critchley, M. (1972). Inter-hemispheric partnership and inter-hemispheric rivalry. In M. Critchley, J. L. O'Leary, & B. Jennett (Eds.), *Scientific foundations of neurology*. London: Heinemann, pp. 216–221.

Efron, R. (1963a). The effect of handedness on the perception of simultaneity and temporal order. *Brain, 86*, 261–284.

Efron, R. (1963b). The effect of stimulus intensity on the perception of simultaneity in right- and left-handed subjects. *Brain, 86*, 285–294.

Efron, R. (1974). Dichotic competition of simultaneous tone bursts of different frequency, duration and loudness. Paper presented at the *Symposium on Central Auditory Processing Disorders*, University of Nebraska Medical Center, Omaha, May 23–24.

Efron, R., & Yund, E. W. (1974). Dichotic competition of simultaneous tone bursts of different frequency—I. Dissociation of pitch from lateralization and loudness. *Neuropsychologia, 12*, 249–256.

Henschen, S. E. (1926). On the function of the right hemisphere of the brain in relation to the left in speech, music and calculation. *Brain, 49*, 110–123.

Jackson, J. H. (1874). On the nature of the duality of the brain. Reprinted in J. Taylor (Ed.), *Selected writings of John Hughlings Jackson* (Vol. 2, pp. 129–145). London: Hodder & Stoughton, 1932.

Levy, J., & Trevarthen, C. (1976). Metacontrol of hemispheric function in human split-brain patients. *J. Experimental Psychology: Human Perception and Performance, 2*, 299–312.

Levy, J., Travarthen, C., & Sperry, R. W. (1972). Perception of bilateral chimeric figures following hemispheric deconnexion. *Brain, 95,* 61–78.

Luria, A. R. (1962). *Vyssie Korkovye Funkcii Celoveka i ich Narausenija pri Lokal'nych Porazenijach Mozga,* Izd. Moskovskogo Universiteta.

Milner, B. (1954). Intellectual functions of the temporal lobes. *Psychological Bulletin, 51,* 42–62.

Milner, B. (1958). Psychological defects produced by temporal lobe excision. *The Brain and Human Behavior,* Vol. 34. Proceedings of the Association for Research in Nervous and Mental Disease, Williams & Wilkins Co., Baltimore.

Rizzolatti, G., Umiltá, C., & Berlucchi, G. (1971). Opposite superiorities of the right and left cerebral hemispheres in discriminative reaction time to physiognomic and alphabetical material. *Brain, 94,* 431–444.

Vallar, G., Bisiach, E., Cerizza, M., & Rusconi, M. L. (1988). The role of the left hemisphere in decision-making. *Cortex, 24,* 399–410.

Vallar, C., Bisiach, E., & Sterzi, R. (1984). Hemispheric lateralization of the decisional stage in choice reaction times. A rejoinder to Heister and Schroeder–Heister. *Cortex, 28,* 277–279.

Vygotsky, L. S. (1962). *Thought and language.* Cambridge, MA: MIT Press.

Yund, E. W., & Efron R. (1975). Dichotic competition of simultaneous tone bursts of different frequency—II. Suppression and ear dominance functions. *Neuropsychologia, 13,* 137–150.

Zingerle, H. (1913). Über Störungen der Wahrnehmung des eigenen Koerpers bei organischen Gehirnerkrankungen. *Monatsschrift für Psychiatrie und Neurologie, 34,* 13–36.

# 8

# The Fate of Some Neuropsychological Concepts: An Historical Inquiry

*Arthur Benton*

*Professor emeritus, psychology and neurology,*
*University of Iowa*

In some essays that appeared in the 1950s and early 1960s the historian, Edwin Boring (1961, 1963), discussed the influence of the *Zeitgeist* on the progress of science in general and on the development of psychology in particular. The term Zeitgeist, which translates into English literally as the "spirit of the time" and more broadly as the "climate of opinion," is the label for the prevailing body of knowledge, beliefs, attitudes, and criteria of judgment that determines what observations and theories are evaluated as correct or incorrect, valid or invalid, credible or incredible, important or not important—in a word, what needs to be taken seriously and what need not be taken seriously.

Boring (1961, p. 330) pointed out that the influence of the Zeitgeist on scientific progress is "sometimes helpful and sometimes hindering." It is helpful (indeed necessary) in that it provides the background of knowledge and experience that is required for sound judgment as new alleged facts and novel conceptions are advanced. Without it, all facts and conceptions, no matter how dubious or far-fetched, would have to receive equal consideration and this could result in a state of confusion resembling, let us say, the state of affairs in modern art or contemporary music. Moreover, the Zeitgeist is not immutable. It does change in the face of substantial empirical evidence and convincing argument that one or another aspect of it can no longer be maintained.

But the Zeitgeist can also be a hindrance to the progress of a science or discipline because by its very nature it offers at least initial resistance to facts or conceptions that challenge it and that later prove to be valid. The history of science is full of examples of delayed recognition of the significance of discoveries and conceptions that were not congruent with the system of theories and beliefs prevailing at the time.

This chapter is a small excursion into the history of neuropsychology that deals with some early studies, each of which was in its way highly original in nature. Decades after their publication, these studies were seen to have provided information of considerable significance. However, at the time when they appeared, the observations contained in them were either ignored by the authors' contemporaries or at best judged to be of little importance. The studies will be described and the possible reasons why recognition of their significance was so long delayed will be explored.

We will deal with three studies, the first published in the 1840s, the second in the 1850s, the third in the 1860s. The paper by Puchelt (1844) offers the first description of what today is called "astereognosis," that is, inability to identify objects that have been palpated without the aid of vision, this failure in identification occurring within a setting of adequate tactile sensitivity. The second paper, by Panizza (1855), presents the first demonstration of the crucial role of the occipital lobes in vision. The third paper, by Quaglino and Borelli (1867), includes the first description of facial agnosia or prosopagnosia, that is, specific loss of the ability to identify the faces of familiar persons.

## ASTEREOGNOSIS

Consider what was known about somesthesis when Puchelt published his paper on "partial paralysis of sensation" in 1844. Aristotle's designation of touch as one of the five primary senses was universally accepted as was his opinion that it was more complex than the other senses in that it probably represented a combination of different types of sensibility. Impairment in skin sensitivity associated with disease of the nervous system (including brain disease) was fairly commonly noted by physicians in early case reports (i.e., in the 16th and 17th centuries) where a patient might be described as having a "paralysis of touch," a "paralysis of feeling," a "paralysis of motion and feeling," or a "paralysis of motion but not feeling." (In those days and for a long time afterward, the term "paralysis" was applied to sensory processes as well as to movement.) In 1826 Charles Bell definitively established the "muscle sense" as a sixth sense whose effective stimulus was in the muscles rather than in the skin. He described what he called "the nervous circle which connects the voluntary muscles with the brain," in which muscular contraction itself sends information along the sensory nerves to the central nervous system, this information then serving as a guide to direct subsequent movements as well as a basis for judgments about weight, size and shape, hardness and softness.

On the other hand, although Ernst Heinrich Weber's Latin monograph which dealt in part with the sense of touch was published in 1834, his far more widely known *Der Tastsinn und das Gemeingefühl* appeared in 1846, that is, 2 years after Puchelt's paper (cf. Ross & Murray, 1978). Moreover, anatomical descriptions of encapsulated nerve endings in the skin, such as Meissner corpuscles, Ruffini cylinders, and the like, which were regarded as sensory end organs, began to appear only in the 1840s.

This was the background of knowledge against which Puchelt made his observations. Quite clearly he applied the term "partial paralysis" to two different phenomena. The first was what today is known as dissociated loss of sensitivity. Thus he described one patient who showed a specific loss of temperature sensitivity with preservation of sensitivity to touch as well as of the ability to identify objects by palpation without the aid of vision. Other patients with loss of pressure sensitivity and the loss of the ability to identify objects by palpation had preserved sensitivity to both pain and temperature. The second phenomenon noted by Puchelt was astereognosis or tactile agnosia. Thus one patient showed preserved sensitivity for all the tactile modalities (pressure, pain, and temperature) but was unable to identify palpated objects. Yet she could report accurately whether the object was warm or cold, large or small, and soft or hard.

Discussing the basis for these "partial paralyses," Puchelt concluded that "the cause of these partial paralyses of sensation is to be found neither in the lamed limb nor in the conducting pathways nor in the spinal cord but in the brain." This is as far as he was able to go, given the knowledge of neuroanatomy of the time.

It can be assumed, I think, that Puchelt's contemporaries were aware of his paper. But evidently they found his observations to be of little interest, because the next investigation of disturbances in tactile object perception did not appear until 39 years later in 1883. This was reported in a monograph by H. Hoffman in Strassburg, who coined the term "stereognosis," and who fully confirmed Puchelt's contention that failure in tactile object identification could occur within a setting of intact basic tactile sensitivity. However, Hoffmann made the further point that stereognostic capacity was related to the muscle sense, that is, kinesthesis or proprioception. Patients with defective proprioceptive sensitivity could identify objects but they did experience difficulty, often taking a long time before they succeeded in the task.

After Hoffmann paved the way, a number of further contributions appeared in the 1880s and 1890s, perhaps the most important of which was made by Wernicke in 1895, when he demonstrated astereognosis with intact tactile sensitivity in two patients with focal cortical lesions and implicated the postcentral gyrus as the locus of the underlying neural mechanism.

Why did it take 40 years before Puchelt's observations were looked into? A reasonable (perhaps oversimplified) explanation is that the time was not ripe. As we saw, sensory end-organs in the skin, muscles, and joints for the reception of somesthetic stimulation had just begun to be described. With respect to the central nervous system, all that Puchelt could say is that he believed that his "partial paralyses" were due to brain disease, possibly because he had not observed them in patients with lesions of the spinal cord or peripheral nerves. But, in the 1870s, physiologists such as Munk and Ferrier parcellated the cerebral cortex into sensory territories or spheres. The visual sphere was in the occipital lobes according to Munk; in the region of the angular gyrus, according to Ferrier. The auditory sphere was in the temporal lobes and the somesthetic sphere was in the parietal lobes. Now disturbances in tactile recognition began to acquire some degree of specific neurological significance and, as we saw, clinical studies on the topic in fact began in the 1880s.

A subsequent development in neuropsychological thought of at least equal importance retrospectively made Puchelt's observations of interest. What he had described was later to be called a form of "agnosia," that is, a failure in recognition or identification that cannot be entirely ascribed to basic sensory deficit. Of necessity, Puchelt and his contemporaries were not aware of this concept which was formulated only in the 1870s. It was then that the Berlin physiologist, Hermann Munk, described the consequences of partial ablation of the occipital lobes in dogs. Complete ablation of the lobes rendered the dog blind. But partial ablations led to a peculiar condition that Munk labeled "mind-blindness." The dog obviously was not blind in the ordinary meaning of the term. It could ambulate freely and would avoid obstacles placed in his path by walking around them or climbing over them or even crawling under them. But it behaved in an oddly stupid fashion. It showed no sign that it recognized his master. It did not react to threatening gestures or even to a flame until the flame was brought close enough so that it felt its warmth. The sight of food did not arouse it but, if the food were brought close enough so that it could smell it, then the animal would snap at it, as any normal dog would.

Munk explained the dog's disability by postulating that the animal had lost its store of visual memory images; in other words, that it had been reduced to the status of a puppy with no background of visual experience, and hence, had to learn the meaning of ongoing visual experience all over again. The fact that typically the "mind-blind" dog recovered from its disability over time was congruent with Munk's hypothesis of relearning. (But it was also congruent with the position of skeptics who believed that "mind-blindness" was nothing more than a partial impairment of vision from which the dog eventually recovered.)

However, in the 1880s ophthalmologists encountered and described patients who showed failure to recognize objects and persons despite seemingly adequate vision and they did not hesitate to classify these patients as cases of mind-blindness or visual agnosia (cf. Lissauer, 1890; Wilbrand, 1887). Now astereognosis could be conceived as the tactile analogue of mind-blindness and cases such as those of Wernicke were designated as instances of tactile agnosia. Retrospectively, some of Puchelt's cases fell into this category.

In summary, the possible significance of Puchelt's observation was not grasped by his contemporaries, who probably regarded it as a not very exciting medical curiosity. This was not because they were particularly obtuse or unimaginative. It was rather a consequence of their ignorance of the neural underpinnings of tactile sensation and perception and the circumstance that the concept of agnosia had not yet been introduced into neuropsychological thought. Thus, they were not prepared to incorporate Puchelt's observations into the structure of their knowledge and understanding. Puchelt himself seems to have had only a vague awareness that there was something special about his "partial paralyses."

## VISION AND THE OCCIPITAL LOBES

In 1854, the French anatomist and anthropologist Pierre Gratiolet, through careful dissection of fixed specimens, was able to demonstrate for the first time the optic radiations arising from the lateral geniculate nuclei and fanning out to the cortex of the occipital and posterior parietal lobes. In the following year (1855), Bartolomeo Panizza, who was professor of anatomy at Pavia, published a paper in which he confirmed the existence of the optic radiations. But Panizza went beyond this purely anatomical determination to investigate the functional significance of this extension from the thalamic level to the cortex. He did this experimentally by destroying the occipital lobes in dogs and finding that bilateral ablation resulted in complete blindness, as Munk was to report 20 years later. Panizza also reported that ablation of a single occipital lobe resulted in blindness in the opposite eye. (He was wrong, of course, and Munk later identified the deficit correctly as visual loss in the opposite half-field or a contralateral hemianopia.) Panizza also described visual loss in some patients with occipital lobe disease and these were the first clinical observations of this type.

It is clear enough that the thrust of Panizza's report was to establish the crucial role of the occipital lobes in the mediation of vision. However, his work was completely ignored. It was only after Munk's definitive studies in the late 1870s that a compatriot, Augusto Tamburini (1880), a neuropsychiatrist, called attention to Panizza's work.

There may have been some incidental reasons why Panizza's observations were ignored. First, it does not seem that he was particularly well known internationally. Secondly, he published in Italian, which may have been a handicap. Finally, his papers were published not in a major journal but in a provincial periodical, which perhaps was distributed as a matter of course to the major libraries of Europe but which probably did not find its way to the desks of the leading researchers of the period.

But there was a more basic reason why Panizza's contentions could have been ignored. The dominant neurological theory of vision at the time stipulated that the cerebral center for vision was at the level of the thalamus—in the lateral geniculate nuclei and in the thalamus itself (hence, the old term, the "optic thalamus"). Panizza's work was, of course, not congruent with this doctrine. Thus, if there were physiologists or physicians who did read his paper, they could well have dismissed it as being outlandish, that is, making no sense. In short, under the influence of prevailing dogma, they were not prepared to consider the implications of Panizza's findings.

## PROSOPAGNOSIA

The paper by Antonio Quaglino (who was professor of ophthalmology at Pavia) and Giambattista Borelli (who was a practicing ophthalmologist in Turin) had to do with the appearance of a triad of symptoms—defective facial recognition, loss of color vision, and impairment in spatial orientation—in a 54-year-old man who had suffered a right-hemisphere stroke. Evidently Quaglino and Borelli considered that this was a very instructive case, since their paper is actually one of a series of three dealing with the same patient. Their primary interest was in the issue of cerebral localization. Here, while they acknowledged that Gall had been in error in a number of respects, such as postulating the existence of cortical centers for complex traits such as "cautiousness," "self-esteem," and "reverence," and assuming that the conformation of the skull coincided with the conformation of the surface of the brain, nevertheless they believed that his fundamental thesis that different parts of the brain mediated different simpler functions was correct. They believed that their case supported the thesis.

Immediately after his stroke this patient had a left hemiplegia and also an apparently complete loss of vision. The hemiplegia disappeared within a month and his vision gradually returned over the course of a few months. When he was first seen by Quaglino and Borelli a year after the stroke, he felt quite well and had no motor disability. His visual acuity was excellent by his own testimony and by examination. He read without difficulty. However, although central vision was intact, he did have a left visual field defect. His main complaints were those that have been mentioned:

First, a loss of color vision. All objects and faces looked pale, white, or gray, and devoid of color. Examination disclosed that he was unable to distinguish colors. In short, the patient showed a bilateral central achromatopsia. (Incidentally, "achromatopsia" is the term used by Quaglino and Borelli.)

Second, some loss of spatial orientation. He retained the concept of orientation and would confidently state that the window of his room faced east. Nevertheless he could no longer indicate the directional arrangements in his apartment, for example, where the east wall stood in relation to the south wall and so on.

Third, there was impairment in facial recognition:

> The patient no longer recognizes the faces of persons, even those familiar to him at home and he has lost his orientation. During the first year he still retained the memory of figures of certain people and he could recall them by listening to their voices. However, for some time now he cannot remember them at all. He sees the figure as in a photograph, but less clearly. . . .

In addition, the authors mention that the patient had forgotten the facades of houses. Whether or not this meant that he no longer could identify specific houses is not clear. In any case, it was this disability that was responsible for the phrase "loss of memory of the configuration of objects" in the title of their paper.

The authors concluded that Gall's postulation of a specific cerebral center for color perception was correct. They diagnosed their case as one of cerebral hemorrhage involving the right hemisphere primarily but possibly extending to parts of the left side of the brain.

Each of the defects noted by Quaglino and Borelli were taken up about 20 years later, in the 1880s, and it was only then that reference was made to their 1867 papers. A case of hemiachromatopsia, or loss of color vision in one visual half-field (in this instance, the right visual field), was described by the French ophthalmologist, Verrey, in 1888. In this case postmortem examination disclosed a lesion in the left occipital lobe. A patient with bilateral or complete achromatopsia, comparable with Quaglino and Borelli's case, was described by MacKay and Dunlop in 1899. In this instance, postmortem study showed infarcts in both occipital lobes. Thus, these case reports provided a more precise determination of the site of the lesions producing loss of color vision than Quaglino and Borelli were able to make.

In 1876 Hughlings Jackson described a patient with fairly serious disturbances in spatial orientation, as reflected in her losing her way as she walked the familiar route from her home to the place where she did her shopping. Sometimes she even became lost in her own house. Almost certainly Jackson was not aware of the Quaglino–Borelli papers. However, in the 1880s and 1890s the topic of loss of spatial orientation within a setting of intact visual acuity and object recognition in patients with brain disease became a topic of considerable interest to ophthalmologists and neurologists and it was then that the papers of Quaglino and Borelli were cited. The site of the lesions producing disorientation were often identified by postmortem study in these later studies and they proved to be in the occipital-posterior parietal territory of the brain.

With respect to the facial agnosia or prosopagnosia that Quaglino and Borelli had noted in their patient, this also was observed some years later. Indeed Jackson's patient who had marked visual disorientation also must have had significant facial agnosia since on occasion she would mistake her niece for her daughter. Jackson considered the defect to be one aspect of a more widespread disability that he called "imperception" and that included visual disorientation and impairment in visual recognition.

As has been mentioned, in the 1880s ophthalmologists described patients with visual object agnosia that was roughly comparable with Munk's mind-blindness. Typically these patients also had lost the ability to identify persons by inspection of their faces. But little was made of the deficit since it seemed reasonable to expect that a patient who could not recognize a familiar object would also have difficulty in identifying a specific face.

The Quaglino–Borelli papers were not completely ignored—at least, not in the sense that Panizza's report was ignored. They were cited as early as 1881 in a book on the brain and vision by a German ophthalmologist, Mauthner. In any case, their description of their patient's facial agnosia was rather sparse and, without postmortem examination, they could only guess at the locus and extent of the underlying pathology.

Yet, despite the limitations of their report, Quaglino and Borelli did think of their patient's failure as representing a specific disability in the identification of individual objects—in contrast to the more general concept of visual object agnosia that was developed a decade later. And this their contemporaries seemed to have missed. Moreover, they related the disability (as well as the accompanying achromatopsia) not to some ocular condition (as they might well have, since they were ophthalmologists) but to brain disease.

It was only in the 1930s that facial agnosia was conceived to be a more or less specific disorder of visual recognition. Two complementary reasons why it was not singled out for special study earlier suggest themselves. On the one hand, facial agnosia was typically observed within a setting of other disabilities—with color blindness and some degree of spatial disorientation, as in the Quaglino–Borelli case, and with pronounced spatial disorientation, as in Jackson's patient. Thus it seemed to be only a number of expressions of a pervasive visual disability, "imperception," as Jackson called it. On the other hand, when facial agnosia presented in more or less isolated form without other obvious signs of cerebral dysfunction, it must have appeared to be such a bizarre complaint that many physicians would have been inclined to regard it as an hysterical phenomenon.

## CONCLUDING COMMENT

This has been the story of three neuropsychological studies whose significance was grasped only decades after they were reported. Apart from incidental factors, the major reason for their neglect would seem to be that the corpus of knowledge and climate of belief at the time of their appearance hindered appreciation of their potential importance.

Can a moral be drawn from this story? One cannot be sure. Of necessity all of us are more or less prisoners of the Zeitgeist. But perhaps we can resolve to be rather "less" than "more" by consciously guarding against the tendency to reject out of hand data and concepts that are not in accord with established doctrine and by giving them a critical but fair reception.

## REFERENCES

Bell, C. (1826). On the nervous circle which connects the voluntary muscles with the brain. *Philosophical Transactions, 116*(Pt. 2), 163–173.

Boring, E. G. (1961). *Psychologist at large: An autobiography and selected essays.* New York: Basic Books.

Boring, E. G. (1963). *History, psychology, and science: Selected papers.* New York: Wiley.

Gratiolet, P. (1854). Note sur les expansions des racines cérébrales du nerf optique et sur leur terminaison dans une région determinée de l'écorce des hémisphères. *Comptes Rendus de l'Academie des Sciences, 29,* 274–278, Paris.

Hoffmann, H. (1883). *Stereognostische Versuche.* Dissertation, Strassburg.

Jackson, J. H. (1876). Case of large cerebral tumour without optic neuritis and with left hemiplegia and imperception. *Royal London Hospital Reports, 8,* 434–444.

Lissauer, H. (1890). Ein Fall von Seelenblindheit nebst einem Beitrag zur Theorie derselben, *Archiv für Psychiatrie und Nervenkrankheiten, 21,* 222–270.

MacKay, G., & Dunlop, J. C. (1899). The cerebral lesions in a case of complete acquired colour-blindness. *Scottish Medical Journal, 5,* 503–512.

Mauthner, L. (1881). *Gehirn und Auge.* Wiesbaden, Germany: Bergmann.

Munk, H. (1878). Weitere Mittheilungen zur Physiologie der Grosshirnrinde. *Archiv für Anatomie und Physiologie, 2,* 162–178.

Panizza, B. (1855). Osservazioni sul nervo ottico. *Giornale, Istituto Lombardo di Scienze e Lettere, 7,* 237–252.

Puchelt, B. (1844). Über partielle Empfindungslähmung. *Medicinische Annalen, 10,* 485–495.

Quaglino, A., & Borelli, G. (1867). Emiplegia sinistra con amaurosi; guaragione; perdita totale della percezione dei colori e della memoria della configurazione degli oggetti. *Giornale d'Oftalmologia Italiano, 10,* 106–117.

Ross, H. E., & Murray, D. J. (1978). *E. H. Weber: The sense of touch.* London: Academic Press.

Tamburini, A. (1880). Rivendicazione al Panizza della scoperta del centro visivo corticale. *Revista Sperimentale di Freniatria e Medicina Legale, 6,* 152–154.

Verrey, D. (1888). Hémiachromatopsie droite absolue. *Archives d'Ophthalmologie, 8,* 289–300.

Wernicke, C. (1895). Zwei Fällen von Rindenläsion. *Arbeiten aus der Psychiatrischen Klinik Breslau, 2,* 33–53.

Wilbrand, H. (1887). Die Seelenblindheit als Herderscheinung und ihre Beziehungen zur homonymen Hemianopsie. Wiesbaden, Germany: Bergmann.

# 9

# Luria and "Romantic Science"

*Oliver Sacks*

*Albert Einstein College of Medicine*

In the autobiography that Luria wrote in the last years of his life, in which he put a whole lifetime, and a lifetime's work, in perspective, the final chapter is entitled "Romantic Science." It is crucial to bring out at the onset that Luria's preoccupation with "romantic science" was not superficial, or a late development, an idiosyncrasy, or extraneous to the vision of science that animated him from his earliest work to his last. Luria wrote his autobiography, *The Making of Mind,* in 1977, but his first book—a critique of psychoanalysis—was written in 1922. A lifetime of expansion and evolution separates these two works, but the vision of science—a complex and (it might seem) contradictory vision—remained constant, and at the heart of his work, throughout these 55 years. He himself tells us this in his final chapter on "Romantic Science," where, after discussing the differences (and even the "dilemmas") between the pursuit of "classical" and "romantic" science, he writes:

> I have long puzzled over which of the two approaches, in principle, leads to a better understanding of living reality. This dilemma is a reformulation of the conflict between nomothetic and ideographic approaches to psychology that concerned me during the first years of my intellectual life. (1979, p. 175)

And yet, despite Luria's own words in the matter—which he expressed not only in his published works, but in innumerable letters to colleagues and friends—there has been a persistent tendency to regard Luria's "romantic" works and preoccupations as light and superficial, scarcely deserving serious scientific and intellectual attention, or even to ignore them altogether. This essay, then, is written to redress this imbalance, to remind readers of the extraordinary complexity and richness of Luria's work and world-view, and of how vital the "romantic" was in his lifetime in science.

Although Luria's preoccupation with Romantic Science was lifelong, it was only relatively late in life that he felt able to express this fully and openly, in his two, late, "neurological novels" (*The Mind of a Mnemonist*, 1968; *The Man with a Shattered World*, 1972) and his posthumously published autobiography, *The Making of Mind*, written in 1977 (he wrote an earlier, more technical intellectual history of Vygotsky and himself, in 1973, which he entitled "The Long Road of a Soviet Psychologist").[1] The most extensive discussion of Romantic Science is to be found in *The Making of Mind*.

The terms "classical" and "romantic," with regard to certain basic attitudes or orientations to sciences, and, equally, the character or temperament of scientists, did not originate with Luria, but with the German scholar Max Verworn, but Luria adopted his terms, and adapted them to his own ends. In Luria's formulation:

Classical scholars are those who look upon events in terms of their constituent parts. Step by step they single out important units and elements until they can formulate abstract, general laws. These laws are then seen as the governing agents of the phenomena in the field under study. One outcome of this approach is the reduction of living reality with all its richness of detail to abstract schemas. The properties of the living whole are lost, which provoked Goethe to pen, "Gray is every theory, but ever green is the tree of life."

Romantic scholars' traits, attitudes, and strategies are just the opposite. They do not follow the path of reductionism, which is the leading philosophy of the classical group. Romantics in science want neither to split living reality into its elementary components, nor to represent the wealth of life's concrete events in abstract models that lose the properties of the phenomena themselves. It is of the utmost importance

---

[1]If we ask why Luria was so tardy in coming out with his Romantic Science, the answer must largely be sought in the repressive atmosphere of Soviet science during his earlier days. Luria tells a vivid and poignant story of how, as a very young man, he presented a copy of his first book, *The Nature of Human Conflicts* to Pavlov, and how the next day the old man, with blazing eyes, tore the book in half, flung the halves at his feet, and roared, "You call this science! Science proceeds from elementary parts and builds up, here you are describing behavior as a whole!" (personal communication, letter of July 19, 1973). Soon after this, Luria (like many others) was officially condemned as "unpavlovian" and "un-Soviet," and forbidden to teach, research, or publish freely—hence the long silence between his first two books (*The Nature of Human Conflicts* was published in Russian in 1928/1929, but *Restoration of Function after Brain Injury* not until after World War II). The research for *Shattered World* dates back to the early 1940s (and of *Mnemonist* even before), but the atmosphere had not thawed enough to allow their publication until 30 years later. It should be added that Luria's work on cultural differences in thinking, initiated with Vygotsky in the early 1930s, could not be published in the Soviet Union until 45 years later (Vygotsky's own works were proscribed after the mid-1930s, and these, indeed, are only receiving their definitive publication now).

to romantics to preserve the wealth of living reality, and they aspire to a science that retains this richness. (1979, p. 174)

Or, to put it another way, as Luria himself often does, the romantic, the naturalist, is content to describe—but the classical scientist is at pains to explain. Both are necessary, both have their shortcomings:

> (On the one hand) . . . romantic science typically lacks the logic and does not follow the careful, consecutive step-by-step reasoning that is characteristic of classical science, nor does it easily reach firm formulations and universally applicable laws. Sometimes logical step-by-step analysis escapes romantic scholars, and, on occasion, they let artistic preferences and intuitions take over. Frequently their descriptions not only precede explanation, but replace it. (1979, p. 175)

It should be very clear that Luria has no impulse to archaism, to espouse an old-fashioned, 19th-century naturalism of a purely descriptive sort—no one sees more clearly the dangers of a *mere* naturalism like this. And yet Luria's own clinical experience, to which he is absolutely faithful, as well as his reading of the great 19th-century clinicians, provides an overwhelming demonstration of the opposite danger—the danger of reductionism, of an analysis which finally loses the very reality it seeks to analyze. Luria sees such reductionism as the very essence of 20th-century science, at least in medicine, physiology, and psychology.

> Since the beginning of this century there has been enormous technical progress, which has changed the very structure of the scientific enterprise. . . . Reductionism, the effort to reduce complex phenomena to their elementary particles, became the guiding principle of scientific efforts. In psychology it seemed that by reducing psychological events to elementary physiological rules, we could attain the ultimate explanation of human behavior. . . . In this atmosphere, the rich and complex picture of human behavior which had existed in the nineteenth century disappeared. (1979, pp. 175–176)

Luria sees this tendency as largely, though not entirely, due to technology— and to the conceptual and emotional atmosphere of technology; he sees this as leading to a scientific, no less than a human and existential decline.

> The medicine of previous years had been based on the effort to single out important syndromes by describing significant symptoms. . . . With the advent of the new instrumentation, these classical forms of medical procedure were pushed into the background. The physicians of our time, having a battery of auxiliary aids and tests, frequently overlooks clinical reality. . . . Physicians who are great observers and

great thinkers have gradually disappeared. . . . In the previous century, when auxiliary laboratory methods were rare, the art of clinical observation and description reached its height. . . . Now this art of observation and description is nearly lost. (1979, pp. 176–177)

The same points are brought out, again and again, with an absolute passion and conviction, in the letters he wrote—and Luria, after a 12- or 16-hour working day, would spend hours more with an enormous scientific correspondence, writing constantly to colleagues, former pupils, and friends, detailed, passionate letters, in half a dozen different languages.[2] In a letter to me, in response to reading *Awakenings,* he wrote:

I was ever conscious and sure that a good clinical description of cases plays a leading role in medicine, especially in neurology and psychiatry. Unfortunately the ability to describe which was so common to the great neurologists and psychiatrists of the nineteenth century . . . is almost lost now. (letter dated July 25, 1973)

Ever conscious, ever sure—Luria always knew where clinical reality lay, the irreducible richness and complexity of the clinical predicament. He always knew the necessity of the *qualitative* in science, and equally, of the historical, the *biographical* in science—at least if one was to study a living being, a human being.

Frankly said, I myself like very much the type of "biographical" study, such as on Shereshevsky *(Mnemonist)* and Zasetski *(Shattered World)* . . . firstly because it is a kind of "Romantic Science" which I wanted to introduce, partly because I am strongly *against* a formal statistical approach and *for* a qualitative study of personality, *for* every attempt to find *factors* underlying the structure of personality.[3] (Letter of July 19, 1973, italics in original)

[2]Luria sometimes felt able to express himself in his letters with a freedom and force not always "permitted" in his published writings. Freud's letters tell us much about Freud the man, but little we do not already know about Freud the thinker. But Luria, in his letters, reveals aspects and dimensions of thought that are scarcely intimated in his published writings. Indeed, we will not have an adequate idea of Luria *as thinker* unless we have a full edition of his letters—and one can only hope that these will be collected before it is too late.

[3]It is an irony, given Luria's aversion to formal statistical approaches and standardized tests that he is now known to many psychologists (and perhaps, to some, *only* known) for the so-called Luria—Nebraska test, a standardized neuropsychological test battery. This was devised in 1979, after Luria's death, and would (I think) have horrified him, as being against the very principles on which his concepts and clinical practice rested. For although Luria was endlessly resourceful in devising cognitive tests of all sorts, he would only administer these *in the context of the individual,* varying them and improvising them, according to the individual and his history.

In a 1973 essay on Luria[4] I had contrasted his "novelistic" or "romantic" works—*Mnemonist* and *Shattered World*—with what seemed to me the much more "scientific" and systematic expositions of other works of his (such as his monumental *Higher Cortical Functions in Man*), but this elicited a heated rejoinder, replete with the emphatic underlinings he so liked, emphases forced from him by the force of his own convictions: "The *style* of these books is different from the others; the *principle* remains the same."

We must not, Luria is here saying, regard *Higher Cortical Functions* et al. as purely "classical," and *Mnemonist* and *Shattered World* as purely "romantic." Both must be seen as "classical" *and* "romantic"; all his work must be seen as embodying the same principle, and thus as—simultaneously—both.

Luria often said (personal communication) that he needed to write "two sorts" of books, but he always saw these two sorts as identical *in principle*. What then is the principle that unites all his work, and that may be regarded as the center, the Lurian point of view? Luria himself spoke of his groping as a young man, of his attempts to reconcile two conflicting viewpoints—and of the "crisis," not only in himself, but in the scientific community generally, to reconcile, or somehow conjoin, an explanatory, physiological psychology with a descriptive, phenomenological psychology—to reconcile a "classical" and a "romantic" approach to the higher cerebral and psychological functions, to Brain-Mind. "One of the major features that drew me to Vygotsky," he writes, "was his emphasis on the necessity to resolve this crisis. He saw its resolution as the most important goal of psychology in our time."

There are many ways in which we can approach the question of what Luria is, and how best to define his point of view and life-work, but I find myself ineluctably drawn to his earliest interests and enterprises—his writing to Freud, at the age of 19; his founding, with Freud's encouragement, a psychoanalytical society in Kazan; and his first book, written as a youth of 20, an appreciation and critique of psychoanalysis (*Psychoanalysis in Light of the Principal Tendencies in Contemporary Psychology*, Kazan, 1922, in Russian, never translated). As his "romantic" case histories have been seen as an old man's aberration, so Luria's early interest in psychoanalysis has been dismissed as a youthful one. This smacks of intellectual laziness, even arrogance, as a start—dismissing some of a man's enterprises and interests because one cannot see how they fit into the pattern, the whole. Everyone, of course, can have "aberrations," but Occam's razor should make one suspicious of such uneconomical hypotheses, should lead one to search for a unity, a pattern—most especially when dealing with a genius, like Luria, for it is characteristic of genius to contain great contradiction and

---

[4]O. W. Sacks, "The Mind of A. R. Luria," *The Listener*, June 28, 1973.

richness, but at the deepest level to resolve these into an ultimate unity.[5] Moreover, we know that Luria's interest in psychoanalysis continued; he wrote the article on psychoanalysis for *The Great Soviet Encyclopedia* in 1940, and showed himself open to psychoanalytical issues and interpretations to the end of his life.[6]

Let us remind ourselves, at this point, of the complex perspective, the multiple perspective, of the Freudian orientation. Leonard Shengold's words, in a recent critique of Freud's drive *(Triebe)* theory, may be quoted here:

> There are currently many psychological theorists who feel that they can and should disregard them ("drives")—disregard not only the drives but any connection between the psychological and the biological. They make a part of our nature into the whole. Man is presented as purely psychological, or social, or as a computer, or as linguistic construct. (There are also those who want to reduce everything to the biological.) (Shengold, 1988, p. 2)

It is suggested by Lionel Trilling (Shengold, 1988) that "the interaction of biology and culture in the fate of man is not a matter which we have begun to understand," and that Freud's emphasis on biology is "actually a liberating idea. It proposes to us that culture is not all-powerful . . . that there is a residue of human quality beyond the reach of cultural control." It might be said, in a complementary way, that Luria's emphasis on culture is also a liberating idea,

---

[5]This is movingly conveyed by Michael Cole, in the epilogue which he appends to Luria's autobiography. At first, Cole acknowledges, he could not see Luria's work—or life—as a whole, but could only see a multitude of seemingly unrelated approaches, styles, and stages:

> What did the cross-cultural work have to do with his work in the Institute of Neurosurgery? Why was he no longer doing conditioning experiments? Why, in his book about S. V. Shereshevsky, the man with an unusual memory, did he spend so much time discussing his personality when his memory was at issue?

Only later, as he came to know Luria as a person, as he immersed himself in Luria's writings and work, and in all the events and books which had influenced him through a lifetime, did a sense of some ultimate unity emerge:

> (Only then did) the otherwise disjointed, zigzag course of Alexandr Romanovich's career begin to make sense. His interest in psychoanalysis no longer appeared a curious anomaly in an otherwise single-minded career. His strong attraction to Vygotsky, his cross-cultural work in Central Asia, the Pavlovian style of his writings in the 1940s and early 1950s, and his apparent shifts of topic at frequent intervals, all took on the quality of an intricate piece of music with a few central motifs and a variety of secondary themes. (1979, pp. 195–198)

[6]Thus in 1976, when I sent him a tape of a patient with severe Tourette's Syndrome, who was prone to sudden tic-like ejaculations of *Verboten!*, uttered in his father's voice, whenever he had "forbidden" impulses of one sort and another, Luria was fascinated, and spoke about "the structuralization of the super-ego," and the "introjection of the father's voice as tic" (letter dated January 29, 1976).

and proposes to us that "biology" is not all-powerful, that man's nature is not fatefully determined by the neurophysiology, the biology, he is born with, but that this itself may be richly modified by his life experiences, by his culture. Luria, indeed, goes much further, and shows from the start an intense sense of the role of the historical, the cultural, the interactive, not merely in modifying, but in actually making higher nervous functions *possible*. Thus the development of language—one of the first subjects studied by the young Luria[7]—was never seen by him as an automatic development of "language areas" in the brain, but as resulting from the interaction of mother and child, from the negotiation of meanings between mother and child, as being in the mode of interaction or "betweenness," and *this* as a prerequisite for, and needing to be structuralized in, the developing neurolinguistic systems of the brain.[8]

Luria's first admiration for Freud was tempered by the thought that Freud was *"too* biological"—but at this time, of course, the "late" Freud had not yet appeared. The young Luria had to separate himself from the dogmatic, physiological "psychologizing" of his time, in particular that of Bechterev and Pavlov, who did not allow the subjective in psychology—did not allow the *psyche* in psychology—and insisted on an objective, reflexological viewpoint.

This, then, was the crisis that faced the young Luria, the crisis that faced every aspiring psychologist of his generation: that the clinical naturalism, the purely descriptive psychology, of the 19th century had collapsed, lacking as it did sufficient conceptual or scientific foundation; and that there had come in its place a reductive new Scientism, a physiological-reflexological-behavioral psychology, which at best could only explain the most automatic of animal reactions, and denied the complexity, the subjectivity, of human nature entirely. There was, in short, no scientific psychology—only the "old" psychology which lacked science, and the "new" psychology which denied the psyche. There existed no science of human nature—nor, it seemed, any possibility of such a science developing. Into this bizarre, forbidding, empty intellectual space, Freud appeared, with his projects, his aspirations, for a scientific psychology.[9] To

[7]See, for instance, A. R. Luria and F. I. Yudovich, *Speech and the Development of Mental Processes in the Child.* London: Staples Press, 1958. Though this book was only published in the late 1950s, the work it describes was done 30 years earlier, when he was working with Vygotsky. Indeed, it was the first "clinical" application of Vygotsky's point of view (as epitomized in Vygotsky's long-suppressed *Thought and Language,* 1962).

[8]Being in the mode of "betweenness" or interaction, language entered the realm of *play*—and this, for Luria, as for Vygotsky, defined the realm of spontaneity or freedom. Strikingly familiar formulations were reached by D. W. Winnicott, the psychoanalyst, who also spoke of the "betweenness" of child and parent, spoke of "transitional" objects and phenomena, of all play and culture as arising in this zone, and of play as the release from instinctual bondage.

[9]Freud's very first such project, his "Project for a Scientific Psychology," was written in 1895, though he turned against it himself almost immediately, as being too exclusively biological (and it was only published, posthumously, in 1950).

Luria, and many other hungry, intellectually starved and disoriented psychologists of his generation, Freud seemed to offer a resolution, a redemption—and even if his actual theories or doctrines were offensive or unintelligible, he offered an orientation, a vision of science, which was liberating, enthralling, because it seemed to promise (if only by analogy, or in principle) the sort of resolution Vygotsky and Luria dreamed of. Whatever objections Luria had to the "biologism" of Freud were minor compared with the immense liberation he afforded: the allowing of the subjective, the conscious, the "mental," as valid, and valid subjects for enquiry, the legitimation of the subjective, in all its richness, as a proper subject for science.

Here, it seems to me, is the key to Luria's early enthusiasm for psychoanalysis, for Freud; here, too, the permanent *heuristic* effect of Freud on his thought, whatever reservations and differences were later to appear. Freud offered a principle—the general principle Luria needed, the only tenable principle for a scientific, human psychology. And this principle was, in essence, an orientation which faced two ways: one which looked down into the biological depths of human nature, but equally and simultaneously up into the events and interactions of social life, a science that looked equally into nature and culture.

And yet the two faces, the two directions, did not develop simultaneously in Luria. There is, indeed, a fascinating contrast here to Freud. Freud started as a biologist, a neurologist, and only later moved up to mental life, to the psyche; whereas Luria started as a cultural relativist and a psychologist with a predominantly social developmental orientation, and only later moved down into neurophysiology and biology. More than half of *The Making of Mind* deals with the early years, the years with Vygotsky, prior to 1935, the years when Luria, with Vygotsky, was studying development—the development of mind, in children, in defectives, in primitive cultures. In this first period, he accused Freud of "biologism," of attaching undue emphasis to purely biological factors in development; but it might equally, or with more truth, be said that Luria himself, at this time, had insufficient "biologism," was insufficiently aware of the role of physiology and biology, insufficiently aware of *the body* in mind. It is a measure of Luria's great courage and clear-sightedness that, seeing this clearly, by the 1930s, he decided that he needed to ground himself in physiology and biology, and although already a professor of psychology, he entered medical school, and became a student again. (Vygotsky, his friend and mentor, did exactly the same, but Vygotsky, tragically, was to die shortly after.) Luria's joy in these (to him) new neurological studies, his sense of being grounded now in the organic (and his sense of adventure), are vividly remembered in his autobiography, where he speaks of these years as "the most fruitful of my life." The two halves of neuropsychology—the "neural" and the "psychic"—started to come together for Luria at this time, above all with his return, in a clinical mode now, to the enigmas of language and, especially, its breakdown in aphasia.

My interest in linguistic phenomena grew naturally out of my early research using the combined motor method and Vygotsky's theory, which emphasized language as a key tool, unique to human beings, for mediating their interactions with the world. But a serious study of language as a highly organized system of human behavior began in earnest only after I had begun work on the problem of the neuropsychology of sensory and semantic aphasia. . . . I found it necessary to continue to study the psychology of language at the same time that I searched for its neurological bases. And just as advances in neurology and neurophysiology were instrumental to our study of brain mechanisms, advances in the study of linguistics were crucial to advancing our understanding of those phenomena of speech which brain pathology was interrupting; *the two enterprises are inextricably bound together.* (1979, pp. 165–169)

It was only when Luria came to grasp the biological aspects firmly—he liked to speak here of the "neurodynamics" of nervous activity, as analogous to the "psychodynamics" of which Freud was speaking—that he was able to achieve the twofold unity which he had so long needed and sought. It was only at this juncture that the "double science" of neuropsychology came into being, as an enterprise analogous to psychoanalysis—neuropsychology dealing with the higher cortical functions and cognitive activities in humans; and psychoanalysis with the "drives" and ego functions; both were rooted, equally, in the biological and the cultural, the interaction of nature and nurture. And it was only at this juncture, finally, that Luria began to see his way to resolving the "crisis" that had haunted him for years: how to reconcile the objective and the subjective, the physiological and the phenomenological, the classical and the romantic, the nomothetic and the idiographic. To see his way to a *conjunction* of the two—that "impossible conjunction" (as the philosopher David Hume once put it) between the modes of anatomy and art. And the key to this was the perception of the individual as a *being,* a living being, containing (but transcending) organic functions and drives, a being rooted in the depths of biology, but historically, culturally, biographically unique. How was one to present such a being, to achieve the "impossible conjunction" of anatomy and art? By creating, if it were possible, a *biological biography,* in which all the determinants of human development and personality would be exhibited as coexistent, coacting, and interacting with one another, in continuous interplay, to produce the final becoming or being. A case history, if you will, but much more than a case history—for a case history merely exhibits a syndrome and its development. What Luria started to envisage was a total portrait, an anatomizing portrait, of the afflicted individual. Here again, it was Freud's example that inspired Luria's movement to a new form, a more-than-classical "romantic" science, to the great portraits (which were equally anatomies or studies) of *Mnemonist* and *Shattered World.* Freud's own masterpieces of anatomizing biography had set the stage:

They provided a concrete model, as psychoanalysis, earlier, had provided the theoretical model.

Luria saw clearly, as Freud did, the shortcomings of a purely descriptive ("romantic") naturalism, and, equally, of a reductive ("classical") science. Both were led, therefore, to a new form of observation, which could combine the virtues and avoid the shortcomings of both. To return, then, to Luria's formulation of this:

> Truly scientific observation is not merely pure description of separate facts. Its main goal is to view an event from as many perspectives as possible. The eye of science does not probe "a thing," an event isolated from other events or things. Its real object is to see and understand the way a thing or event relates to other things or events. . . . Truly scientific observation, further, has nothing in common with the reductionism of the classicist . . . (rather) it seeks out the most important traits or primary basic factors that have immediate consequences, and then seeks the secondary or "systemic" consequences of these basic underlying factors. *Only after these basic factors and their consequences have been identified can the entire picture become clear.* The object of observation is thus to ascertain a network of important relations. When done properly, observation accomplishes the classical aim of explaining facts, while not losing sight of the romantic aim of preserving the manifold richness of the subject. (1979, pp. 177–178)

And it is *this* that Luria means when he speaks of Romantic Science—not the unbridgeable gulf between naturalism and reductionism (which is the irresoluble conflict aroused by Max Verworn's concepts of "romantic" and "classical")—this is how he resolves the crisis. And it must be emphasized that this entails a redefining of both "romance" and "science," in a way that allows them to be complementary, to be conjoined together.

There can be no resolution, no conjunction, between the concepts of "whole" and "parts" unless both concepts are radically related and redefined. "Totality," "allness," "completeness," "wholeness," all of these are words which, at different times, Luria uses. Words such as "global" or "holistic" are carefully avoided, because they deny the notion of differentiation. It is only when everything (significant) is shown in relation to everything else (significant) that a complete, but also analytical, picture of reality can be obtained. This, of course, can never be wholly achieved—but it is the aspiration of Romantic Science—and perhaps of all science.

> The more we single out important relations during our description, the closer we come to the essence of the object, to an understanding of its qualities and the rules of its existence. And the more we preserve the whole wealth of its qualities, the closer we come to the inner laws that determine its existence. . . . It was this perspective which led Karl Marx to describe the process of scientific description with the strange-sounding expression, "ascending to the concrete." (1979, pp. 177–178)

Now, at last, we are getting to the homestretch, toward the destination of "the long road" of which Luria often speaks, and which he himself had to traverse from the beginning to the end. Observation starts with the concrete; but it is precisely this which we then tend to lose, as soon as we analyze, or dissect, or "scientize" it. What is needed is a third stage—a stage of synthesis—in which the concrete and the analytic are truly fused. In this way the concrete is recovered, re-apprehended—not just as a datum, a thing-in-itself—but in relation to everything else: an exemplar of, a key to, an entire conceptual universe.[10] This long road, this threefold process, is discussed by William James in a famous memoir on his teacher Agassiz. Agassiz came to Harvard, in the middle of the last century, with a genius for description, a passion for the concrete; but by the end of the century, as James saw it, both he and his naturalism had become outmoded, were replaced—but this (so it seemed to James) led to an aridity and an impoverishment, a reductionism which formed a hazard in itself:

> The truth of things is after all their living fullness, and some day, from a more commanding point of view than was possible to anyone in Agassiz' generation, our descendants, enriched with the spoils of all our analytic investigations, will get round to that higher and simpler way of looking at nature. (James, 1911, p. 15)

I once quoted this passage, in our correspondence, to Luria, and he liked it, was moved by it, and said he agreed with it, provided, he cautioned, that "higher and simpler" was not taken to connote anything "beyond" or "transcendent," but only the total principles of a man's living, his "plight," his being-in-the-world.

"Ascending to the concrete" was Luria's final aim: ascending to the concrete *is* Romantic Science. And if one's subject is a human life (not atoms or stars) then it is not just "life," in some general theoretical sense, but *a life*—the living and structure of an actual human life—that must become the subject of the fullest scientific observation. The depiction, the scientific depiction, of an actual human life, such as Luria attempts in *Mnemonist* and *Shattered World*—becomes, therefore, the apex of his aspiration and achievement; the "ascent to the concrete" to which his entire lifetime of scientific work ascends and tends.

As a very young man, Luria tells us, he loved Walter Pater, especially his book *Imaginary Portraits,* and the idea of a portrait, not an imaginary but a real one, was to haunt him throughout his life. But to make it real, to give it its fullest

---

[10]One might exemplify these three stages in Darwin's work: his early work on barnacles is purely descriptive. There is, as yet, no central, theorizing core; this has yet to develop, and only appears, years later, in the *Origin*. But the most magical of Darwin's books is the book that came after this—on the *Fertilization of Orchids*. It is here, above all, that we see the re-apprehension of the concrete, in relation now to a vast conceptual whole. Darwin, manifestly, was in love with orchids—the lyrical is very evident in this book; but they are shown, and live for him, not just as fixed, static objects, but as wonderful, resourceful exemplars of evolution. Thus the concrete is recovered, transfigured, in Darwin.

scientific underpinnings and structure, he had first to make a huge scientific and analytic investigation, the enormous biological and cultural investigation which is neuropsychology. Only then, using the spoils of all his analytical investigations, could he think of going back and creating the dream of his youth.

> In both books (*The Mind of a Mnemonist* and *The Man with a Shattered World*) I describe an individual and the laws of his mental life. . . . But since it is impossible to write an analytical description of the personality of someone taken at random from a crowd, I choose to write about two men each of whom had one feature that played a decisive role in determining his personality and which set him apart from all other people. In each case I tried to study the individual's basic trait as carefully as possible, and from it deduce his other personality traits. . . . Thus S. V. Shereshevsky (the hero of *Mnemonist*) had an outstanding memory which dominated his personality. But it was not his memory itself, but rather its influence on his life and personality, which formed the subject of the book. . . . By contrast my second book using the approach of romantic science began not with an outstanding capacity, but with a catastrophe that had devastated a man's intellectual powers. . . . I observed this patient for thirty years. The book about him is in no sense an "imaginary portrait" . . . (but rather) a true portrait which is also an attempt to come closer to understanding some psychological facts through the use of neuropsychology. (1979, pp. 179–187)

Luria adds, at the very close of his autobiography, that there were many times when he would have liked to write a third book, or even a short series of such books:

> I could describe a man with a complete loss of memory and all that happened to his personality as a result of this loss.[11] Or I could write about a patient with a frontal lobe lesion which caused a complete breakdown of his ability to formulate plans and goals and how this affected him. . . . One has to find individuals with exceptional qualities—an overdevelopment of some trait or a breakdown of some primary function—which have caused a complete change of personality. Then one has to spend decades following up that "unimagined story," singling out decisive factors and step by step constructing the whole syndrome. (p. 187)

The use of the term "constructing" (which might better be "reconstructing") is crucial here, and reminds one of the title and theme of Freud's great, late (1937)—and almost final—paper, "Constructions in Analysis." The final function of psychoanalysis is to allow "constructions" of human nature, with particu-

---

[11]It was largely in consequence of Luria mentioning this to me, in our correspondence, that I myself came to write such a story, "The Lost Mariner" (in *The Man who Mistook his Wife for a Hat*, New York: Summit Books, 1986).

lar reference to the "psychodynamics" involved; the final function of neuropsychology is wholly analogous, to allow "constructions" of human nature, with particular reference to the "neurodynamics" involved. Such constructions, at once actual, paradigmatic, and dramatic, are the very acme of Romantic Science.

The constructions of physical science, or biology, may be lyrical, but are impersonal and theoretical. There is no "story" in the life of an orchid or earthworm—no *personal* story, no drama, no plight, no predicament. Therefore the art of storytelling, of narrative, is not necessary for its description. But with human life, human nature, it is wholly different: there is drama, there is intentionality, at every point. Its exploration demands the seeing and telling of a story, demands a narrative structure and sensibility and science. Two modes of thought are always required here—Jerome Bruner calls them the "paradigmatic" and the "narrative,"[12] and these, though so different, must be completely intertwined, to produce a unity greater than either could alone. This is the unity we sense in Luria and Freud.

"The proper study of mankind is Man." To write true stories, to construct true lives, to present the essence and sense of a whole human life—in all its living fullness and richness and complexity—this must be the final goal of any human science or psychology. William James saw this, in the 1890s, but could only dream of its accomplishment. (The three-stage movement, from naïve naturalism, through analysis, to a "higher and simpler way" would take, he estimated, a century or so.) We ourselves are very privileged, because we have seen, in our own century, with the profound "unimagined portraits" constructed for us by Freud and Luria, at least the beginnings of this ultimate achievement. "This is only the beginning," Luria would always say, and, at other times, "I am only a beginner." Luria devoted the whole of a long life to reaching this beginning. "It has been my life's wish," he once wrote, "to found or refound a Romantic Science." (personal communication, letter dated July 19, 1973) Luria, surely, accomplished his life's wish, and indeed founded or refounded a totally new science—the newest science in the world, in a way, and yet the first, and perhaps the oldest of all.

## REFERENCES

Bruner, J. S. (1986). "Two modes of thought," in *Actual minds, possible worlds,* Cambridge, MA: Harvard University Press, pp. 11–43.
Freud, S. (1937). "Constructions in Analysis," In J. Strachey (Ed. and Trans.), *The Standard Edition* (Vol. 23).

[12]See "Two Modes of Thought," in Jerome Bruner, *Actual Minds, Possible Worlds* (Cambridge, MA: Harvard University Press, 1986), pp. 11–43.

James, W. (1911). "Louis Agassiz," In *Memories and studies,* London: Longmans, Green, pp. 3–16.

Luria, A. R. (1973). "The long road of a Soviet psychologist," *Int. Soc. Sci. J., 25*(1/2).

Luria, A. R. (1978). *Psychoanalysis in light of the principal tendencies in contemporary psychology* (in Russian), Kazan, 1922. Never translated into English; but see "Psychoanalysis as a system of monistic psychology," in (Ed.), Michael Cole *The selected writings of A. R. Luria.* White Plains, NY: Merle Sharpe.

Luria, A. R. (1979). *The making of mind: A personal account of Soviet psychology,* M. Cole & S. Cole (Eds.). Cambridge, MA: Harvard University Press.

Luria, A. R. (1987a). *The man with a shattered world,* reissued with a new foreword by O. Sacks, Cambridge, MA: Harvard University Press.

Luria, A. R. (1987b). *The mind of a mnemonist,* reissued with a new foreword by J. S. Bruner, Cambridge, MA: Harvard University Press.

Luria, A. R., & Yudovich, F. I. (1958). *Speech and the development of mental processes in the child,* London: Staples Press.

Sacks, O. W. (1973). "The mind of A. R. Luria," *The Listener,* June 28.

Shengold, L. (1988). *Halo in the sky: Observations on anality and defense,* New York: Guilford Press.

Vygotsky, L. S. (1962). *Thought and language,* Cambridge, MA, and New York: MIT Press and Wiley.

# 10

# Preliminaries for a Theory of Mind

*Jason W. Brown*

*New York University Medical Center*

## INTRODUCTION

You see an apple in a dish, decide to reach for it, bring it to your mouth and take a bite. Simple? Yes, but consider the problems that are raised. There is a motivation to act that provides an impulse or a drive leading to an action and there is a decision that an action is or is not forthcoming. The action may be propelled by the drive but you have the feeling of initiating a movement, a willed or purposeful movement, that leads outward to a real object in a real physical world. You reach for the object which is independent of your Self and you ingest it as a foreign body.

From a purely neurological standpoint it seems that activity in an appetite center motivates or is initiated by the sight of an apple in the visual center. There is a concatenation of a drive and a perception, of a state of hunger that arises internally and the sight of an apple in the environment, and this association rouses the motor centers for limb action. Mechanisms serving these functions are located in different parts of the brain and are connected by pathways. At the same time, standing behind or embedded in these mechanisms, perhaps integrating them, a conscious Self observes and supervises the events that are happening. Unlike these mechanisms, however, consciousness is not localized in the brain though it is presumed to be elaborated by brain activity. This, in a nutshell, is the thrust of most neurological speculation on the matter.

There is much research on the different components of this behavior, on the perception of a round red object, an apple, distinct from but superimposed on a round flat one, the plate, positioned at some distance in external space. There is work on the nature of appetite and satiation, on motor initiation, ballistic reaching and grasping, and there are even studies on the neurology of consciousness. However, as each of these components is examined in detail we seem to move further from an understanding of the behavior as a whole. We learn, for example, that there are cells in the cortex tuned to edges and colors, perhaps even sensitive to certain shapes. There are cell columns for stereoscopy. There is a representation of the visual field in several regions of cortex. We are told that an object is assembled in serial and/or parallel fashion from the features that constitute it and that a configuration or code corresponding to the object is relayed to memory banks for identification. The logic is that a behavior is explained when it is fractionated into constituent operations which are separately interpreted and then reunited. The behavior is understood by an analysis of its parts and the parts, like pieces in a puzzle, satisfy the explanation when they exhaust the content of the behavior.

As we proceed in this way, the elements comprising even the simplest performance turn out to be incredibly complex, indeed, a world unto themselves. The color sensitive cells that are presumably involved in seeing the apple's redness are a vast topic with controversy on the most banal observation. How color-specific are the cells, how localized and where? How is color coding effected, in what way do the color cells at various levels in the nervous system enter into the perception of the red apple, what are the effects of damage to these cells at different points in the visual pathway, and how is color vision integrated with other visual functions? For those who would speculate on the way the brain elaborates color as an attribute of objects, or for that matter how any object comes to be represented in the mind, the existence of such cells does not appear to be decisive with regard to almost any position one could take. This is not because our knowledge of color coding in the nervous system is incomplete but because we lack a general theory within which this knowledge has a place. There is always a context around a local theory which is the area of its weakness. The more local the theory—and scientific theories tend to be extremely local—the less the theory explains. A complete theory of color vision is also a theory of object and space perception. A theory on the nature of perceptual space is a theory on action in that space, and any theory of action or perception requires a concept of the observer for whom acts and objects exist. In a very real sense, everything needs to be explained before anything can be understood.

General concepts dissolve in the process of analysis and are replaced by a mosaic of elements. The hope, of course, is that the analysis will provide a solid foundation for the next round of general concepts. Yet there is a nagging doubt as to the relevance of any scientific demonstration to the development of a scientific theory. Theory does not spring from data but arises as an insight about the context within which the data appear. Data, facts and observations limit the scope in which theory can develop but are more neutral in relation to the development of the theory than is commonly recognized. Theories help to organize experience; they are not waiting to be discovered when all the facts are known, but are engaged in the process of discovery as covert motivations. A theory is not an outcome but an intuition about the concepts that are quietly guiding the research.

Karl Popper argues that the role of science lies in the negation of theory and not the generation of new data that inevitably fall within one or another existing paradigm. This is because the method of investigation determines the data that are collected. A researcher is often unaware of the paradigms by which his own studies are driven. The local model at risk in a given investigation tends to fall within such a paradigm, one that may be so removed from the field of research that it seems to belong to another domain of study. For example, the study of color sensitivity as an element in object perception independent, say, of shape or space perception implies that separate components underlying color, shape and space interact or combine in the process of object formation. This seems a rather straight-forward idea but it is intelligible only in the context of a theory on the limits of mind in the world, one that assumes that the constituents of a perceived object are elements in its reconstruction. The concept of color detection as a building block in the representation of coloured objects in external space is part of a concept of what the world is. In this case, the concept is that a real world provides the raw material out of which objects are constructed. This larger concept gives rise to the local model which in relation to it is only a kind of tributary.

In sum, there is a tacit bias in any observation or experiment rooted ultimately in collective assumptions on the nature of mind and externality. The concepts driving the research are more important than the concepts which the research seems to be generating. Fundamental ideas implicit in the research shape it in ways that are often inapparent. This is especially important in the study of psychological function.

## THE APPROACH TO MIND

What concepts should guide our understanding of the human mind? An account of mind could begin in one of several ways but the starting point is important. The first step establishes the type of account to be elaborated and lays down the basis for all future research and observation.

A common-sense starting point is with the sensory experience of the objects of the world around us. The world seems real enough, and an ingested world seems to be the basis for all of our ideas and behavior. Mind is shaped by the world to such an extent that even ideas which seem novel can be traced to events that are learned. In fact, it is difficult to imagine a mind that is rooted in a world other than the one we share.

Mind undergoes growth and change. In the infant, growth is rapid; mind develops in a few short years while a change in the world is imperceptible. With age and disease mind decays and objects remain indifferent. The survival of the world does not depend on the growth, the decay or even the existence of mind, while the vitality and continuance of mind are always at risk. How can we escape the conviction that mind is a local phenomenon in a world of other objects and other minds? Perhaps the world that mind embraces is part of a larger sphere of creation, one beyond the comprehension of any human mind. Perhaps the world is a fleeting thought in the mind of the Creator. But for the individual, a mere cipher overwhelmed by the physical expanse, the world is a sea of solid objects in an endless dispassionate space.

We can begin with this world, the world of independent objects, and move in to the subjective. When we do, however, the path we travel is not purely a road to understanding but is part of the picture we obtain. It leads to a mind that is built on sensory or experiential events, a mind of constituents, an assemblage of the bits and pieces of externality.

A theory of mind centered in the world is a theory of mind as a construction. It is a theory that entails that physical objects impinge on mind and that mind reconstitutes the object from its elements and attributes. This means that sensory impressions flowing from the object form the basis of the object in awareness. That is, sensory impressions not only instigate the process leading to the object but are direct components of the object formation. Specifically, if an object is an end result of a concatenation of sensory events, sensory elements are intrinsic links in this sequence. This much seems required by an input or experientially-based theory of mind, that a perception, a mental state, is a *direct* product of the raw material of the physical world.

But an object in perception is not an actual object, it is an event in a brain in a perceptual state. The physical object corresponding with the perceptual object is the brain state that generates the perception, not the physical presentation of the object that is actually seen. In other words, the true referent of the perception is not the physical object "out there", but the more proximate brain state correlated with that perception. When we begin with sensory experience it seems that the physical state of the external object, not the neural state responsible for the object perception, is the correlate of the mental state through which the object is represented. In some manner the "projection" of an object into the world entails a contrast between Self and object that is so compelling we have difficulty maintaining the thought that the objective world is not quite as it appears. We are drawn irresistibly to the idea of two separate domains of existence, a private world of mental states, imagery, inner speech and awareness, and an in-dependent physical world that is scrutinized in perception.

When we give ourselves up to this view, the object of perception is a real object in a real external space presented to and surveyed by the mind. The neural correlate of mind seems distinct from the neural correlate of the object. That is, the object in perception does not seem to be part of a mental state but is rather a content which that state can observe. As a result, the neural correlate of the mental state is taken to exclude the physical underpinnings of the object. Instead, the Self and its awareness, the feeling and knowledge brought to bear on the object, in a word, the *consciousness* of the object not the object representation, becomes the central expression of the mental state. The mental state comes to apply to what is going on inside the head and not what is happening "out there in the world".

On the other hand, if we begin with mind as primary and seek to explain objects from inner states and private experience, the discontinuity between inner and outer evaporates: mind is everywhere, a universe. An object is an extension of the mind of the perceiver. Mind reaches out to articulate a world that is limitless like a dream and the real world is a reality beyond mental representation. The world that is scrutinized in perception is simply part of the extrapersonal extent of mind.

On this view, wherever we look we see cognized objects. Whereas before we thought to perceive objects, now we understand that we think them. Objects are pieces of the mind of the perceiver. The *extension* of object space is no longer an obstacle to a material theory of mind but a characteristic of mind distributed over the objects of its own making. The private space of dream, the unextended moment of awareness, the brief duration of an act of reflection, these are other worlds that mind deposits on the way to object representations. This also pertains to intention which is not the coping of the Self as it strives after meaning but a feeling that arises with the object that is sought after. Intentions are descriptions of what happens in the representing of objects, not cognitions applied to the objects with which the Self is confronted. There is no Self that is waiting for an object. The Self is generated in the course of the object development. The Self is another type of object, an intrapersonal object that appears side by side with other perceptual contents.

When objects are interpreted from this standpoint, the physical correlate of the object in perception—indeed, the entire object world—is linked to the underlying brain state and is not the physical counterpart of the external object, while the real object, the thing in itself, is a type of creation myth on the origins of object representations. Is the world my dream, or am I a dream in the mind of the Creator?

From this point of view we struggle to understand the world itself, the richness and diversity of the world. As the unity of a mind built on physical stimuli is a problem for sensory theories, the diversity of the world is a problem for mental theories. We have to explain how mind is shaped by the world; mind could not invent a world such as this! Sensory experience figures in the growth of mind and object representations, which develop in relation to that experience as a type of model. This model is so faithful to the world it represents that whether an object is mental or not is of little concern in day to day behavior. Mind articulates a world of such objectivity that no theory can avoid the problem of its sensory determinants. The physical world, the world of sensation, has to be accounted for even if it is beyond the reach of mental representation. We also have to account for our knowledge of other minds, for as we infer an independent status to inanimate objects we attribute mind to animate ones. The major issues are the activity and ontogeny of a mind contingent on but independent of sensation, and the belief in "other" objects and "other" minds though these co-occur in the purely mental space of one perceiver.

It seems a choice is involved that depends on a certain perspective, the stand we take on the nature of the world around us. We can begin with the physical and work our way up to the mental, or we can begin with mental representation and try to reclaim the physical. According to the choice we make, the physical world approaches mind from either of two directions: from brain states underlying mentation; or from a world embedded in object representations.

The problem of the physical basis of mental events arises from each of these directions, the link between mind and brain state, and the link between object and object representation, usually framed in terms of learning and the sensory determinants of mental states. The relation between the physical brain state and the physical object has to do with two events of the same order. When we move inwards from object to brain state, as we must whatever our theory, we seem to be closer to the physical basis of mind. But here there is another interface, that between the resultants of sensations in the brain and brain states actualizing as mental states. Mind is encapsulated, and neural states underlying mental states are also encapsulated; they are not the termini of complex sensory transformations. Mind is not built on sensory information and does not appear at some point in the elaboration of sensation. There is no transition to mind over levels of sensory processing, no compounding of reflex arcs. There is, in fact, a fundamentally different principle at work (see Brown, 1988).

Regardless of where we begin, with objects, brain activity or cognition, we need a theory of a mind sensitive to physical constraints but centered in the subjective for this is ultimately what the theory has to explain. Without inner states there is no need for a theory; indeed, there is no mind to theorize with!

## MIND WITHIN OBJECTS

We are constantly reminded of the fragility of objects. A case of vertigo in which objects rotate around the viewer should be sufficient to convince one that the stability of the object world is precarious. Vertigo places the existence of objects in doubt. Object motion and stability depend on the state of the nervous system, they are not unchanging features of the object. Why is this not the case for object form? If the stability of objects is an illusion, perhaps the solidity of objects is a mirage. Illusions of object shape and size occur in drug or toxic states and brain damage but are far less common than illusory movement. Such phenomena lead one to ask whether objects prone to illusory change may be illusory objects, whether a world that swims around the viewer does so because it is a world the viewer has created.

Every day we have the feeling that the boundaries between objects and images are indistinct. An object that is incompletely perceived is like an image at the threshold of perception. There is a constant flow between image and object and a given perception can settle at any point. How many of us have wondered whether we have just heard a name whispered or a voice in the wind? Did we think our "mind was playing tricks" on us? Was that a train in the distance or are we imagining things? Russell (1921) says, "When we are listening for a faint sound—the striking of a distant clock, or a horse's hoofs on the road—we think we hear it many times before we really do, because expectation brings us the image, and we mistake it for sensation. The distinction between images and sensations is, therefore, by no means always obvious to introspection." In this example, the point is not that expectation makes a difference—it does regardless—but the fine line between image and object.[1]

These are minor distortions in a perceptual process that is otherwise reliable. But they do signal the presence of a mind within objects. They are signs that an object is not a neutral entity that engages the mind from outside but is through and through a product of cognition. Objects are apparitions in the extrapersonal extent of mind. The intuition of mind in objects is engraved in superstition, in the fear that unkind thoughts will come to pass, in the power of the word, in prophecy and the belief that events are forecast in dream. Part of the basis of myth is the intuition that mind is at work in the shaping of reality. One can also point to constancy effects, for example the fact that objects do not undergo changes in perceptual size predicted by the geometry of object distance, optic illusions, impossible objects, phenomena which all indicate a cognition within the object. Not only do we not see things as they are, we do not see them as they could possibly be.

## IMAGINATION AND PERCEPTION

Imagination fills and elaborates the object experience and persuades us that objects develop in the context of mind. The presence of an image in every object perception and the potential of every image to approximate an object, are the basis for thinking that objects are images of a different type. We can peel away

---

[1]This can also be demonstrated with tests of brain function. If one gives a series of diminishing tactile stimuli to the hand, and measures blood flow in the opposite "sensory" cortex, there is activation of brain at the point where the subject imagines he has been touched by a subthreshold stimulus that was not applied. In other studies (Phelps et al, 1982; Buchsbaum et al, 1982) an increase in brain metabolism in the visual and auditory cortices has been shown during visual and auditory hallucination, respectively. These studies confirm the clinical evidence that brain events underlying imagery involve the same areas as, and presumably are similar to, those underlying perception.

the surface of the world and discover the hidden realm of imagery, while contents in the imagination, horse's hoofs or a distant train whistle, can take on an object-like clarity.

Images and objects can be thought of as points on a continuum. Objects grow out of images, images can resolve to the threshold of an object perception. An image is like an object that is arrested in its development, it is a preliminary object. The mental space of imagery (and hallucination) is a preliminary space. Images and objects do not just share mechanisms in common. The image is part of the formative process leading to the object. Vertigo, for example, involves not only objects but dream imagery and 'objectless space'. Someone with vertigo can close his eyes and "see" the diffuse visual gray spin like a solid object. Patients with vertigo have rotatory dreams.

Dream is an object experience that is pure imagination. Dreams are not like objects but for the viewer they are as real as any perception. It is rare—less than 5% of dream experiences—that one apprehends the dream as unreal *during* the dream. The feeling of reality for dream does not arise from the approximation to an object but from an inability to affirm the unreality of the dream image through alternative perceptual systems. In dream as in perception, an image is seen, heard and experienced in other ways. In dream and perception the senses reinforce one another. The feeling of reality for objects in waking life and dream is the result of a conspiracy of the senses. This is why Dr. Johnson's famous "refutation" of Berkeley by kicking a stone is so fatuous. Tumor cases with hallucination apprehend the image as hallucinatory until there is an auditory or tactile element, at which point the image is taken for a real object.

Dream would be our only reality were it not for waking life. When we awake we regain the world of objects. The dream that lies beneath the surface of wakefulness dissolves like a waking experience that has long been forgotten. Waking objects struggle out of dream and the dream content fades to a memory that is only dimly recollected. Now we understand that a moment ago we were "only dreaming". But we are unsettled. Is the world of waking objects a dream that seems real, as real as a dream that is happening? How would we know if it were not? How can we escape the impression that the perceptual world is a dream of objects, a dream from which we too could awaken, a dream that in death slips away perhaps in expectation of yet another dream to follow?

For most of us there are two worlds, that of dream and that of wakefulness. Could we as well say we live in two dreams only one of which seems real? For the psychotic, there is one dream that embraces both worlds, a single world where dreams exteriorize and objects become like thoughts. The shift from dream to wakefulness is not an alternation between two parallel states but a process of emergence. We apprehend a dream as unreal because on waking we pass to an intentional awareness where the dream content is given over to reflection. This is not the case in dream, though dream cognition weaves its way through fragments of the preceding day. Were it possible to reflect intentionally in dream on the contents of wakefulness, we might see more clearly the delicate balance on which hangs the supposed reality of waking cognition.

In sum, there are many reminders in everyday life that the world of waking objects is not as stable and independent as it seems but that it bridges into a private world of dream and imagery. Conversely, the world of the imagination threatens to expand beyond mind into the objects that surround us. In spite of this, we behave as if the world of perception is a real world. Whatever an object is conceived to be is of little consequence in relation to the commonsense view that objects are physical entities owing nothing to the onlooker, who is in any event an accidental feature of the landscape. One challenge that is set to a theory of the world as mental representation is to explain this paradox, the firmness of belief in a world of real objects and actions that effect those objects, and the conviction that mind is independent of the objects of its own making.

## NATURE AND NURTURE

Mind is not filled but shaped by experience to replicate one of many possible worlds. Evolution delivers a mind that is prepared to replicate the world we live in. Patterns of brain activity generate mental states before the brain's encounter with sensory experience. These patterns and the mental states which correspond to them are pre-set at birth to engage a slice of the physical world. A change in these patterns or in the world for which they are designed is incompatible with survival. The brain of a bat is adapted to the world in which the bat lives. An infant bat borne into a world other than that for which it evolved, a world, say, with continuous jamming of sonar, would perish as surely as if it were borne with a defective brain.

The human mind:brain is equally ready to be shaped by the world. Patterns of neural activity configured in the brain arise spontaneously to mediate instinctive behavior, even prior to birth, for example thumbsucking in the fetal infant. In older children and adults, such patterns are the basis for concepts guiding actions that are planned for the future. They form a nucleus for the derivation of conscious representations. We see this in sucking and grasping in the infant, automatisms that lay down a structure for the development of fine articulatory and digital movements. Handedness emerges out of an orientation bias about the body midline reflected in the tonic neck reflex. Actions undergo specification out of older motor systems that are spontaneously active. It seems that archaic systems in the brain elaborate spontaneous activity underlying preliminary stages in cognition.

Regions of the cortex are also prepared to respond at birth. The presetting of visual cortex for lines and angles dissolves if visual sensation is abolished or these features are not encountered. The pre-setting for lines would not appear in the visual system of other life forms that engage a different perceptual world.

The brain of a bat is presumably pre-set for sonar. Other "primary" cortices, including motor cortex, are similarly pre-wired. Many aspects of bird song are innate, as well as the response to the songs of other birds. The picture that emerges is one of spontaneous activity at deep levels in the brain generating the foundations of perception and behavior and a pre-setting of sensory systems linked to features in that sector of the physical world for which the organism is designed. Levels in mind:brain are primed at birth to receive and respond to impressions from the world.

There is a nucleus of native ability not only in moods and motivations, and motor synergies like breathing and walking, but in complex skills such as grammar and the rhythms of dialogue. How can we describe what is innate in these behaviors? Are innate rules or instructions applied to symbols that are acquired? Are concepts inborne? What is given by nature is at least a preparedness to respond to the environment. What is less clear is the character and extent of this endowment and the interface of cognitive primitives with sensory experience.

Roman Jakobson (1968) commented that the development of speech out of babbling proceeds from the universal to the specific. Babbling contains the sounds of the many languages of the world, and all save those of the mother tongue are lost as proficiency is gained. The native language is not constructed but carved or selected into elements. This is also true for the development of the language areas of the brain. The asymmetry which is present at birth is due to fractionation, not accentuated growth. Continued development through life may occur through regional specification. Other sensory systems develop through selective loss of connections. Edelmann (1987) describes competition for survival at the neuronal level. Cells that are unfit or maladaptive disappear. Nurture is the reinforcement of systems pre-set by nature and the channeling of the varied possibilities of behavior into those which advantage the organism in its environment.

Such observations show that mind is not waiting to be enlarged by experience but flows into the crevices that experience makes possible. Nature provides the organism with a predisposition to act and react in a certain way. The predisposition is a structure that confronts and challenges the physical world, an image of the world that is refined and articulated through adaptation to the constraints of sensation. The mind of the infant is like the sprout of a tree just beginning its journey through life.

## THE IDEA OF STRUCTURE

We would not say that the structure of a building is in the face it presents to a viewer. This is its appearance, its form; its structure consists in the pattern and composition of its elements. Structure means internal structure, not just surface form. Internal structure, however, is more than the concatenation of parts; it includes the functional relations between the parts. If one element depends on another, that relationship has to be incorporated. If one element is required to support or activate another it becomes a part of its structure. For example, one could say the structure of a bee includes its position in the hive. The bee does not exist independently but is like a cell in an organ like a brain. These contextual effects apply to any system which is part of a larger organization.

Structures are not static arrangements but dynamic patterns. A structure changes with a change in state. The structure of a lamp changes when it is illuminated. The activation of quiescent elements, the current flow, creates a new system. The gross morphology of the brain a moment after death is identical to that during life but there is a momentous difference. Structure is defined by active processes. The real structure of a brain is not in the parts and circuitry but the configurations that dance over the living cellular elements.

In this way the idea of process enters the concept of structure. Process is not the output of structure; process neither drives structure nor is instantiated through structure, as for example a computer program drives or is realized through the hardware. In organic systems, structure is stasis imposed on the dynamic of process. Process applies to internal activity and differs from function, which is a super-ordinate term for the action of a system as a whole. Function serves to unite internal components which are otherwise dissimilar or discontiguous; function provides a label for variation in a system, for example, the function of respiration, or digestion, or cognition.

Function accounts for the design of a system but structure is independent of a functional description. Respiration or digestion occur in different ways in different organisms. In a physical system such as a building, functional values influence design but are not inherent features. In organic systems, growth is constrained by functional demands. The functional requirements of a lung or intestine determine their structure, like the resistance of soil determines the growth pattern of roots. In evolution, adaptation has a shaping effect on structure; the system is altered by the environment. Structure is affected by functional demands that are external to the process through which the structure is elaborated. One can say that function constrains growth and outlines process but is not an intrinsic part of structure.

Process leaves behind a physiological change as a type of structural marker. The activation of nerve cells results in growth, a lack of stimulation in atrophy. Structure is built on functional activity. An accent in the native language, the effects of knowledge on perception, athletic and instrumental skill, depend on physiological processes which are etched into the structure of the brain. These processes lay down the structure so that in a complex network such as a brain it is really the physiological flow, the relationship between components, not the arrangement of parts that determine what the structure is.

Structure, therefore, is the illusion of stability in a system in continuous transformation. For any mind:brain state, there is a temporal context, a before and an after, within which that state is embedded. The state is configured by the context and cannot be extracted as an independent event. There is no brain state that corresponds to a word or a percept. Nor is there a psychological state that corresponds with a word or a percept. A word has to be considered in relation to its elicitation from the mental lexicon and stages in its phonological realization. Where in this process is the state corresponding to the word? One can isolate neither the brain state nor its psychological counterpart. Perhaps a segment of brain activity can be mapped to a segment of mental flow, but this is not the same as mapping one state to another. In a process model, structural units are like mental snapshots, moments in the life of process artificially frozen in time.[2]

With process there is the opposite problem, we are lost in a sea of continuous change. Flow has to be punctuated into resting points from which we can get a bearing. A grain of sand is a whirl of active particles. There is a subatomic dynamic in any physical system. Solid objects are built on movement and activity. This is true at all levels of observation. Structure in mind:brain is a conceptual anchor in the unending flow of process.

A central feature of mind:brain is the capacity to segment flow into chunks such as words, objects and categories and elaborate these into more complex groupings. Categories imposed on an acoustic stream create words and meanings. Two dimensional shapes superimposed are seen as distinct objects, not as a single complex form. Consciousness is populated by short-term memory, images, attentional devices, a self-concept and other mental entities which emerge out of continual flux. Functions are assigned to these entities in both neural and psychological components; this is part of our everyday approach to mind and the world and needs careful thinking to overcome. The structure of the brain, like that of mind and world, is not a rigid framework but a fluid arrangement of dynamic processes. The fact that mind:brain partitions flow into stable configurations does not mean these configurations are constitutive elements.

## PROCESS IN RELATION TO LOCALIZATION THEORY

The idea of centers in the brain as sites for specific functions—whether storehouses of images, processes, strategies, procedures or representations—entails a set of structural components which interact through connecting path-

---

[2]The distinction between being and becoming, or permanence and change, goes back to Parmenides and Heraclitus. This distinction, as that between qualia and relata in physical systems, is similar to that between state and process or object and context in psychological systems. There is likely a deep inner relation to such problems as wave:particle duality. We identify a thing at the expense of its dynamic, or we focus on the dynamic and lose sight of the thing itself.

ways. Modularity theory is a contemporary version of functional localization but one that is relatively immune to the usual criticisms because the modules are largely psychological concepts. Modularity does not require fixed centers; it is compatible with distributed, even overlapping, networks so that the impact of this theory for brain study is unclear. Certainly, its proof or disconfirmation is unlikely to come from traditional brain-behavior correlation methods.

Modularity theory assumes that cognition is partitioned into "central" or general cognitive system(s) and various "peripheral" components (Fodor, 1983). The peripheral components are modular in that they are highly specific both to the domain in which they operate and the vocabulary of that domain, they are automatic and obligatory in their action and "impenetrable" to influence from central systems. In other words, the "peripheral" modules, e.g. language (syntax), face recognition, perhaps musical or mathematical abilities, have the autonomy and inevitability of programs containing all the information required for their enactment, with the brain analogous to a computer through which these programs, modules, are implemented.

The theory proposes that certain functions reflect the operation of distinct "organs" or dedicated components that may or may not be pre-wired or genetically encoded and need not be localized. Such issues as the nature of what goes on "within" the module and discontinuities between modules and "central" systems, not to mention the relation to non-modular capacities or such hobgoblins of psychology as awareness, agency and affect are rarely addressed.

As interpreted by cognitive psychologists, the theory entails the existence of discrete units at successive stages in processing which experimental studies seek to tease apart. For example, there are relatively independent sub-systems within, say, the language module that output information to other processors, rather than language perception and production being laid down through a continuous wave-like flow. One might ask at what point in the process does a segment in a processing chain constitute a sub-system or a module, in other words what are the boundary conditions between the sub-system and the module, and the module and its output phase?

Considered as a general theory of mind, modularity is a step in the analysis of mind into elements, requiring a decision as to what the natural elements are going to be. From this point of view, the theory may seem innocuous. But once the approach takes hold it easily runs amuck when confronted with the diversity of the behavior that needs to be explained. One can speak of the modularity of the grammar as well as the modularity of a graphemic output buffer (in writing). What constitutes a module, how independent are the sub-systems within modules—are these sub-systems also modules—and do all sub-systems within a module share the characteristics of the module as a whole? Once we begin to analyze the internal structure of a module, elements in a performance get uncoupled from larger neighboring phenomena and become so distanced from the parent domain that they take on a life of their own. The graphemic output buffer is not just a hypothetical phase between the lexicon and a writing system but is psychologically (and neurologically) real! One could say that the analysis leads away from the overall structure of the phenomenon being analysed so that ultimately it is the analysis rather than the phenomenon that is understood.[3]

The many technical problems with modularity have been discussed elsewhere (Schweiger and Brown, 1988). Some of these are in brief:

- the organization and breakdown of putative modular systems (e.g. face recognition) show the same patterns as occurs in presumably non-modular systems (e.g. object recognition);
- pathology does not induce the restricted loss of elements that modularity theory entails. The failure to demonstrate other inwardly related non-modular defecits is due to the failure to look for them;
- in the brain, "modular" systems—e.g. language—are organized in relation to perceptual and action components. The evolutionary continuum to and relation with these components remains unspecified.
- the organization of some modules is claimed to be encoded in the genome— this is plausible—but it is far-fetched to maintain this is true for modular systems in general (e.g. reading), so that genetic specification is a weak link in modular theory;
- many performances, for example juggling or playing the piano, become "modularized" with practise. These skill-based "modules" fulfill most if not all the criteria for those which are genetically specified. This points again to the lack of any overarching theoretical motivation for proposing a given function as a module;

More generally, the idea of modularity is deeply antithetical to evolutionary theory, which assumes the gradual appearance of new formations out of pre-existing ones. Modularity is discontinuous over evolution since links between modular and other systems are not specified and because certain modules, such as language, are claimed to be uniquely human without precursors in other species. A theory of language should be grounded in a theory of vocal action and auditory perception; these are complex systems, not just input and output functions for cognitive maps.

Moreover, not only is there an evolutionary or longitudinal discontinuity, but there is a horizontal or synchronic discontinuity across modules. The parsing of cognition into a collection of elements does not account for the blending of elements in a given behavior, nor the unitary nature of mind across those elements. Theorists attempt to deal with this problem by postulating "central"

---

[3]The objection here is to the stasis imposed on components arising artificially through the analysis, not as natural elements. For further arguments, see Ackermann (1971).

systems which receive and elaborate input from different modules. Since the nature and boundaries of central systems are undemarcated, new modules can proliferate unchecked. In fact, the very assumption of modularity necessitates the postulation of vague central systems to account for the continuity and unity of normal behavior.

## EVOLUTION AS THE BASIS FOR A THEORY OF MIND

Local theories of mental function such as modularity posit discrete centers or subsystems for different aspects of mentation and behavior. The functional component—whether a knowledge system such as that presumed for grammar or mathematical knowledge, or a physiological module such as that linked to color vision or ballistic movement—is *ad hoced* from a performance and the performance reconstructed from a network of inferred components. In spite of the many problems with this approach, it appears to promise an explanation of the diversity of normal and abnormal mental phenomena through the assumption of (damaged) modules underlying various abilities (impairments). Indeed, it is difficult to conceive of another approach that so well explains the richness of mental content and the variety of psychopathological states.

Evolutionary theory is also an account of diversity. It is a theory in which the environment has a shaping effect on the emergence of new form. The mechanism of variation relates to the genetic material of the organism. Even minor changes in the genome may translate into major deviations in phenotype. The principles of variation are only one element of evolutionary theory. The other is the concept that variation is pruned by environmental pressure so that only the fittest survive. This component of the evolutionary process is extrinsic to the organism and non-lawful, in that it depends on changing aspects of the surround. The parsing of unfit organisms is the basis of natural selection which is a constraint on variation through the elimination of disadvantageous features and the survival and propagation of those best suited to the external conditions in which the organism will live. Variation throws out alternative forms and the environment inhibits or sculpts these forms to select out those features that are uniquely adapted for a particular niche in the world. In other words, variation elaborates, the environment eliminates, the result being a selective growth by way of inhibition. Intrinsic laws of development determine patterns of growth but the external environment has the final say in what survives.

Evolution requires competition among organisms for survival. The drive to prevail is crucial but not central to the theory. The drive for self-preservation is a given. What counts is the struggle among the many forms prior to the emergence of the one that is successful. Evolution requires competition. The environment does not passively shape the selection process by elimination. Competition is necessary to establish the fitness of the adaptation.

This pattern of a developmental growth process guided by intrinsic laws generating a variety of forms that struggle to prevail in a slice of the external world, a world in which the selection of organisms occurs through an active, competetive pruning of those less well adapted for the conditions of life, constitutes the basic framework of evolutionary theory. The question is, can this framework also serve as a model for the process of cognition?

## REFERENCES

Ackerman, R. (1971). The fallacy of conjunctive analysis. In E. Freeman & W. Sellars (Eds.), *Basic issues in the philosophy of time*. Chicago, IL: Open Court.

Brown, J. W. (1988). *The life of the mind: Selected papers*. Hillsdale, NJ: Lawrence Erlbaum Associates.

Buchsbaum, M., et al. (1982). Cerebral glucography with positron tomography. *Archives of General Psychiatry, 39*, 251–259.

Edelmann, G. (1987). *Neural Darwinism*. New York: Basic Books.

Fodor, J. (1983). *The modularity of mind*. Cambridge, MA: MIT Press.

Jakobson, R. (1968). *Child language, aphasia and phonological universals*. The Hague: Mouton.

Phelps, M., Mazziotta, J., & Huang, S.-C. (1982). Study of cerebral function with positron computed tomography. *Journal of Cerebral Blood Flow and Metabolism, 2*, 113–162.

Russell, B. (1921). *The analysis of mind* (eighth printing, 1961; p. 145). London: Allen & Unwin.

Schweiger, A., & Brown, J. W. (1988). Minds, models & modules. *Aphasiology, 2*, 531–543.

# 11

# Chronotopic Localization of Cerebral Processes: The Temporal Dimension of Brain Organization

*Herbert G. Vaughan, Jr.*

*Albert Einstein College of Medicine*

The temporal dimension has historically played a subsidiary role in theories of brain function, often notable by its absence. Despite the fact that contemporary formulations of brain mechanisms recognize their dynamic nature, the temporal aspects of neural processes have not been explicitly integrated into an overall theoretical treatment in modern cognitive science. Neuropsychology, the discipline most closely devoted to the analysis of relations between the brain and psychological processes, should be in the forefront of efforts to elucidate the dynamic aspects of brain mechanisms. This unfortunately, has not been the case. Over the more than a century since Broca's original description of motor aphasia due to a lesion of the left third frontal convolution, the principal empirical and theoretical concerns of neuropsychology have been with the spatial extent and location of the neural mechanisms that underlie psychological processes, rather than with the nature of the mechanisms themselves. Professor A. R. Luria, whose extraordinary contributions to this discipline we honor with this book, took note of the dynamic and spatially extensive nature of the brain systems that were required for specific psychological functions, but he did not explicitly address the topic of temporal sequencing and interaction within and among the brain systems he discusses (Luria, 1973).

Even in neurophysiology, most dynamic of the neurosciences, spatial data and concepts predominate. Neuronal receptive fields are defined in terms of the magnitude of neural response, with little or no attention being paid to their temporal properties. There is, for example, little information on the distribution of response latencies of single neurons within the primary and secondary sensory cortical areas. Although some timing data are available in the form of poststimulus time histograms, these are often used as a graphical convenience for depicting neural response magnitude, rather than for analysis of temporal relationships among neural responses. Such data are necessary, however, to determine whether neural processes in sensory cortex are occurring sequentially or in parallel. Elucidation of the dynamic pattern of local circuit activation within each cortical region also requires a quantitative analysis of the spatiotemporal pattern of intracortical neuronal activity. Such data have only recently begun to be sought in a systematic manner (viz. Arezzo, Vaughan, Kraut, Steinschneider, & Legatt, 1986; Mitzdorf, 1985).

It is puzzling that temporal factors have been so sparsely represented in theories of brain organization. This deficiency may reflect in large measure a fundamental spatial bias in our perception of the world. In everyday experience we are dominated by the spatial features of the environment. Our egocentric space is principally a visual one. We identify up, down, left, and right; and less definitively, nearer and farther. This information is given through vision, supported by kinesthetic and auditory spatial information, all of which are ordinarily referred to the gravitational vertical defined by the vestibular system. It is not difficult to formulate principles upon which the spatial features of the external world and of our body image might be mapped onto the brain (e.g., Pellionisz & Llinas, 1985).

When we turn to the appreciation of time, however, we find it to be both experientially and conceptually elusive. In marked contrast to the immediacy and almost palpable nature of our spatial impressions, which lend themselves readily to description and to quantification, the time domain is difficult both to experience clearly and to measure subjectively. We have many cues to tell us about perceived spatial relations, so that we are ordinarily reliably informed of the shapes of objects and spatial relations among them. In the appreciation of time, however, we must rely on noticing the order of discrete events or changes in the environment to signal that time has elapsed. Spengler articulated the matter:

> All of us are conscious as being "aware" of space only, and not of time. Time is a discovery which is made only by thinking. . . . Only the higher cultures, whose ideas have reached the stage of a mechanical nature, are capable of deriving from the idea of a measurable and comprehensible spatial, a projected image of time, the phantom time, which satisfies their need of measuring and explaining all things. (1962)

This formulation points up the fact that our scientific concepts reflect a primarily spatial view of the world. Furthermore, according to Spengler, the concept of time currently accepted by modern literate societies was alien to the classical Greeks, whose ideas have so heavily influenced the logical framework of modern science. These circumstances may account in large measure for the subsidiary position of the temporal dimension in the traditional neural and behavioral disciplines.

During the past 2 decades, there has, however, been an extraordinary development of three interrelated research areas concerned with the dynamic features of human psychological and brain processes: namely Cognitive Psychology, Neural Network Theory, and what I shall call Cognitive Neurophysiology. These approaches all recognize the temporal dimension as a necessary part of their empirical and theoretical structure, although each deals with different aspects of the mind-brain question. Of these disciplines, cognitive neurophysiology affords the most direct empirical approach to the relation between brain physiology and mental processes. As yet, however, this relatively young enterprise has not yet achieved widespread recognition of its accomplishments and promise. In this chapter, I shall briefly outline some of the opportunities afforded by human cognitive neurophysiology to elucidate the spatiotemporal organization of psychological processes within the brain.

## THE TIMING OF MENTAL PROCESSES

Despite the ephemeral nature of our experience of time, the temporal aspects of mental processes can be measured objectively. However, until Helmholtz measured the conduction velocity of motor nerves in 1850, neural transmission and mental processes were generally believed to be instantaneous. Since the earliest recorded history, the passage of time had been principally defined by the periodicities of astronomical events: the rising and setting of the sun and the apparent movement of celestial bodies. The scale of time afforded by astronomical periodicity is so slow in comparison with the timing of mental operations that the instantaneous nature of these processes seemed almost self-evident.

It is interesting, therefore that the initial attempts to measure the speed of human perception were provoked by the nuisance of individual differences in determining the precise timing of astronomical events. The notion that it took some finite amount of time to perceive a visual stimulus led to the early efforts by Helmholtz to measure the conduction velocity of sensory nerves, using voluntary motor reaction time (RT) to tactile stimulation of body locations at different distances from the brain. He reasoned that the difference in RT would be the conduction time along a sensory nerve corresponding in length to the distance between the stimulated points. His estimates were in error, apparently due to the fact that the central components of the RT were considerably more variable than the peripheral ones, which made it difficult to measure peripheral nerve conduction velocity reliably using the RT method. Helmholtz's experiments led his friend F. C. Donders, the eminent Dutch ophthalmologist and physiologist, to employ the RT method to measure "the speed of mental processes" (Donders, 1868). His experiments were designed not only to measure the total RT to individual visual and auditory stimuli, but to estimate the time required for a sensory discrimination between two stimuli, and the time required to generate one of two alternative responses to the stimuli. Donders explicitly viewed this method of "mental chronometry" as a means of determining the duration of individual brain processes that underlie specific psychological processes. Despite Donders's prominence within the European physiological community, and the espousal of his method by the laboratories of Wundt and Catell, the assumption of temporally discrete processing stages was strongly criticized by Kulpe. In the absence of an effective rebuttal, the RT method fell into disuse soon after the turn of the century.

The failure of psychologists to recognize the importance of temporal factors in mental processes was not corrected until the middle of this century when interest in the temporal aspects of human performance was reawakened. Several important experimental studies of human performance using the RT method were published during the 1950s and 1960s, culminating in an influential paper by Sternberg, "The Discovery of Processing Stages: Extensions of Donders' Method" (1969). With this renascent interest in the temporal aspects of human mental processes and performance the field of Cognitive Psychology was born.

The basic idea behind Donders's method is that the total time between stimulus and response (RT) is made up of discrete sequential processing stages. A major criticism of Donders's original experiments was that one cannot be certain that the postulated processing stages are independent of one another, so that experimentally introduced stages are simply added to the total RT. Sternberg (1969) endeavored to meet this criticism of the "stage insertion" technique of Donders, by proposing a method that manipulated the duration of individual stages without addition or deletion of stages. However, this Additive Factors Method (AFM), can likewise be faulted in that it assumes that individual stages can be independently manipulated without affecting the duration of other stages. Like Donders's method, AFM assumes that processing stages are strictly serial.

A number of other models of human information processing have been proposed to circumvent some of the problems inherent in the AFM. In considering these models it is especially important to note that there are fundamental differences between models that assume serial ordering of processing stages, and those that involve parallel processing. The mathematician John von Neumann pointed out that in many respects the information-processing capabilities of the brain could be mimicked by digital computers. The digital computers of that day, and the preponderance of those currently in use are "von Neumann machines," that is, computers that are strictly serial in their central processing mechanism. Similarly, until fairly recently, most cognitive models of human information were serial as well. Sternberg's (1969) influential experiments involved the time required for a serial search of memory, which was considered a separate store that would be serially addressed like a computer memory.

During the past decade or so, it has become increasingly evident that the serial conceptualization of brain mechanisms that is inherent in Donders's method, the AFM, and some more recent information-processing models, is not consistent with known principles of brain organization. It is clear, from neuroanatomical considerations alone, that many operations within the central nervous system are performed in parallel. The brain receives massive parallel inputs through the sensory pathways, and a number of cortical sensory areas are believed to process at least some of this information concurrently.

A major theoretical divergence from serial computation occurred with efforts to develop models of visual perception. Rosenblatt (1962) developed a computational model of visual processing that, like living visual systems, carried out its transactions in parallel. Despite criticisms of this approach (e.g., Minsky & Papert, 1969), a number of neural network models that involve parallel distributed processing (PDP) have subsequently been developed (viz. Rumelhardt, McClelland, 1986, for an introduction to this work). The importance of PDP, which must be incorporated into any realistic model of brain function, lies in the very different manner in which brain operations are conceptualized, compared with serial processing models. Not only are many operations carried out simultaneously, but the principal locus of computing is no longer at a "central processor," but at the nodes of the PDP network, which can be considered to correspond to individual neurons within the nervous system. Changes in facility of synaptic transmission at each neuron within an active network determine the input-output transformations of the network as a whole. Memory is no longer a physically separate store that must be serially addressed, but is distributed throughout the nodes of the processing network itself, residing in the total pattern of learned synaptic modifications. Perceptual processing, memory, and response organization are all intrinsic properties of the neural network architecture. Thus, PDP models of neural and psychological processes differ fundamentally from the conventional serial processing models.

Given the necessary complexity of realistic models of the brain mechanisms that underlie specific perceptual, cognitive, and motor operations, a large number of operational features must be clearly specified. Among these are the following examples:

(1) What are the functionally specifiable processing stages in a given information-processing task? (2) Do these stages make sense in terms of what is known about the anatomy and physiology of the relevant brain structures? (3) Which stages in a given information-processing task operate in parallel. (4) How does the output from each stage provide the information required for the next stage(s) to be initiated? (5) Does the input to a stage begin at the end of the preceding stage, or is information from the earlier stage provided to the later one before all processing is completed? and (6) Do the processing stages pass their output to the next stage discretely or continuously? Several of these issues have been addressed experimentally by cognitive psychologists over the past decade or so, but are not yet resolved, even for rather simple discriminative tasks such as those employed by Donders (viz., e.g., Miller, 1988). It has become in-

creasingly recognized that behavioral (RT) data alone are insufficient to resolve conclusively important questions on the mechanisms of human information processing (Taylor, 1976).

The seminal formulation of distributed brain processing was made by Hebb (1949), who proposed that the brain operates through activation of more or less localized "cell assemblies," dynamically linked into neural networks called "phase sequences" that can be widely distributed within the brain. A major implication of Hebb's ideas is that, although a dynamic psychological process can involve large portions of the brain in the course of activation of a particular phase sequence, this activation must occur over a period of time, and must involve the linkage of many cell assemblies. This formulation of brain operations requires that information processing models incorporate both serial and parallel mechanisms.

Despite the undoubted need for direct information on brain physiology in elucidating the mechanisms underlying mental processes, such data were not available to students of brain and behavior until quite recently. Nearly a century passed after Donders's original experiments before reliable methods became available for directly observing some of the human brain processes that Donders had examined by behavioral techniques. Therefore, most of our information on the localization of brain mechanisms has been derived from clinical observations of psychological impairment following localized brain lesions. Some of the limitations of this approach must be noted before proceeding to a consideration of the methods of cognitive neurophysiology.

## NEUROPSYCHOLOGICAL CONCEPTS OF CEREBRAL LOCALIZATION

A large body of evidence on cerebral localization, derived from observations on patients with focal brain damage, was collected after the seminal report by Broca in 1860. These data added substance and detail to Gall's basic idea of functional localization within the cerebral cortex. But these elaborations remained essentially spatial and static. Gall proposed isolated cortical centers that were virtually independent "mental organs," and the possible interactions among them were not considered. Wernicke added anatomical interconnections between receptive and motor cortical regions, by way of the subcortical white matter, to account for the dependence of meaningful speech on the functional integrity of the posterior temporal region. Various schemes of cortical interconnection were developed during the latter half of the 19th century to account for the functional relations among the various expressive and receptive components of speech, reading, writing, and other kinds of complex motor behavior as well. Considerable dispute surrounded the facts and interpretations of the available clinical observations. These controversies reflect the uncertain nature of evidence provided by brain lesions that are inherently variable and poorly defined in their anatomical locus and extent. Nevertheless, the basic notion of specialized brain centers interconnected by cortical pathways remains a central feature of modern neuropsychological doctrine (Geschwind, 1965; Luria, 1973).

It is noteworthy that formulations of functional localization within the brain, as well as the opposing view of the brain as a diffusely organized equipotential structure, were mainly concerned with spatial issues. At no time during the 19th, or the first half of the 20th century did concepts of functional localization within the brain intersect with Donders's idea of mental chronometry. The virtual absence of temporal factors in neuropsychological theories is remarkable. Almost alone, von Monakov (1911) called attention to the "chronological localization of function" within the brain. But as with Donders, neither the conceptual atmosphere nor the necessary physiological techniques were available to support empirical studies of the temporal aspects of brain function.

Some neuropsychological formulations appear to equate the localized processing carried out within a particular cortical structure with a processing stage, for example, visual word recognition. However, Luria (1973) pointed out that psychological processes should not be considered the function of a circumscribed tissue, but rather of an extended system, each part of which carries out various aspects of the process under consideration. This formulation clearly implies a temporal sequence of brain activation, in which a number of more or less localized brain areas carry out specific operations that are linked dynamically within the overall psychological process. If methods were available to observe the moment-to-moment activity within the brain, these dynamic patterns of local activation could be visualized. Indeed, evidence obtained by modern techniques for measuring local metabolic changes associated with neural activity, such as regional blood flow and positron emission tomography, have conclusively demonstrated the correctness of cortical localization, not only of sensorimotor processes, but of complex linguistic and cognitive activity (e.g., Lassen, Roland, Larsen, Melued, & Soh, 1977; Mazziota, Phelps, Carson, & Kuhl, 1982). Thus, during speech or reading, for example, multiple cortical areas increase their metabolic activity in the course of these mental and behavioral processes. The location of these circumscribed regions conforms quite well with the conventional cortical localization schemata derived from clinical observations on the impact of focal brain lesions.

However, the temporal sequencing and dynamic interactions among the active brain regions are not disclosed by these techniques of noninvasive mapping of brain metabolism. By contrast to the "steady state" mapping of cerebral metabolism, the electrical signals generated by neurons within the brain provide a real time manifestation of their activity. The idea that operations of the brain could be manifested in the massed electrical signals generated by groups of neurons during specific perceptual, cognitive, and motor activities formed the basis for the research program that my colleagues and I began in the early

1960s.[1] The expectation that specific brain processes could be delineated both in time and space within the brain was the cornerstone of this research into the neural basis of mental functions.

## ELECTROPHYSIOLOGICAL MANIFESTATIONS

The electrical activity of the brain was first observed by Richard Caton in 1875, when he noted fluctuations of currents recorded directly from the cortex in awake animals (viz. Caton, 1887). Responses to visual and auditory stimuli were found over the occipital and temporal cortex, respectively, and fluctuations were also seen over motor cortex when the animal moved its extremities. These briefly reported observations were not followed up, despite a few later reports that confirmed some of his observations. Sustained study of the brain's electrical activity in alert, behaving organisms did not begin until the remarkable series of experiments by Hans Berger during the 1920s. He discovered and described many of the properties of spontaneous electrical activity of the human brain, recorded from the intact scalp (Berger, 1929). The electroencephalogram (EEG), following its validation by Adrian and Matthews in 1934, became an important clinical tool in neurology by virtue of the characteristic electrical manifestations of epilepsy and other forms of brain pathology that it disclosed. Efforts to use the EEG for study of mental processes, which had been Berger's original intent, were not very fruitful. Although changes in brain rhythms could be observed in normal humans when visually stimulated or engaged in mental activity, specific brain responses to stimulation and with voluntary movement could not be readily discerned in the EEG. A few observations of potentials elicited by visual and auditory stimuli were reported during the 1930s, and one study, recording from the exposed motor cortex during epilepsy surgery, noted electrical responses from sensorimotor cortex that followed, but did not precede voluntary movements (Bates, 1951). The English physiologist George Dawson is credited with the invention of methods to record reliably sensory evoked potentials from the intact scalp. By averaging the brain activity following a series of identical stimuli, the more reliable time-locked brain responses evoked by the stimuli are progressively enhanced relative to the random background EEG. The introduction in the early 1960s of small averaging computers that could be used in the laboratory made the technique widely available, and a surge of investigation of human sensory evoked potentials (EP) were exploited both as a clinical tool and as a method for examining the cortical processing of stimuli in normal individuals.

[1]The initial studies of human brain activity associated with RT tasks were planned and carried out with Dr. L. D. Costa throughout the 1960s. We were joined in 1965 by Dr. Walter Ritter, who remains a principal collaborator in this work.

Observations of the electromagnetic manifestations of neural activity are capable in principle of depicting the moment-by-moment pattern of activity within the brain during sensorimotor and mental processes. Modern techniques of recording and signal analysis permit a detailed examination of the patterns of neural activity that are manifest during various psychological processes in both experimental animals and humans. Because microelectrode recordings from single neurons became the procedure of choice in animal neurophysiology by 1960, due to their greater specificity, averaged evoked potentials have been studied principally using human scalp recordings. The inferences concerning brain operations that could be drawn from these studies were initially severely limited by the lack of detailed information on the brain regions and specific neural processes that produce the scalp-recorded waveforms. During the past two decades the gap between scalp-recorded potentials and the detailed observations of brain physiology that can only be carried out in experimental animals has begun to be narrowed. This permits us to make increasingly confident statements regarding the cerebral origins of, and in some instances the neural mechanisms that underlie the scalp-recorded human brain potentials (viz. Vaughan & Arezzo, 1988).

The following brief remarks present a highly selective account of our quest for the chronotopic localization of specific brain processes that underlie certain mental operations. It emphasizes some of the work done by my colleagues and me, and is by no means a comprehensive review of work done by ourselves and others.

## "EVENT-RELATED POTENTIALS"[2]

We began our studies of human scalp-recorded potentials in 1961, when averaging computers first became commercially available. We believed that using the signal averaging technique we might be able to record averaged brain potentials specifically associated with sensory, motor, and cognitive processes. Our first experiments were directly designed after those of F. C. Donders. Initially, in simple RT tasks, we sought to identify the onset of cortical activity following visual or auditory stimulation, using the latency of the cortical evoked potentials (EP), and the onset of potentials overlying motor cortex prior to the response as indexes of cortical processing time. The time between the stimulus and onset of the sensory EP would define the duration of the afferent limb of the RT, whereas the time between motor cortex activation and the muscular response delineated its efferent limb. By subtracting these afferent and efferent transmission times from the total RT, we could measure the time utilized for central

---

[2]The term Event Related Potentials or ERP (Vaughan, 1969) was coined in order to encompass all types of brain potentials averaged in synchrony with a discrete stimulus or motor act.)

processing of the stimulus and initiation of the motor response (Vaughan, Costa, Gilden, & Schimmel, 1965). This "central delay" was between 20 and 60 msec. in simple RT tasks.

The potentials recorded in visual RT tasks were maximum in amplitude overlying the occipital visual cortex, and the "motor potentials" (MP) were localized to the central part of the scalp overlying motor cortex. This topographic localization made us confident that we were observing manifestations of the activation of visual and motor cortex respectively. However, the maximum auditory EP (AEP) overlies frontocentral cortex, rather than the temporal lobe nearest to auditory cortex. Furthermore, large components of the VEP, AEP, and SEP (somatosensory EP) that peak at about 200 msec. after the stimuli are all largest over the central scalp. Most investigators took this apparently common topography as evidence that these late "vertex" potentials were generated by the nonspecific thalamocortical projections that had received prominent attention in the cortical physiology of the 1950s and early 1960s.

We realized that interpretation of the physiological significance of the sensory EP, and other ERP discovered in association with discriminative and cognitive tasks was dependent on knowing where they were generated within the brain. Our search for evidence of "chronotopic localization" was critically dependent on reasonably accurate estimates of the location and configuration of active intracranial generators. This requirement led us to a series of topographical analyses, supplemented by a spatially extended dipole generator volume conduction model[3] that allowed us to estimate the surface potential distributions that would be expected with cortical generators of known location, size, and shape (Vaughan, 1974).

Our early studies of the topography of the various sensory EP and the MP demonstrated scalp distributions consistent with their generation within primary and secondary cortex of each sensory modality, and in the case of the MP, in motor cortex (Vaughan, 1969; Vaughan, Costa, & Ritter, 1968). Both the SEP and the MP had distributions along the mediolateral direction over the central scalp that were consistent with the sensory and motor homunculi delineated by Penfield and colleagues by electrical stimulation of the sensorimotor cortex. The scalp topography of the AEP was puzzling, in that it was largest near the vertex, far from primary and secondary auditory cortex. It had been suggested earlier by Wolfgang Köhler in his early studies of cortically generated currents, that the auditory cortex would generate currents flowing perpendicular to its surface, and thus would be maximal at the top of the head, where the axis perpendicular to the auditory cortex within the supratemporal plane reached the scalp. We showed that the AEP inverted in polarity at the approximate level of the sylvian fissure (Vaughan & Ritter, 1970), which was consistent with the postulated dipolar generator within the auditory cortex. This conclusion was controversial for many

---

[3]This model was developed in collaboration with Herbert Schimmel.

years, but a substantial body of converging evidence from lesion studies, magnetoencephalographic localization and quantitative generator modeling has settled the issue in favor of primary and secondary auditory cortical generation of the AEP (Vaughan & Arezzo, 1988).

The onset latency and duration of the sensory EP vary somewhat depending on the specific stimulus parameters, but the cortical EP to brief stimuli of moderate intensity generally have an onset latency of about 20–50 msec. and persist for about 250–300 msec. Thus, in general, passively repeated stimuli that do not require a discriminative response elicit a characteristic obligatory series of potentials that are apparently restricted to primary and secondary sensory cortex.[4]

Psychological studies suggest that perceptual duration, and the duration of iconic and echoic storage as well (Haber & Standing, 1969; Massaro, 1972), fall within the 250–300 msec. duration of the sensory EP. It seems likely in view of the timing and topography of the sensory EP that these obligatory cortical responses are manifestations of a part of neural activity that underlies the conscious perception of the stimuli.

An important early discovery in cognitive neurophysiology was made by Sutton and his colleagues (Sutton, Braren, Zubin, & John, 1965) when they noted a large, long latency evoked potential component that they labeled "P3" or P300[5] because it was the third positive peak of the ERP, occurring at around 300 msec. This wave was found in a task in which the subject did not know the identity of each successive stimulus, but had to guess before each trial. Sutton suggested that P3 might reflect resolution of uncertainty about the identity of each stimulus. We observed similar potentials in a passive stimulation situation in which either expected or unexpected pitch changes occurred within trains of identical stimuli (Ritter, Vaughan, & Costa, 1968). P3 was seen with the unexpected, but not the expected pitch changes. We then sought to learn whether P3 might occur in active discriminative tasks, with the idea that it might signal the discriminative brain process itself. We found that P3 was recorded whenever a discriminative response occurred, but not when two stimuli failed to be differentiated (Ritter & Vaughan, 1969).

We soon realized that P3, although an apparently ubiquitous component of the ERP in discriminative tasks, occurred too late to be a manifestation of the brain processes underlying the discriminative process itself (Ritter, Simson, & Vaughan, 1972). This circumstance led us to pay greater attention to the changes

---

[4]In primate physiology we identify as primary cortex those cytoarchitectonic areas that receive their principal thalamic input from the phylogenetically newer dorsal lateral geniculate nucleus, lateral medial geniculate nucleus and the VPL and VPM somatosensory thalamus. Secondary areas receive inputs both from primary sensory cortex and from other modality specific thalamic nuclei.

[5]ERP are traditionally labeled by their polarity and either their sequential position or latency with respect to the averaging event.

in the ERP waveform that preceded P3. We noticed that ERP elicited by the target stimuli in a two-stimulus discrimination task exhibited a negative deflection that immediately preceded P3. This "N2" or N200 component was especially distinct in trials with a longer RT due to the fact that, although N2 moved in latency with RT, the obligatory EP components, including the long latency P2 component, remained stable in latency. Thus, with longer RT the N2 component that was obscured by the concurrent P2 in short RT trials was unmasked. Inasmuch as the latency of N2 covaried with RT and its timing was consistent with a role in the discriminative process, we surmised that it might be a manifestation of target selection (Ritter, Simson, Vaughan, & Friedman, 1979). N2 was also found to be modality-specific in its topography, consistent with generators in secondary visual or auditory cortex. By contrast, P3 has a modality nonspecific topography overlying parietal association cortex, and in some conditions, frontal cortex as well. (Simson, Vaughan, & Ritter, 1977).

N2 is present in the target ERP in various kinds of discriminative tasks, regardless of whether the differentiation is based on the physical characteristics of the stimuli or upon some categorical rule, such as semantic classification (Ritter, Simson, & Vaughan, 1983). Differences in the onset and duration of N2 reflect both the difficulty of the discrimination and the type of discrimination required. For example, in a task that required discrimination of visual stimuli that differed in the complexity of their geometrical properties, the onset of N2 was about 175 msec. for the easier discrimination and 220 msec. for the harder one. By contrast, N2 onset in the semantic classification task was approximately 275 msec. In line with the interpretation that N2 represents target selection, these latencies would represent the time at which the discriminative process has provided sufficient information to differentiate the target from the nontarget stimuli. If we subtract the approximately 50 msec. required for the stimuli to arrive at visual cortex, we see that 125–170 msec. is the longest probable duration of the processes involved in the differentiation of the geometrical properties of the visual stimuli used in these tasks, whereas about 225 msec. is required for the more complex processes involved in identifying each word and deciding whether it fit the target semantic category. In either case, the brain processes required for each discrimination must be occurring prior to the onset of N2, that is, during the course of the obligatory sensory EP.

We should, therefore, be able to identify an ERP manifestation of these discriminative processes still earlier in the waveform than N2. When we compared the waveform of the nontarget ERP in the visual discriminative task with the ERP elicited by the same stimuli when no discrimination was required, we observed another negative component, which we called Na. This potential began at about 140–160 msec. after stimulus onset in all three of the discriminative tasks. Its duration, however, increased across tasks by somewhat less (about 30 msec. per task) than the increments in N2 latency. Furthermore, N2 began in all cases before the termination of Na. N2 began about 40 msec. after the onset of

Na in the easy geometric discrimination, approximately 70 msec. later in the harder discrimination, and at 120 msec. in the semantic classification. Thus, since the onset of N2 represents the time at which the target has been differentiated from the nontarget stimulus, the difference between the onset of Na and N2 can be taken as the duration of the discriminative process itself. Inasmuch as the semantic and the geometrical discriminations involve rather different neural mechanisms, we would anticipate that further electrophysiologic distinctions could be made within them. We would anticipate topographic differences between the Na recorded in the two geometric discriminations and that in the semantic classification task. Although a detailed topographic analysis of this potential has not yet been done, we find that the geometrical discriminations yield an Na topography restricted to the occipital and posterior temporoparietal scalp, whereas Na in the semantic task extends somewhat further anteriorly (Ritter et al., 1983). This result would implicate more of the posterior parietal cortex in the semantic discrimination process, in line with conventional neuropsychological localization of visual word meaning. The spatiotemporal diversity of the early cortical processing of visual stimuli is indicated by the fact that detailed analysis of the Na has disclosed no fewer than three subcomponents that overlap temporally but have different scalp topographies (Ritter, Simson, & Vaughan, 1988). It is our belief that Na and a number of relatively short latency negative potentials that have been reported by others reflect various aspects of the perceptual analysis of stimuli in discriminative tasks.

In an experiment with particular relevance for the spatiotemporal cortical localization of linguistic processes, we compared the ERP recorded with a set of letters, half of which, such as "D," had curved segments, and half of which rhymed with the letter "V" (Lovrich, Simson, & Vaughan, 1986). One task, "FORM," required a response to the letters with loops, which involved a geometrical discrimination. The other task, "RHYME," was to respond to the letters that rhymed with "V," which required that the letters be identified visually and then matched with their appropriate phonetic representations. The analyses in this experiment involved a comparison of the timing and topography of the ERP recorded during each discrimination condition with the ERP elicited by the letters when no discrimination was required. In both the RHYME and the FORM conditions a negative potential was present that began over the occipital region at about 150 msec. and continued until about 400 msec. This potential lasted longer in the RHYME condition, and its topography, while identical in the two conditions during the initial part of the waveform, extended anteriorly over the posterior temporal lobe in the RHYME condition. RT was longer for the RHYME than the FORM condition, consistent with the longer duration of the processing required in this task. The N2 potentials, which represented the differential processing of the target stimuli following the discrimination, also were longer in latency for the RHYME condition and had an anterior extension of their scalp distribution. These data provide direct physiological manifestations of the cortical processing involved in the visual identification of a letter, and the additional cortical processes required for retrieving its phonetic representation.

In another experiment, we compared the processing of auditory words identified according to their acoustic features, with a task that required their semantic classification (Lovrich, Novick, & Vaughan, 1988). Here, we found that acoustic processing manifested in the ERP involved auditory regions both within the sylvian fissure and on the lateral surface of the temporal lobe. When the topography of the ERP associated with acoustic processing was compared with that obtained in the semantic processing task, the latter extended into the posterior temporal and inferior parietal region, in contrast to the former, which were more restricted to the midtemporal region. These ERP localizations were again in conformity with clinical inferences on the cortical regions involved in phonetic versus semantic processes, derived from patients with focal lesions (Cappa, Cavallotti, & Vignolo, 1981).

## CHRONOTOPIC CORTICAL LOCALIZATION

The foregoing examples illustrate the possibility of using the timing and topography of ERP to define spatial and temporal sequences of cortical neural activity during the performance of specific perceptual and cognitive operations. Nevertheless, a number of empirical and theoretical limitations of ERP studies must be emphasized. First and foremost, scalp-recorded ERPs do not represent a full picture of the neural activity within the brain. It is obvious that they provide only a limited representation of the complex neural activity within active cortical regions. They must be complemented by neurophysiologic data obtained in experimental animals, which can, however, serve only as limited models for human cognitive processing. Nevertheless, a number of perceptual and cognitive processes do have their animal counterparts, especially in primates. Thus, it is possible that many of the detailed neural processes that underlie specific ERP can be disclosed by appropriate primate intracranial recordings.

It is also extremely important that proper methods of topographic recording and analysis be used to obtain optimal information from studies of scalp ERP distribution. Among the key requirements are an adequate number of scalp-recording sites, a method of reference-independent topographic mapping, and a suitable model to assist in the localization of intracranial generators (viz. Vaughan & Arezzo, 1988, for further discussion).

Careful attention must be paid to the design of the behavioral experiments themselves. It is important to employ a well-defined set of experimental conditions that tap the process under study, and that compare the brain responses to the same stimuli when they are passively received. Comparisons of several processing requirements in the same experiment are particularly valuable. Many of the experimental paradigms studied by cognitive psychologists can be directly adapted for ERP studies. Such direct comparisons can be of considerable value in clarifying a number of important issues regarding human information processing models that are of current concern in Cognitive Psychology (viz. Meyer, Osman, Irwin, & Yantis, in press; Miller, 1988).

I have not discussed the important question of how ERP components are related to processing stages, nor what the implications of parallel processing may be for the interpretation of ERP features. It is probably correct, however, to state that ERP can be localized to specific brain structures during those intervals of time defined by a stable topographic distribution of the ERP waveform. However, many processes of interest to cognitive neurophysiology will involve adjacent, concurrently active cortical regions. As yet we do not know the limits of spatial resolution of ERP topography. The success of magnetoencephalographic localization of cortical areas that are quite closely spaced, suggests that using proper analytic techniques, it will certainly be possible to resolve cortical localization of ERP generators to a centimeter or so (Kaukoranta, Hari, & Lounasmaa, 1987). Given the ability to define activation of a specific cortical region or regions over a defined time period, it is an empirical question as to whether a specific experimentally defined operation can be directly related in time to a concurrent ERP feature with a well-defined topography. This experimental enterprise offers great promise for future research in Cognitive Neurophysiology.

It must be emphasized that ERP may not disclose all active brain sites. Despite the fact that potentials generated within the brainstem and deep within the hemispheres can be detected at the scalp, due to volume conduction, many brain structures are not organized or oriented in a manner that permits recording of their activity at the scalp. For this reason, we must be extremely cautious in drawing negative conclusions regarding the extent of brain activation from scalp-recorded ERP. In most tasks of interest to cognitive science, we can assume, on the basis of connectivity alone, that many brain regions will participate during some portion of the information-processing task. We will have to pay particular attention to brain regions of known behavioral significance, such as deep limbic system structures, that may not manifest their activity at the scalp. Here, again, animal studies, as well as well-planned human studies in those instances in which intracranial recording can be carried out, can provide invaluable information unobtainable by noninvasive scalp recordings.

In conclusion, I feel confident in predicting that the cognitive sciences will soon begin to incorporate physiological insights into brain operations afforded by ERP studies in humans and experimental animals into more comprehensive and realistic models of human information processing. The merging of concepts and techniques from Cognitive Psychology, Neural Network Modeling, and Cognitive Neuroscience should presage new insights into the cognitive operations of the human brain.

# REFERENCES

Arezzo, J. C., Vaughan, H. G., Jr., Kraut, M. A., Steinschneider, M., & Legatt, A. D. (1986). Intracranial generators of event-related potentials in the monkey. In R. O. Cracco & I. Bodis–Wollner (Eds.), *Frontiers of clinical neuroscience. Vol. 3, Evoked potentials.* New York: Alan R. Liss, pp. 174–189.

Bates, J. A. V. (1951). Electrical activity of the cortex accompanying movement. *Journal of Physiology,* (Lond.), *113,* 240–257.

Berger, H. (1929). Über das Elektrenkephalogramm des Menschen. *Arch. Psychiatr. Nervenkr., 87,* 527–570. *Archic fur Psychiatrie und Nervenkrankheiten.*

Cappa, S., Cavallotti, C., & Vignolo, L. A. (1981). Phonemic and lexical errors in fluent aphasia: Correlation with lesion site. *Neuropsychologia, 19,* 171–177.

Caton, R. (1887). Researchers on electrical phenomena of cerebral grey matter. *Tr. Ninth Internat. Med. Congr. 3,* 246.

Donders, F. C. (1868). Over de snelheid van psychische processen. Onderzoekingen gedaan in het Physiologisch Laboratorium der Utrechtsche Hoogeschool, Tweede reeks, *2,* 92–120. (Trans. W. G. Koster), *Attention and Performance II,* 412–431.

Donders, F. C. (1969). On the speed of mental processes. In W. G. Koster (Ed.), *Attention and performance, 30, Vol. II.* pp. 412–431. Amsterdam: North Holland.

Geschwind, N. (1965). Disconnexion syndromes in animals and man. *Brain, 88,* 585–644.

Haber, R. N., & Standing, L. G. (1969). Direct measures of short-term visual storage. *Quarterly Journal of Experimental Psychology, 21,* 43–54.

Hebb, D. (1949). *The organization of behavior. A neuropsychological theory.* New York: Wiley.

Kaukoranta, E., Hari, R., & Lounasmaa, O. V. (1987). Responses of the human auditory cortex to vowel onset after fricative consonants, *Experimental Brain Research, 69,* 19–23.

Kulpe, O. (1909). *Outlines of psychology: Based upon the results of experimental investigation* (Third edition). New York: Macmillan. Translation of original work published in 1893.

Lassen, N. A., Roland, P. E., Larsen, B., Melmed, E., & Soh, K. (1977). Mapping of human cerebral functions: A study of the regional cerebral blood flow pattern during rest, its reproducibility, and the activations seen during basic sensory and motor functions. *Acta Neurol. Scand. Suppl. 64,* 262–263. Acta Neurologica Scandinavica Supplement.

Lovrich, D., Simson, R., Vaughan, H. G., Jr., & Ritter, W. (1986). Topography of visual event-related potentials during geometric and phonetic discriminations. *Electroencephalography and Clinical Neurophysiology, 65,* 1–12.

Lovrich, D., Novick, B., & Vaughan, H. G., Jr. (1988). Topographic analysis of auditory event-related potentials associated with acoustic and semantic processing. *Electroencephalography and Clinical Neurophysiology, 71,* 40–54.

Luria, A. R. (1973). *The working brain.* New York: Basic Books.

Massaro, D. W. (1972). Preperceptual images, processing time, and perceptual units in auditory perception. *Psychological Review, 79,* 124–145.

Mazziotta, J. C., Phelps, M. E., Carson, R. E., & Kuhl, D. E. (1982). Tomographic mapping of human cerebral metabolism: Auditory stimulation. *Neurology, 32,* 921–937.

Meyer, D. E., Osman, M. A., Irwin, D. E., & Yantis, S. (in press). Modern mental chronometry. *Biological Psychology.*

Miller, J. (1988). Discrete and continuous models of human information processing: Theoretical distinctions and empirical results. *Acta Psychologica, 67,* 191–257.

Minsky, M., & Papert, S. (1969). *Perceptrons.* Cambridge, MA: MIT Press.

Mitzdorf, U. (1985). Current Source-Density Method and Application in Cat Cerebral Cortex: Investigation of Evoked Potentials and EEG Phenomena. *Physiological Reviews, 65*(1), 37–100.

Pellionisz, A., & Llinøs, R. (1985). Tensor network theory of the metaorganization of functional geometries in the CNS. *Neuroscience, 16,* 245–273.

Ritter, W., Simson, R., & Vaughan, H. G., Jr. (1972). Association cortex potentials and reaction time in auditory discrimination. *Electroencephalography and Clinical Neurophysiology, 33,* 547–555.

Ritter, W., Simson, R., & Vaughan, H. G., Jr. (1983). Event-related potential correlates of two stages of information processing in physical and semantic discrimination tasks. *Psychophysiology, 20,* 168–179.

Ritter, W., Simson, R., & Vaughan, H. G., Jr. (1988). Effects of the amount of stimulus information processed on negative event-related potentials. *Electroencephalography and Clinical Neurophysiology, 69,* 244–258.

Ritter, W., Simson, R., & Vaughan, H. G., Jr., & Friedman, D. (1979). A brain event related to the making of a sensory discrimination. *Science, 203,* 1358–1361.

Ritter, W., Vaughan, H. G., Jr., & Costa, L. D. (1968). Orienting and habituation to auditory stimuli: A study of short term changes in average evoked responses. *Electroencephalography and Clinical Neurophysiology, 25,* 550–556.

Ritter, W., & Vaughan, H. G., Jr. (1969). Averaged evoked responses in vigilance and discrimination: A reassessment. *Science, 164,* 326–328.

Rosenblatt, F. (1962). *Principles of neurodynamics.* New York: Spartan.

Rumelhart, D. E., & McClelland, J. L. and the PDP Research Group. (1986). *Parallel distributed processing, Vol. 1.* In J. A. Feldman, P. J. Hayes, & D. E. Rumelhart (Eds.), *Parallel distributed processing,* Vol. 2. Cambridge, MA: MIT Press.

Scherg, M., & Von Cramon, D. (1986). Evoked dipole source potentials of the human auditory cortex. *Electroencephalography and Clinical Neurophysiology, 65,* 344–360.

Simson, R., Vaughan, H. G., Jr., & Ritter, W. (1976). The scalp topography of potentials associated with missing visual or auditory stimuli. *Electroencephalography and Clinical Neurophysiology, 40,* 33–42.

Simson, R., Vaughan, H. G., Jr., & Ritter, W. (1977). The scalp topography of potentials in auditory and visual go/nogo tasks. *Electroencephalography and Clinical Neurophysiology, 43*, 864–875.

Spengler, O. (1962). *The decline of the West*. New York: Knopf.

Sternberg, S. (1969). The discovery of processing stages: Extensions of Donders' method. In W. G. Koster (Ed.), *Attention and Performance* (Vol. 2, pp. 276–315). Amsterdam, London: North Holland.

Sutton, S., Braren, M., Zubin, J., & John, E. R. (1965). Evoked-potentials correlates of stimulus uncertainty. *Science, 150,* 1187–1188.

Taylor, D. A. (1976). State analysis of reaction time. *Psychological Bulletin, 83,* 161–191.

Vaughan, H. G., Jr. (1969). The relationship of brain activity to scalp recordings of event-related potentials. In E. Donchin & D. B. Lindsley (Eds.), *Averaged evoked potentials: Methods, results, evaluations*. Washington, D.C.: National Aceronatics and Space Administration (NASA No. SP 191), pp. 45–94.

Vaughan, H. G., Jr. (1974). The analysis of scalp-recorded brain potentials. In R. F. Thompson & M. M. Patterson (Eds.), *Bioelectric recording techniques, Part B: Electroencephalography and human brain potentials*. New York: Academic Press, pp. 157–207.

Vaughan, H. G., Jr., & Arezzo, J. C. (1988). The neural basis of event related potentials. T. W. Picton (Ed.), *Human event-related potentials* (EEG Handbook, Vol. 3), Amsterdam: Elsevier Science Publishers.

Vaughan, H. G., Jr., Costa, L. D., Gilden, L., & Schimmel, H. (1965). Identification of sensory and motor components of cerebral activity in simple reaction-time tasks. *Proceedings of the 73rd Conference of the Amer. Psychol. Assn., 1,* 179–180.

Vaughan, H. G., Jr., Costa, L. D., & Ritter, W. (1968). Topography of the human motor potential. *Electroencephalography and Clinical Neurophysiology, 25,* 1–10.

Vaughan, H. G., Jr., & Ritter, W. (1970). The sources of auditory evoked responses recorded from the human scalp. *Electroencephalography and Clinical Neurophysiology, 28,* 360–367.

von Monakov, C. (1911). Localization of brain functions. In W. W. Nowinski (Ed.), *The cerebral cortex*. Springfield, IL: Charles C. Thomas, pp. 231–250.

# 12

# Higher Cortical Functions in Humans: The Gradiental Approach

*Elkhonon Goldberg*

*Medical College of Pennsylvania and Institute for Advanced Studies, Hebrew University of Jerusalem*

## MAIN APPROACHES TO LOCALIZATION

Attempts to understand the principles of cortical localization of functions in humans have resulted in two basic types of approaches.

The first such approach is aimed at the formulation of fundamental dichotomies and has taken two forms. One of them, along the left–right dimension, emphasizes the distinction between linguistic, analytical, sequential, categorical, routinized, processes associated with the left hemisphere, and visuospatial, holistic, parallel, apperceptive, orienting and novel processes associated with the right hemisphere. The other fundamental dichotomy is concerned with the anterior–posterior dimension. This distinction, most succinctly formulated by Luria (1974, 1980), emphasizes the leading role of the anterior (frontal) cortex in sequential processing and the leading role of the posterior (parietal, temporal, and occipital) cortex in simultaneous processing. It can be said that these two dichotomies emphasize horizontal aspects of cortical organization.

The second basic approach to cortical brain-behavioral relations emphasizes what may be called the vertical aspect of cortical organization. It views the cortex as consisting of three types of functionally distinct regions with distinct hierarchic relationships among them. Usually, three fundamental levels of the cortical hierarchy are specified: Level 1 includes areas of primary cortico-subcortical interface characterized by stimulotopic organization (retinotopic, tonotopic, or somatotopic) and modality specificity. These include primary visual, auditory, and somatosensory cortices and the motor cortex. Level 2 involves cortices which are still modality-specific but are devoid of the stimulotopic organization and are critical for higher-order integration. Level 3

**229**

involves supramodal associative cortices which provide integration of various modalities and sensorimotor integration. Prefrontal cortex and posterior associative cortices (inferotemporal and inferior parietal) are usually assigned to this highest level of the cortical hierarchy. It has been argued, however, that further subdivision should be made within level 3, in the sense that prefrontal cortex is hierarchically higher than the temporo-parieto-occipital associative cortex (Goldberg, 1985; Goldberg & Bilder, 1987).

The hierarchic approach to cortical organization bears clear hereditary relationship to the work of Hughlings Jackson (1931/1932). Luria (1980) and Bernstein (1967) are among the most prominent contemporary advocates of this approach. The cognitive psychological theory developed by Miller, Galanter, and Pribram (1960) is clearly kindred to this approach although it does not focus on the cerebral substrates.

The purpose of this chapter is to introduce another approach to the brain-behavioral relations in the neocortex. I will refer to this approach as the gradiental approach.

Like the first, dichotomous approach, it emphasizes the horizontal aspect of cerebral organization. It emphasizes, however, the continuous aspect thereof rather than the oppositional, discrete aspect.

Like the second, hierarchic approach, the gradiental approach to be developed here makes substantial use of the concept of three levels of cortical hierarchies. It emphasizes, however, relations across these hierarchies rather than the vertical structure of the hierarchies.

It is proposed that the gradiental approach to cortical localization captures certain principles of cerebral organization which are as fundamental as the ones reflected in dichotomous and hierarchic approaches. It is *not* implied that the proposed gradiental approach should replace the other two. The three approaches, dichotomous, hierarchic, and gradiental, are not viewed as mutually exclusive. It is assumed, rather, that they capture different aspects of cerebral organization, and that all three have to be taken into account if one hopes to have a complete picture of functional cortical organization in humans.

In the subsequent discussion the principles of the gradiental approach will be formulated and an attempt will be made to substantiate it empirically.

This will be done with the full awareness of the fact that existing empirical evidence does not permit a complete, detailed substantiation of this approach at the time. There is enough evidence, however, to justify the formulation of this approach at least as a heuristically promising way of looking at cortical localization of functions if not as a fully verified theory.

In my attempts to substantiate the notion of the cognitive gradient, I will take the route common to neuropsychology and cognitive neuroscience. I will use findings of focal brain damage as the empirical basis, while attempting to reconstruct normal functions of corresponding cortical areas.

No attempt will be made to provide an exhaustive review of cortical neuropsychological syndromes. Only those syndromes will be reviewed that are particularly pertinent to the evaluation of the validity of the gradiental approach to localization.

## THE CONCEPT OF A COGNITIVE GRADIENT

Central to the gradiental approach to be developed here, is the premise of the high degree of consistency between the spatial and the functional metrics of the neocortex. By the spatial metric I mean the physical distribution of various cortical regions and physical distances between them. By the functional metric I mean a set of "distances" that characterize the relationship between various cortical areas in terms of their functional characteristics, in other words, in terms of the cognitive characteristics of the functions mediated by them.

It is proposed that an isomorphic or near-isomorphic relationship exists between these two metrics. This means that any two cortical regions are functionally close (in terms of their respective cognitive characteristics) if and only if they are also spatally close. The extreme formulation of this principle (which has to remain within the domain of mental experimentation) is as follows: Assuming that we can ordinally arrange spatial distances between every pair of cortical regions, and ordinally arrange cognitive distances between every pair of cortical regions, we would arrive at two identical arrangements.

The subsequent review will attempt to demonstrate that close relationships indeed exist between the spatial and functional cortical metrics.

Fundamental to the view of brain-behavioral relations to be developed here is the notion of a cognitive gradient. It will serve as the basic unit of analysis and is comparable in this sense with the concept of a level in the hierarchic model.

The notion of the cognitive gradient is only as viable as the notion of the cortical spatial-functional isomorphism is valid. By a cognitive gradient I mean an array of functionally distinct cortical regions aligned along the axis defined at its extremes by two areas of primary sensory cortical projections (A, B). It is presumed that the cortical regions along the axis thus defined adhere to the rule of spatial-functional isomorphism: Areas physically closest to the sensory projection area A are also functionally dominated by that sensory modality. As one moves away from pole A, one encounters areas which can be functionally described in terms of intermodal integration between modalities A and B. As one proceeds farther along the axis toward the other pole B, one encounters cortical regions dominated by sensory modality B.

It is clear that this definition of a cortical gradient is immediately applicable only to the posterior cortex. In the review of the evidence related to the concept of the cognitive gradient, I will consider the posterior cortex first. I will then attempt to extend the concept to include also the anterior cortex. The schematic, invariant structure of a posterior cognitive gradient is illustrated in Figure 1.

Further, it is clear that the cognitive gradient thus defined invariably consists of three types of areas as described in hierarchic terms (Figure 1). Any gradient by definition includes two primary cortical sensory projection areas at its extremes (level 1). Adjacent to each of them is an area which if described in hierarchic terms would be labeled as a level 2 area, that is, an area of higher-order but still modality-specific integration. Finally, in the center of the gradient a level 3 area is found, which can be characterized as associative, modality nonspecific. This establishes the relationship between the vertical, hierarchic, and the horizontal, gradiental dimensions of cortical localization: the hierarchic stratification can be applied to every gradient individually.

By the definition of cognitive gradient, there should be three of them in each of the posterior halves of the two hemispheres: occipitotemporal, occipitoparietal, and temporoparietal. These gradients are defined by the three corresponding areas of primary sensory cortical projections: the occipital striate Brodmann area 17 ($O_1$), the parietal, postcentral gyrus Brodmann areas 3, 1, and 2 ($P_1$), and the temporal Herschl area, corresponding to Brodmann areas 41 and 42 ($T_1$) (Carpenter, 1976). These extreme points of the gradients are presumed to be functionally equivalent in the left and the right hemispheres.

Symbols $O_1$, $P_1$, and $T_1$ will be used to denote the extreme points of the three gradients. To be entirely explicit, the occipitotemporal gradient is defined by the $O_1$–$T_1$ pair; occipitoparietal gradient by the $O_1$–$P_1$ pair; and the temporo-parietal gradient by the $T_1$–$P_1$ pair.

As mentioned before, there is a clear relationship between the horizontal, gradiental and vertical, hierarchic dimensions of cortical localization. Every gradient has level 1, level 2, and level 3 components. We will refer to modality-specific level 2 components as $O_2$, $P_2$, and $T_2$, respectively. We will refer to associative, level 3 components involved in intermodal integration as $OP_3$, $OT_3$, and $PT_3$, respectively. Figure 2 provides a schematic representation of the posterior cortical gradiental structure and the hierarchic composition of each

Schematic representation of a cognitive gradient

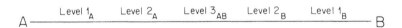

A ——— Level $1_A$ ——— Level $2_A$ ——— Level $3_{AB}$ ——— Level $2_B$ ——— Level $1_B$ ——— B

*FIGURE 1* Schematic representation of a cognitive gradient. A and B—two sensory modalities. Levels 1A and 1B—corresponding cortical primary sensory projection areas. Levels 2A and 2B—corresponding secondary, modality-specific cortical areas. Level 3AB—associative, tertiary cortex. (Reproduced from the *Journal of Clinical and Experimental Neuropsychology*).

Gradiental structure of posterior cortex

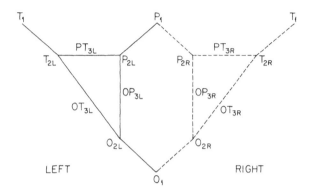

*FIGURE 2* Gradiental structure of posterior cortex. O1—primary visual cortex (Brodmann area 17); T1—primary auditory cortex (Brodmann areas 41 and 42); P1—primary somatosensory cortex (Brodmann areas 3, 1, and 2). O2—secondary visual cortex (Brodmann areas 18 and 19); T2—secondary auditory cortex (Brodmann area 22, or posterior partion of the superior temporal gyrus); P2—secondary somatosensory area (Brodmann areas 5 and 7, or superior parietal lobule); OT3—associative inferotemporal cortex; PT3—associative cortex (supramarginal gyrus division of the inferior parietal lobule); OP3—associative cortex (angular gyrus division of the inferior parietal lobule). These abbreviations refer to corresponding areas in the left hemisphere when amended by L, and the right hemisphere when amended by R. Damage to O2L produces visual object agnosia; OT3L—lexical deficit of Wernicke's type (when more anterior) and anomic aphasia (when more posterior); T2L—acoustic agnosia and semantic associative auditory agnosia; PT3L—semantic aphasia and acalculia of spatial type; P2L—tactile agnosia; OP3L—ideational apraxia and spatial apractagnosia. (Reproduced from the *Journal of Clinical and Experimental Neuropsychology*).

gradient. In this schematic form, the diagram applies both to the left and to the right hemispheres.

## THE POSTERIOR LEFT HEMISPHERE

Having defined the concept of the cognitive gradient, I will now defend its reality. We will begin our review with the posterior aspect of the left hemisphere.

The extreme points of the three left posterior gradients have already been defined since it is presumed that they are functionally equivalent for the left and the right hemispheres.

I will now specify secondary, level 2 components of the cognitive gradients of the posterior left hemisphere. It is proposed that all three level 2 areas of sensory modality-specific higher-order perceptual integration in the left hemisphere can be characterized in similar terms. All three are critical for categorical stimulus identification, in other words for recognizing specific exemplars as members of generic categories. When damage occurs to any of these three areas, a particular form of "symbolic" agnosia occurs. Although some of these syndromes are quite rare, their theoretical value for the understanding of brain-behavioral relationships should not be underestimated.

## Visual Object Agnosia

This syndrome (or "associative blindness," or "psychic blindness") was first described by Lissauer (1890) and Freud (1891), who in fact introduced the term "agnosia." Although the existence of this syndrome in its pure form has been questioned (Bender & Feldman, 1972), combined work by numerous investigators leaves no doubt about the reality of this syndrome (Albert, Reches, & Silverberg, 1975; DeRenzi & Spinnler, 1966; Hecaen & Albert, 1978; Hecaen & Angelergues, 1963; Hecaen et al., 1974; Luria, 1980; Rubens & Benson, 1971; Warrington, 1975). The syndrome is characterized by the dissociation between visual sensory and perceptual analysis which is intact, and the ability to assign the visual stimulus pattern to a generic category, to discern its "meaning," which is severely deranged. Upon visual examination of the object, the patient can accurately describe its sensory and perceptual attributes and even copy it but he or she is unable to identify it by name, through pantomime, or through functional description. The deficit is not a linguistic one, since (a) not only the ability to name the object but also the ability to convey its meaning through nonverbal means is impaired and (b) the deficit is limited to the visual sphere. As soon as the patient is allowed to examine the object tactilely, to smell its characteristic odor, or to hear its characteristic sound, the identification becomes easily available. It is not, on the other hand, an elementary sensory or perceptual deficit, since the perceptual pattern analysis is intact or near intact. What is defective, however, is that the patient treats the object as a meaningless stimulus pattern, unable to identify it as a member of a generic category. The syndrome can be naturally characterized as a higher-order integration deficit within visual modality.

The neuroanatomy of visual object agnosia has been invariably associated with the periphery of the occipital lobe, close to its border with the temporal and parietal lobes (Albert et al., 1975; Benson, Segarra, & Albert, 1974; Hecaen et al., 1974; Rubens & Benson, 1971; Warrington, 1975).

Although in the present context the intrahemispheric localization of the critical lesion is more important than the issue of its lateralization, the latter question can also be resolved on the basis of the available literature. Although some authors emphasized the bilateral nature of the lesion (Albert et al., 1975; Hoff & Pötzl, 1935), most authors associate the syndrome with left lateralized lesions (Benson et al., 1974; Hecaen et al., 1974; Lhermitte, Chedru, & Chain, 1973; Neilsen, 1937; Rubens and Benson, 1971; Warrington, 1975). There are only very few reports, on the other hand, associating the syndrome of visual object agnosia with the isolated right lateralized lesion (Nielsen, 1937).

In the probably most authoritative review up to date, Nielsen summarizes his extensive review of cases in the following fashion: "Within the occipital lobe the cortex of the second and third convolution represents an area which is essential for the recognition of objects" (1937, p. 133). Further examination of the diagram provided by Nielsen leads one to the conclusion that Brodmann area 19 and possibly also in part area 18 have to be involved in order to produce visual object agnosia.

On the basis of the aforedescribed clinical material, I will infer the normal function of the left occipital periphery (Brodmann areas 19 and in part 18) on its junction with the temporal and parietal alobes in the following fashion: It is involved in categorical identification of visual percepts which is a form of higher-order visual perceptual integration. This area corresponds to area $O_2$ in the schematic diagram of the left posterior gradiental structure (Figure 2).

## Tactile Agnosia

This syndrome (or "pure astereognosia," or "tactile asymbolia") is, in a cognitive sense, the tactile equivalent of the visual object agnosia. It was originally described by Wernicke (1894) and more recently by Hecaen and Albert (1978), Lhermitte and de Ajuriaguerra (1938), Luria (1980) and Bauer and Rubens (1985). The patient is unable to identify the object by touch, although he can easily do so with reliance on other sensory systems. Although some authors argued that the deficit is rooted in the impairment of elementary somesthesis (Dejerine, 1914), the existence of "pure astereognosia," a higher-order deficit unaccompanied by elementary sensory components, is currently accepted (Bauer & Rubens, 1985; Hecaen & Albert, 1978; Luria, 1980). "Pure astereognosia" implies an inability to make tactile identification of an object as a member of a meaningful generic category, even though the ability to describe separate tactile properties of the stimulus is preserved.

While some cases of pure astereognosia allow an essentially linguistic interpretation in terms of anomia (when astereognosia is limited to the left hand and the corpus callosum is damaged), others do not. These latter cases are of particular interest here. These are the cases of bilateral pure astereognosia (affecting both hands) in the presence of a unilateral lesion (Foix, 1922; Goldstein, 1916; Lhermitte & de Ajuriaguerra, 1938).

Cases of bilateral pure astereognosia unassociated with elementary sensory deficits or aphasia and secondary to a unilateral lesion can be best interpreted as deterioration of and/or impaired access to somatosensory generic engrams which provide categorical representations of open classes of equivalent objects. The anatomy of this form of astereognosia implicates the posterior part of the left hemisphere, in its parietal aspects, as the critical lesion (Lhermitte & de Ajuriaguerra, 1938). More specifically, Luria (1980) proposed that the secondary parietal areas are implicated. These correspond to Brodmann areas 5 and 7, or in other words, the superior parietal lobule.

On the basis of aforedescribed clinical material, I will infer the normal functions of the left parietal periphery (superior partietal lobule, Brodmann areas 5 and 7) in the following fashion: It is involved in categorical identification of tactile and proprioceptive percepts, which is a form of higher-order somatosensory perceptual integration. This area corresponds to area $P_2$ in the schematic representation of the left posterior gradiental structure (Figure 2).

## Acoustic Agnosia

This term is used by Luria (1980) to denote a clinical syndrome closely resembling Wernicke's aphasia (Goodglass, 1980; Goodglass & Geschwind, 1976). Although "acoustic agnosia" and "Wernicke's aphasia" refer to very similar entities, in terms of neuropsychological descriptions, as well as postulated mechanisms and neuroanatomical loci (Goodglass, 1980; Goodglass & Geschwind, 1976; Luria, 1980), they are not quite identical. This is not surprising, given the multitude of alternative taxonomies of aphasias. In effect, Luria emphasizes the phonological aspect of Wernicke's aphasia and treats it as a separate syndrome. In our subsequent discussion we will also treat the phonological and lexical (anomic) aspects of Wernicke's aphasia as two separate entities. Following Luria, we will refer to the former one as the "acoustic agnosia" and to the latter one as the "Wernicke's anomia." They are presumed here to have adjacent neuroanatomical territories but distinct, although related neuropsychological mechanisms, the first being essentially phonological, the second lexical. The specific location of the two respective neuroanatomical territories and their relative positions in the gradiental scheme will become clear from the subsequent discussions. Our subsequent discussion will be based on Luria's concept of "acoustic agnosia" but close parallels with Wernicke's aphasia will be obvious.

Acoustic agnosia is a deficit of phonemic hearing in the absence of elementary hearing deficits or primary articulation deficit. Luria (1980) argues that the deficit is rooted in an inability to apply dichotomous phonematic oppositional distinctions implicit in the distinctive features as described by Jakobson and Halle (1956). This assertion is based on the observation that in moderately severe cases of acoustic agnosia, phonematically distant (in terms of

Jakobson's metric of the number of distinguishing dichotomous features) sound pairs can be repeated but phonematically close ones cannot be repeated. In severe cases of this syndrome, phonemic differentiation is affected both for close and distant pairs.

The very term "acoustic agnosia" implies the postulated mechanism. Luria considers it a categorical disorder, whereby the "physical identity" of the sound may be intact but the ability to classify it as an allophone belonging to a particular phonemic class is impaired. The deficit is therefore categorical in the sense that it entails deficient sorting of allophones as members of generic, phonemically defined categories. Luria (1968, 1980) views the comprehension deficits and abundant literal paraphasias present in the verbal output of these patients as secondary to the fundamental impairment of categorical phonemic hearing. Deficits of reading and writing reveal the same phonematic basis as the underlying mechanism, and the errors parallel those present in the patient's oral output.

This description is not that different from the one of Wernicke's aphasia. In explaining the mechanism of florid paraphasias of Wernicke's type, Goodglass invokes the notion of breakdown of the phonological retrieval (1980).

The neuroanatomical descriptions of the critical lesions responsible for "acoustic agnosia" and "Wernicke's aphasia" are virtually identical: both implicate the posterior partion (the posterior third, according to Luria) of the superior temporal gyrus in the left hemisphere.

A related syndrome of "semantic associative" auditory agnosia has also been described (Faglioni, Spinnler, & Vignolo, 1969; Spinnler & Vignolo, 1966; Vignolo, 1982). The deficit involves an inability to understand the "meaning" of nonverbal sounds and noises, that is, to associate them with the correct source. Purely auditory perceptual aspects of analysis are, however, intact and the patient's capacity for "same-different" judgment with respect to nonverbal sounds is intact, nor does he or she suffer from amusia. Vignolo (1982) contrasts this syndrome to "discriminative" auditory agnosia in which auditory perception per se suffers.

Semantic associative auditory agnosia usually co-occurs with Wernicke's aphasia and the neuroanatomical territories associated with the two conditions strongly overlap. Semantic associative auditory agnosia is also invariably associated with left temporal damage. Unlike in "discriminative" auditory agnosia, same-different judgment with respect to meaningless sound pairs is intact both in semantic associative auditory agnosia and in Wernicke's aphasia (Vignolo, 1982). The latter observation is of particular interest, since it supports Luria's notion that auditory discrimination per se is intact in Wernicke's aphasia and that the deficit is categorical.

It is not entirely clear whether acoustic agnosia/Wernicke's aphasia and semantic associative auditory agnosia represent two different entities with different mechanisms but adjacent neuroanatomical territories, or whether they represent two aspects of the same syndrome with the same fundamental underlying mechanism which can take two different forms of expression. I tend to favor the latter possibility and think of both deficits as two manifestations of the same fundamental impairment of auditory categorization which transcends the traditional linguistic-nonlinguistic dinstinction.

On the basis of aforedescribed clinical material, I will infer the normal function of the secondary temporal area (posterior part of the superior temporal gyrus, or Brodmann area 22) of the left hemisphere in the following fashion: It is critically involved in categorical recognition of auditory stimulus patterns, which is a higher-order form of auditory perception. This unitary mechanism is critical both in the linguistic context where it provides the basis for phonemic hearing, and in nonlinguistic contexts where it provides the basis for categorization of environmental sounds. The area discussed corresponds to $T_2$ in the schematic representation of the left posterior gradiental structure (Figure 2).

In terms of the vertical, hierarchic approach to cortical localization, we have completed the review of secondary modality-specific, level 2 areas of the posterior portion of the left hemisphere. All three of them share the same fundamental property. They are involved in modality-specific categorical perception. They ensure, in other words, the capacity to identify a specific stimulus pattern as a member of a prespecified category. Each of the three areas ensures this capacity in a particular, single sensory modality: visual, somatosensory, or auditory, respectively. The concept of categorical perception as used here is not limited to linguistic perception; it is broader and is viewed as more fundamental on cognitive, developmental, and evolutional grounds.

I view the fundamental property of categorical perception as being the basic description of the posterior left-hemisphere function (Goldberg; in press-A). This point of view is distinctly different from the one regarding language as the fundamental attribute of the left hemisphere. I will further comment on the difference between these points of view in the latter parts of this chapter.

The secondary areas, together with previously reviewed primary modality-specific, level 1 areas (cortical projection areas) constitute the building blocks of the cognitive gradients to be introduced.

We are now ready to review the associative, level 3 areas and by so doing complete the cognitive gradients of the posterior left hemisphere. The neuroanatomical territories of the middle parts of the postulated occipitoparietal and temporoparietal gradients are adjacent and together they occupy the territory of the inferior parietal lobule, which is known to be a major part of the tertiary, associative cortex. It consists of two subdivisions, the supramarginal gyrus and the angular gyrus. On strictly geometrical, anatomical grounds, the angular gyrus can be readily assigned to the occipitoparietal gradient and the supramarginal gyrus to the temporoparietal gradient. Theoretically, then we will view the angular gyrus as the associative $OP_3$, area, and the supramarginal gyrus as the associative $TP_3$, area.

In reality, however, neuroanatomical descriptions of various neuropsychological syndromes do not clearly distinguish between the two subdivisions of the inferior parietal lobule. This is likely to be due to the very close proximity of the two gyri and their relatively small size. Most etiologies produce lesions which are too large to be contained within either one of these two areas.

## *Syndromes of the Left Inferior Parietal Lobule—Angular Gyrus*

Several major categories of deficit have been prominently associated with lesions in this area.

## Ideational and Ideomotor Apraxias

The notion of "ideational apraxis," introduced by Liepmann (1900, 1908), refers to the disintegration of skilled, overlearned, object-oriented movements. Although individual motor components are intact, their integration into coherent motor programs fails (Hecaen & Albert, 1978). Liepmann's definition of "ideational apraxia" requires that it occur without associated paresis or ataxia, and the presumed mechanisms is that of the disintegration of "motor engrams." The deficit is bilateral and general rather than segmental with respect to body parts (Hecaen & Albert, 1978), but it is produced by a unilateral, circumscribed lesion limited to the posterior part of the dominant hemisphere (De Renzi, Pieczulo, & Vignolo, 1968). Posterior parietal and temporoparietal regions of the left hemisphere appear to be the critical locus for this syndrome (de Ajuriaguerra, Hecaen, & Angelergues, 1960; Hecaen & Albert, 1978). More specifically, Foix (1916) and Heilman and Gonzales Rothi (1985) associate it with the damage to the left angular gyrus.

Ideomotor apraxia is variably defined as being limited to simple, single gestures (Hecaen & Albert, 1978), or as deficit of imitation of object use (as opposed to actual object use) (Morelaas, 1928). It is also a bilateral, whole-body (nonsegmental) deficit usually caused by a unilateral, left parietal lesion. Some authors regard ideomotor apraxia as a severe form of ideational apraxia (Denny-Brown, 1958; Sittig, 1931; Zangwill, 1960) but others view the two syndromes as distinct although highly related (De Renzi, Pieczulo, & Vignolo, 1968; Foix, 1916; Morelass, 1928). Hecaen (1967) proposed that the difference between the two syndromes may be related to two types of gestural behavior: conventional symbolic and expressive gestures vs. gestures descriptive of object use (with or without the real object). Like ideational apraxia, ideomotor apraxia is also associated with lesions of the angular gyrus (Foix, 1916) or supramarginal gyrus (Heilman & Gonzales Rothi, 1985).

## Spatial Apractagnosia

Luria (1980) used this term to denote a group of deficits of processing asymmetric, meaningful spatial arrays, such as maps, clocks without numbers on the clock face, letters, and digits. What appears to be the common denominator among the stimuli whose processing is affected in this condition is (a) their symbolic, representational nature; (b) visual input modality; (c) asymmetrical space being critical in representing the meaning of the symbols. "Spatial apractagnosia" arises following inferoparietal lesions in the occipitoparietal junction, in the area of angular gyrus. Luria claims that either left or right side of the lesion can produce the deficit with the left occipitoparietal lesions producing a more severe deficit.

Whereas Luria regards "apractagnosia" as a unitary syndrome which is likely to encompass all the aforementioned components, other authors consider its different aspects separately. Thus Hecaen and Albert (1978) and Benton (1985) talk about loss of *topographical concepts* (mental maps) as a separate clinical entity, distinct from the disturbance of processing letters and digits.

The postulated neuroanatomy of this syndrome is at variance with the one proposed by Luria in terms of its lateralization but also implicates the parietooccipital junction. According to Hecaen and Albert (1978), deficits of topographical concepts (map reading) are usually seen following bilateral or right-sided lesions in the posterior parietal areas. However, Benton (1985) questioned these data because of the likely confounding effects of the fixed left hemifield visual neglect associated with the damage to the right hemisphere. He suggests that both hemispheres may play a role in the topographical orientation deficits. This appears to be the most plausible conclusion.

The other component of Luria's complex syndrome of "apractagnosia" is known as "alexia with agraphia," or "parietal alexia" (Friedman & Albert, 1985; Hermann & Poetzl, 1926; Hoff, Gloning, & Gloning, 1954). It is characterized by the absence of obvious aphasia, but is highly associated with apraxia and acalculia. Left angular gyrus is commonly regarded as the cortical lesions responsible for this syndrome (Benson & Geschwind, 1969; Hecaen, 1967; Nielsen & Raney, 1938), in agreement with the location of Luria's "apractagnosia." A related deficit, alexia/agraphia for numbers is also associated with the territory of the left angular gyrus (Henschen, 1925; Levin & Spiers, 1985).

The two types of deficits—(1) ideational/ideomotor apraxias; and (2) the group of deficits involving processing of visually presented, spatially asymmetrical, meaningful layouts—appear to share the same neuroanatomical territory, that of the angular gyrus in the left hemisphere. Neuroanatomically, this is a subdivision of tertiary, associative, supramodal cortex (Carpenter, 1976) on the parieto-occipital junction. Geometrically it is located in the middle of the occipitoparietal gradient, or area $OP_3$, in Fig. 12.2.

It is proposed here that both the ideational/ideomotor apraxia and the "apractagnosia" (including alexia and agraphia) seen following lesions of the left angular gyrus area represent two clinical forms of the same fundamental deficit: disintegration of the visuospatial synthesis with respect to categorical processing.

"Apractagnosia" by definition involves impairment of visual arrays for which the appreciation of asymmetrical properties is fundamental (e.g., letters, clock hands). In this respect, symbols are radically different from real objects. In object recognition, only the vertical axial asymmetries are important whereas horizontal ones by and large are not. In symbol recognition, both types of asymmetries are often relevant. Deficit of spatial analysis is therefore more central to "apractagnosia" than it is to visual object agnosia as described previously.

Ideational and ideomotor apraxias entail disintegration of visuosomatosensory synthesis, since object manipulation is usually involved.

This generalization regarding the common basis between apraxia and "apractagnosia" is supported by the fact of their usual co-occurence (Luria, 1980; Friedman & Albert, 1985).

Both deficits involve disintegration of categorical representations. "Apractagnosia" is by definition characterized by the deficient processing of symbolic, generic representations. Apraxias of the aforementioned types should be regarded as deficits of categorical representations since the "motor engrams" affected describe motor programs invariant across a variety of specific conditions, applicable to any object of a given class and executable by any limb.

On the basis of the aforementioned clinical material, I infer the normal function of the left parieto-occipital junction (angular gyrus) in the following fashion: It is critical for intermodal, associative integration between higher-order visual and somatosensory/spatial information which is symbolic, representational in nature. In terms of our notation, this area is $OP_3$, the associative, level 3 component of the occipitoparietal gradient. The cognitive characterization of this area is in complete agreement with its neuroanatomical geometry. Both cognitively and spatially it is situated between the visual modality-specific and the somatosensory/spatial modality-specific areas of higher-order integration. The rule of cognitive-neuroanatomical isomorphism appears to hold along the occipitoparietal axis, and we have completed the left occipitoparietal cognitive gradient. It can be otherwise referred to as the visuospatial gradient of symbolic representations.

I characterized it in terms of two fundamental characteristics: First, it is organized in the continuous, level 1–level 2–level 3–level 2–level 1 fashion. This is the general, invariant structure of all the cognitive gradients of the posterior cortex.

Secondly, the components of these gradients were characterized as being involved in symbolic, generic representation. This is the specific property of the left hemisphere. It is proposed that the right hemisphere occipitoparietal gradient does not share the latter property.

## *Syndromes of the Left Parietal Inferior Lobule—Supramarginal Gyrus*

### Semantic Aphasia

Following Head (1926), Luria (1980) maintains that lesions of the left parieto-occipital areas lead to a particular language disorder. The disorder consists of difficulties in comprehending and expressing asymmetrical relational constructions ("complex logicogrammatic constructions," according to Luria). Luria terms the deficit "semantic aphasia." It is characterized by the preservation of phonological and lexical (nominative) aspects of language (which sets it apart from Wernicke's or amnestic aphasia), and severe disruption of the comprehension and expression of a wide range of relational constructions. These include spatial relations ("below" vs. "above," "to the right of" vs. "to the left of"), temporal relations ("before" vs. "after") and other comparative relations ("smaller" vs. "larger," "taller" vs. "shorter"). The patient suffering from semantic aphasia cannot differentiate between reversible constructions derived on the basis of such relational terms (e.g., between "Bob arrived before Jim" and "Jim arrived before Bob"). Comprehension of passive voice and possessive case is affected in a similar fashion, so that the patient cannot differentiate between "father's brother" (i.e., "uncle") and "brother's father" (i.e., "father"), or between "Jim was hit by Bob" and "Bob was hit by Jim."

Luria (1970, 1980) maintains that the syndrome of "semantic aphasia" as well as its association with the lesions of the left inferoparietal area has been well documented in large numbers of cases. Luria distinguishes it from the agrammatism secondary to the anterior (Broca's) lesions. It is quite puzzling that the linguistic propositional deficits described by Luria under the rubric of "semantic aphasia" have received so little attention in the contemporary Western aphaseology. It is not mentioned in taxonomies of aphasias provided by such authorities as Goodglass, Geschwind, Benson, or Hecaen. I assume, however, that the syndrome is real.

### Acalculia

Various types of acalculia have been described; among those "acalculia of the spatial type" (Levin & Spiers, 1985) is of particular relevance here. Description of this type of acalculia correspond closely to the definition of acalculia provided by Luria (1980). It is characterized by the disintegration of the decimal structure of numbers and of the appreciation of the spatial asymmetries implicit in the decimal number structure. The patients cannot properly align compound multidigit numbers in written computations or, in severe cases, even understand their meaning. It is different from alexia/apraphia for numbers in that the ability to read or write separate digits is preserved. Spatial acalculia is usually associated with the inferoparietal, post-Rolandic lesions (Levin & Spiers, 1985; Luria, 1980). There is no consensus regarding the lateralization of the critical lesion. Hecaen, Angelerques, & Houillicr (1961) maintain that isolated spatial acalculia is consistent with an isolated right-hemisphere lesion. However, acalculia in the context of Gerstmann's syndrome and/or in combination with the features of "semantic aphasia" have been associated with left inferoparietal lesions (Gerstmann, 1940; Luria, 1980). It may be reasonable to conclude that damage to the inferoparietal area on either side can contribute to the disintegration of computational skills. The two hemispheres may provide different contributions and their relative roles may vary as the function of individual differences (Goldberg & Costa, 1981).

Luria (1980) proposed that the cognitive mechanism of "semantic aphasia" is related to the disintegration of the spatial basis of relational constructions. This implies that normal cognitive representations of a wide range of relational concepts are spatial or "quasispatial" in nature. This is true, according to Luria, not only for spatial relations, but also for temporal, quantity comparison relations, as well as for those expressed by passive voice and possessive case.

Likewise, Luria (1980) regards acalculia of the spatial type to be secondary to the disintegration of the spatial basis of numerical concepts. This implies that normal cognitive representations of numbers and numerical operations have a very strong spatial component. Luria bases this conclusion on cultural-anthropological and developmental considerations.

If one accepts these interpretations as I do, then one has to conclude that the syndromes of "semantic aphasia" and "acalculia of the spatial type" represent two manifestations of the same fundamental cognitive deficit: disintegration of the spatial aspect of cognitive representations underlying linguistic and otherwise symbolic (e.g., numerical) codes. Indeed, "semantic aphasia" and acalculia are highly correlated phenomena, according to Luria (1980).

What is the nature of the presumed unitary cognitive dimension whose disintegration leads to "semantic aphasia" and acalculia of the spatial type? I propose that the cognitive dimension in question is that of the interface between linguistic (and quasilinguistic) and spatial representations. It is the cognitive capacity for linguospatial integration. In this sense we are dealing with an intrinsically intermodal integration between the auditory-based linguistic systems and somatosensory-based spatial schemata.

In terms of its cognitive status, the proposed cognitive dimension of "linguospatial interface," or "spatial basis for linguistic representations," adheres closely to the properties expected of the middle, level 3 segment of the left temporoparietal gradient, or area $PT_3$, in our notation (Fig. 12.2). Distintegration of this cognitive dimension is indeed associated with damage to the left inferoparietal area.

In our idealized gradiental scheme, it is tempting to differentiate between the angular gyrus, which is viewed as the associative, level 3 segment of the occipitoparietal cognitive gradient, and the supramarginal gyrus, which is viewed as the associative, level 3 segment of the temporoparietal cognitive gradient.

Unfortunately, this distinction is not made in the neuroanatomical descriptions of spatial acalculia or semantic aphasia. Instead, more general terms such as "retro-Rolandic" or "inferoparietal" are used. This is understandable in view of the fact that most etiologies produce lesions too large to be contained within but one subdivision (angular or supramarginal) of the inferior parietal lobule.

The cognitive gradiental theory predicts that the postulated cognitive dimension of the "spatial basis of symbolic representations" is specifically associated with the supramarginal gyrus more than the angular gyrus, since it is the former which constitutes the geometrical center of the temporoparietal gradient. This prediction will have to await an empirical verification or refutation by neuroimaging means in normal individuals. Functional neuroimaging techniques, such as position emission tomography (PET), regional cerebral blood flow (rCBF), or computerized multiple recording electrophysiological imaging (BEAM), under conditions of appropriate cognitive activation seem like the potentially most promising techniques to assess the differential contributions of the angular gyrus and supramarginal gyrus. A considerable amount of time may elapse, however, until the spatial resolution of these neuroimaging techniques will begin to approach the required degree of precision.

## Neurolinguistic Digression I: Cortical Representation of Lexicon

In order to be able to proceed further with the discussion of cortical cognitive gradients, we must first discuss the cerebral representation of lexical knowledge in general terms. Logically, two extreme possibilities should be considered: (a) that cerebral representation of lexical knowledge is compact and distinct, separated from the cerebral representations of those aspects of the physical world which it is supposed to denote; (b) that cerebral representation of lexical knowledge is distributed and is in close relationship with cerebral representations of the various aspects of the physical world which it is supposed to denote. The distributedness of lexical representation will then follow from the fact that various aspects of the physical world are represented in different parts of the cortex. Cerebral representations of the corresponding lexical domains will be expected to be distributed in a similar way.

The fundamental assumption of "separateness" of lexical vs. perceptual cerebral representations was implicit in the "disconnection" view of anomia (Geschwind, 1965, 1967; Geschwind & Kaplan, 1962). While this point of view is easily capable of explaining anomia on confrontation, in particular its modality-specific forms (Beauvois, Saillant, Meininger, & Lhermitte, 1978; Freund, 1889; Lhermitte & Beauvois, 1973), anomia in spontaneous speech, in particular phenomena such as semantic (verbal) paraphasias cannot be explained by the disconnection approach nearly as easily. The disconnection theory-based view of anomias as a retrieval deficit (Gardner, 1973; Goodglass & Geschwind, 1976; Weigel–Crump & Koenigsnecht) against the background of intact semantic representations has also been questioned recently.

The alternative point of view, namely that semantic knowledge, or the "mental dictionary" itself is impaired, has been gaining prominence, and it offers powerful, albeit indirect, support for the idea of the distributed nature of cerebral representation of lexical knowledge.

The "semantic deficit" hypothesis implies that in anomic patients the organization of the *physical world* representations through hierarchically related categories is disrupted. Presumably, the distinction between semantically critical and incidental perceptual features is blurred, and the ability to select and apply such perceptual features for categorical recognition of objects is compromised. Three lines of evidence support this conclusion. First, it has been demonstrated that categorization processes are impaired in patients with anomia both with respect to pictures of objects (Grober, Perecman, Kellar, & Brown, 1980) and words-nouns (Grober et al., 1980; Zurif, Caramazza, Myerson, & Galvin, 1974). The deficit is particularly pronounced for low-typicality items. Secondly, it has been demonstrated that in tasks requiring classification of pictorial representations into two (or more) functionally defined categories, anomic patients fail to use what Caramazza, Berndt, and Brownell (1982) call "semantically guided, perceptual parsing ," in other words, to base their classification selectively on semantically salient perceptual properties (Caramazza, Berndt, & Brownell, 1982; Whitehouse, Caramazza, & Zurif, 1978). Finally, it has been demonstrated that perceptual degradation of pictorial images exacerbate anomia in aphasic patients even when they retain the ability to recognize the images (Benton, Smith, & Lang, 1972; Bisiach, 1966; North, 1971).

This evidence implies that under normal conditions, lexical-semantic and perceptual-categorical "dictionaries" are intertwined and are likely to be built of the same units of encoding (Miller & Johnson–Laird, 1976), and that the process of "evoking" a verbal label entails discerning in the object of perceptual properties which are salient in terms of it categorical attribution, which is what is meant by "semantically guided perceptual parsing."

To the extent that one believes in the essential unity of perceptual and semantic "dictionaries," one is tempted to infer that the cerebral representations of the two also strongly overlap, or may even be the same. Although indirectly, this reasoning provides strong support for the hypothesis of the distributed nature of cerebral representation of the lexicon.

This means, in a nutshell, that lexical-semantic representations of certain concepts are localized in close proximity to the areas in which the representations of corresponding aspects of the physical world are localized. It is obvious that most representations of things and events are multimodal, but it is likely that representations of certain types of objects or events are more dependent on certain modalities than on others. Thus, one would assume that representations of static objects are more visually based than based on other modalities (this assertion is supported by the work of Beauvois, 1982; Goodglass, Barton, & Kaplan, 1968), and that representations of actions are more based on motor images than are representations of, shall we say, colors. This means, among other things, that cerebral representation of nouns (the lexical domain which denotes objects) is expected to be in intimate proximity to the cortical areas involved in visual processing (i.e., occipital cortex) and cerebral representation of verbs is expected to be in intimate proximity to the cortical areas involved in the control over motor sequences (i.e., premotor cortex).

My reasoning here is deliberately crude to emphasize the main points. In reality, of course, one has to think in terms of shades of gray rather than stark black-and-white distinctions. Neither "objects" nor "actions" constitute cognitively homogeneous classes, let alone "nouns" and "verbs." First, both nouns and verbs differ in terms of their degree of "physicality." The verb "idealize" is certainly less directly linked to motor images than verbs "punch" or "kick." Likewise, the noun "republic" does not nearly as readily correspond to a physical object as the noun "table" does. Secondly, even for those lexical items which are readily related to distinct physical objects or events, their representations may be characterized by different combinations of sensory modalities. Thus, on a priori grounds, one may expect that tool-objects may have more complex representations than nonfunctional objects in that they would rely not only on visual but also on proprioceptive and motor representations. Likewise, object-oriented (transitive) actions may be based on more complex representations than intransitive actions, the latter being more purely motor and the former involving visual and kinesthetic representations in addition to motor ones.

In spite of these complicating factors, the hypothesis of the distributed nature of lexical representations and its link to cerebral representations of the denoted aspects of physical world, is a testable hypothesis, since it leads to certain predictions and is falsifiable on the basis of already available data.

The concept of "distributedness" of lexicon in the above sense was implicit in the work of Luria (1980), who maintained that posterior, temporal lobe aphasias are characterized by a greater degree of impairment of nouns and to some extent adjectives than verbs or prepositions; that posterior, parieto-occipital aphasias are predominantly characterized by the impairment of prepositions and adverbial clauses; and that anterior aphasias are characterized by particular disintegration of verbs, with nouns being more intact. The latter claim is made both with respect to "efferent motor" aphasia which in Luria's taxonomy roughly corresponds to Broca's aphasia, and to Kleist's dynamic aphasia which can be understood as the deficit of the executive control over linguistic behavior, rather than as disintegration of linguistic structures per se.

This point of view has not found much support in North American and European neuropsychology, and it is in direct contradiction with the work of Goodglass et al. (1966), who failed to find any differences in noun-versus-verb utilization when anterior and posterior aphasias were compared. Most Western authors associate lexical deficit with posterior, Wernicke's and amnestic aphasias. Vast literature exists to support this notion (Coughlan & Warrington, 1978; Damasio, McKee, & Damasio, 1979; Yamadori & Albert, 1973, to quote a few). Furthermore, several studies directly compared posterior and anterior aphasias and concluded that lexical knowledge is deranged in the former and relatively intact in the latter (Grober et al., 1980; Whitehouse, Caramazza, & Zurik, 1978; Zurif et al., 1974). All these findings, however, are inconclusive in the context of our discussion because usually only nouns were assessed, and the status of verbs is left unexplored. These studies certainly demonstrate quite convincingly that lexical knowledge *for nouns* is impaired in posterior but not in anterior aphasias. This is a very important finding in its own right, but it sheds no light on the possibility of verb-noun, anterior-posterior double dissociation because these experiments were not designed to detect it even had it existed. The available studies therefore fail to provide any basis for choosing between these two possibilities: that the double dissociation indeed exists, or that all lexical knowledge is associated with the posterior brain.

There are but very vew quantitative, experimental studies known to me where nouns and verbs were explicitly compared with respect to anterior-posterior distinction. As mentioned before, Goodglass, Klein, Carey, & Jones, (1966) failed to find any verb-noun lexical proficiency difference between anterior and posterior aphasis. Miceli et al. (1983), however, described massive omission of main verbs but no comparable omission of nouns in a case with a documented focal lesion in the Broca's area. Furthermore, Miceli et al. (1984) demonstrated a *double dissociation* between verbs and nouns, and between agrammatical and anomic aphasics. In the former, naming actions was more impaired than naming objects. The latter demonstrated the opposite picture. Consistent with these findings is the report by Brown, Lehman, & Marsh (1980), of the noun-verb, anterior-posterior double dissociation in normal subjects. They studied the topography of the CNV-like preparatory, slow negative wave during a listening task. Two types of stimuli were used, both involving homophones. The first type involved verb phrases, the second noun phrases (constructed of the same set of homophones, e.g., "sit by the fire," vs. "ready, aim, fire"). It was found that the preparatory wave was shifted anteriorly during processing of verb phrases and posteriorly during listening to noun phrases.

Given the sparsity of experimental studies of the issue, we have to resort to more clinical reports.

## "Posterior Aphasias"

It is universally agreed that speech of posterior, "fluent" aphasics is characterized by the emptiness of content, the lack of object-words (Goodglass & Geschwind, 1976; Luria, 1980). Luria (1980) noted that verbs are better preserved in their spontaneous speech and that they tend to resort to the description of actions, that is, to verbs in their circumlocutory attempts to name an object. This implies a specific dissociation: a specific impairment for nouns but not verbs in posterior aphasias. In relating it to the underlying mechanisms, one is tempted to attribute this dissociation to the fact that the lexical domain most impaired in posterior aphasias (secondary to lesions on the temporo-occipital axis) is that which denotes (predominantly) visually represented aspects of physical world. This interpretation finds its support in two observations. Warrington (1975) reported a case of anomia associated with visual object agnosia due to a posterior lesion. The anomia was characterized by a greater impairment of concrete (i.e., sensory-based) nouns than abstract nouns (i.e., those unrelated to a distinct sensory image). Goodglass, Heyde, and Blumstein (1969) reported that highly picturable nouns are the ones most impaired in fluent (Wernicke's and amnestic) aphasias. The authors were reluctant to use the visual imagery-based explanation of the phenomenon since they concluded that it would entail "construction of an ad hoc neurological model." The general concept of the distributed nature of cerebral representation of lexical knowledge is certainly more than an ad hoc model; in fact, it would predict the findings of Goodglass and his associates.

In a very insightful single case study, Yamadori and Albert (1973) described a patient with a left posterior dysfunction and anomia for nouns. The lexical deficit was selective, since it affected bodily parts and room objects but not tools (whose representations are likely to have a stronger motor component). The patient's circumlocutions were characterized by resorting to action words, for example, "to help people walk" for "cane," "to sit on" for "chair."

## "Anterior" Aphasias

Broca's aphasia (or in Luria's nomenclature, "efferent motor aphasia") is commonly characterized as "telegraphic" or "agrammatical" (Goodglass & Geschwind, 1976; Luria, 1980). While appreciating the agrammatical nature of spontaneous speech in this syndrome, Luria (1980) was equally impressed by the lack of verbs in the patients' spontaneous speech. He viewed the deficit as related to the disintegration of the predicative structure of language. The concept of internal speech introduced by Vygotsky (1962) is of central importance to this line of reasoning. Vygotsky viewed "internal speech" as the level of deep structure, a condensed plan of a narrative utterance. Internal speech was essentially *predicative,* according to Vygotsky. The underlying mechanism of Broca's aphasia is therefore viewed as distrubance of internal speech, in other words, disturbance of predicative in nature, internal plans of the discourse. Agrammatism, which characterizes Broca's aphasia, is viewed as the manifestation of the disintegration of the predicative structure. It is therefore the disintegration of predicative, action-based aspects of language which underlies the agrammatism of Broca's type, according to Luria. This point of view was shared also by Roman Jakobson (1964).

Evaluation of samples of nonfluent aphasics' spontaneous speech provided by other authors also strikes one as being more devoid of verbs than of nouns, even when this feature is not emphasized by the authors themselves (as in examples provided by Goodglass & Geschwind, 1976). These authors do, however, note that in highly inflected languages, such as German, there seems to be a shift to nominalized use of verbs. This finding was confirmed by Saffran, Schwartz, & Marin, (1980). A similar observation was made by Luria with respect to Russian, also a highly inflected language. The nominalization of verbs in nonfluent asphasics seems to be a phenomenon complementary to the heavy reliance on verbs in fluent aphasics' circumlocutions.

The so-called Kleist's dynamic aphasia, which is observed following damage to a somewhat more anterior (than in Broca's aphasia) division of the left hemisphere, has been characterized as a deficit selectively affecting language behavior rather than disintegration of linguistic competence per se. It will be discussed in greater detail later in this review. At this point I will only mention that it is also characterized by a conspicuous *paucity* of action words and predicative forms (Luria & Tsvetkova, 1968).

Although some authors view the disruption of the action-words and the predicative structure in anterior aphasias as a manifestation of or a consequence of general agrammatism, I propose the opposite direction of causation: The disruption of the grammatical structures in nonfluent aphasics is due to the disruption of the predicative basis of language which is essentially verb, action-based.

To summarize our neurolinguistic digression, the point of view advanced here is that the cerebral representation of lexical, semantic knowledge is not compact, but that it is distributed throughout the neocortex. This distribution of various lexical domains parallels the distribution of cortical representations of corresponding aspects of the physical world denoted by these lexical domains.

This approach has to be viewed as hypothetical at this point. I feel, however, that it is sufficiently substantiated to serve as the basis for our further discussion of some of the cognitive gradients to be considered.

## *Syndromes of the Left Temporo-occipital Junction*

### Fluent Aphasias

The middle part of the temporo-occipital cognitive gradient, its level 3, $OT_3$, part, should occupy the associative part of the temporal lobe in close proximity to the temporo-occipital junction. This is the cortical territory whose damage leads to "fluent" aphasias: the Wernicke's anomia (posterior part of the superior temporal gyrus) and in particular the anomic aphasia (posterior part of the middle temporal gyrus). According to the rule of cognitive-structural isomorphism, the function of this posterior temporal area should be intermodal and intimately related to the integration of visual and auditory modalities. In the left hemisphere, the function of this area should be symbolic, representational in nature.

It has been proposed in the previous section that the lexical deficit implicit in fluent aphasias is specific to those lexical domains which denote the aspects of the physical world represented with the maximum reliance upon the visual modality. It has been further proposed that such a selectivity of lexical deficit in posterior aphasias is a reflection of the distributed nature of the cerebral representation of lexicon.

I now propose that the normal function of the middle part of the left occipito-temporal gradient (posterior part of the temporal lobe at the temporo-occipital junction) is related to those aspects of linguistic representations which denote the visually based aspects of the physical world. The role of this area, therefore, consists of auditory-visual integration within the linguistic context.

Comparison of Wernicke's aphasia and the anomic aphasia reflects their relative positions along the temporo-occipital gradient. The former is closer to the auditory, modality-specific temporal end of the gradient (due to lesions in the posterior part of superior temporal gyrus) and it has a strong phonological component manifested as deficient auditory comprehension. Many paraphasias seen in Wernicke's anomia are literal, also reflecting the phonological basis of the deficit. Anomic aphasia is associated with a more posterior territory; it is usually seen following lesions in close proximity to the temporo-occipital junction. The deficit here does not have a distinct phonological components, and the lexical deficit appears to be more purely semantic (Goodglass, 1980; Goodglass & Geschwind, 1976).

### Extinction of Word Meaning

Luria (1980) described this phenomenon of an inability to evoke a visual image following a verbal label. The patient is able to draw objects from samples and to name them on confrontation. He is unable, however, to draw common objects from memory. The "extinction of word meaning" phenomenon is seen following lesions in the same middle area of temporo-occipital gradient which cause anomic aphasia. It also usually co-occurs with anomia (Luria, 1980; Yamadori & Albert, 1973). Although the latter is the case, it is important to stress that the "extinction" phenomenon can be seen even with respect to those words which are available to the patient in confrontation naming. This is what justified treating it as a distinct phenomenon. This is also why a "disconnection" model of the deficit cannot readily explain the word-meaning extinction phenomenon.

I propose that the "extinction of word meaning" phenomenon is another manifestation of the breakdown of linguovisual integration following damage to the middle part of the temporo-occipital gradient in the left hemisphere.

We have thus completed the review of the left temporo-occipital gradient. As the two previously described gradients, it abides by the rule of functional-structural isomorphism. Fluent aphasias and the word meaning extinction represent the consequences of the breakdown of its level 3, associative segment $(OT_3)$. Anomic aphasia is the clear manifestation of the damage to the level 3 $(OT_3)$ area, whereas Wernicke's aphasia can be conceptualized as resulting from lesions of the junction of level$^2$ $(T^2)$ and level 3 $(OT_3)$ areas.

### Summary of Posterior Cognitive Gradients

We have completed the review of cognitive gradients of the posterior part of the left hemisphere. A rather distinct triangular structure emerges with a continuous distribution of functions along each of its sides: occipitoparietal, occipitotemporal, and temporoparietal. To restate these gradients in cognitive terms, one may refer to them as visuospatial, visuolingual, and linguospatial gradients, respectively.

It should be clear that this description reflects two properties: One is the fundamental property of intermodal interaction along the gradients. In this sense, the occipitoparietal gradient is the visuospatial one; the temporoparietal gradient is the auditory-spatial one; and the occipitotemporal is the visual-auditory gradient. This basic gradiental structure is presumed to be symmetrical, identical in the two hemispheres.

Superimposed upon the basic symmetrical gradiental structure are hemispheric elaborations. In the context of this discussion, hemispheric asymmetries are clearly viewed as secondary, elaborative features which are superimposed on a fundamentally symmetrical neurocognitive architecture. It is precisely for this reason that ambiguities of the lateralization of several syndromes central to this discussion were dealt with somewhat lightly in this discussion. Spatial acalculia and "spatial apractagnosia" are examples of such syndromes. It was implicitly assumed in this discussion that temporoparietal and occipitoparietal associative areas of both hemispheres play a role in calculations and in spatial analysis, but that they contribute different aspects to them in accordance with the hemispheric elaborations. The issue of the exact weights of the lateralized contributions of these areas to the corresponding functions is not regarded as central to this discussion, since we are concerned here predominantly with the fundamental *symmetrical* properties of cerebral organization. It is felt that the gradiental principle is the main expression of these fundamental symmetries.

Although this is a secondary issue in our context, we have to deal with the issue of hemispheric elaborations nevertheless. The left posterior hemisphere is viewed as being central to categorical processing; in other words, to the processing which relies on generic classifications and rules of sorting specific items of the physical world in terms of generic categories. This point of view is articulated in greater detail elsewhere (Goldberg, in press-a). When this elaboration is superimposed on the posterior cortical cognitive gradients of the left hemisphere, the occipitotemporal, visual-auditory gradient becomes linguovisual; the temporoparietal, auditory-spatial gradient becomes linguospatial; and the occipitoparietal, visuospatial gradient turns out to be specifically involved in processing representational, symbolic stimuli. Although we do not have a special name to distinguish it from its right-hemispheric counterpart, one can think about it as the visual-symbolic gradient.

We will not dwell on the right posterior cognitive gradients in detail. The purpose of this chapter is not to present an exhaustive account of neuropsychological phenomena and syndromes, but to introduce a certain principle of cerebral organization. My views regarding the relationships between the two hemispheres have been stated elsewhere (Goldberg & Costa, 1981). Here, it will suffice to say that the basic triangular gradiental structure is probably elaborated in the right hemisphere in terms of physical identity processes as opposed to categorical identity mechanisms. Indeed, the comparison of left- and right-hemispheric agnosias have led various researchers to believe that whereas the former are symbolic, associative in nature, the latter are "apperceptive" in that they consist of an inability to identify a specific object as its own physical self at various conditions of observation (Vignolo, 1982; Warrington, 1982). This point of view has a definite appeal to me, too. Although the perceptual judgment implicit in establishing the object's physical identity also requires generalizations, these are first-order generalizations, compared with the second-order generalizations implicit in categorical recognition. These first-order generalizations probably rely on more basic, and to a greater extent, innate (as opposed to learned) codes, which are probably more atomic compared to the more molar codes of the left hemisphere. Goldberg and Costa (1981) proposed that the two are related the way the compiler (the left-hemisphere codes) is related to the machine language (the right-hemisphere codes). Of course, this computer analogy is only a metaphor.

It is possible to explicate the syndromal composition of the right posterior cognitive gradients in a fashion similar to the one employed in this review for the left hemisphere, but I will reserve it for future publications.

I feel that there is enough empirical evidence to entertain the concept of the cognitive gradient as a plausible one. One has to understand, however, that there was a considerably hypothetical, speculative element in our review. The proposed breakdown of associative, level 3 syndromes into their gradiental affiliations was based on the fundamental conceptual premise entertained here, that of structural-functional cortical isomorphism, and has to be regarded as hypothetical. Indeed, most of the corresponding syndromes are traditionally associated with the "angular gyrus area" without further attempts at more precise, differential neuroanatomical descriptions. In fact, the "angular gyrus area" designation is meant as "anywhere on the temporo-parieto-occipital interface." Given that the whole area is relatively small, it may seem reasonable to defer any attempts at more precise localization within that area. Our gradiental model, however, provides the basis for such precise localization. Although it may look at a first glance as reverting back to Gall-style mosaic localizationism, the real conceptual outcome of this more precise localization is exactly the opposite. This argument will be developed in the concluding part of the chapter.

Although hypothetical to a large degree, our breakdown of the "angular gyrus" syndromes into distinct subsets, each with its own gradiental affiliation, finds at least partial support in Mishkin's (1972) notion of the "what" and the "where" systems in monkeys. The first one deals with the object identity, the second one with its space localization. According to Mishkin's theory, the "what" system is distributed along the temporo-occipital axis, and the "where" system along the parieto-occipital axis. Both their functional and neuroanatomical descriptions are in a virtually ideal agreement with our temporo-occipital and parieto-occipital cognitive gradients, respectively.

## ANTERIOR COGNITIVE GRADIENTS

Every cortical lobe, occipital, parietal, temporal and frontal, can be viewed as consisting of three types of cortices: primary, organized in a stimulotopical fashion (level 1), secondary, which is still modality-specific but does not exhibit stimulotopical properties (level 2), and tertiary, associative cortex which is considered supramodal (level 3).

In the posterior cortex, the primary level 1 areas of the three lobes (occipital, temporal, and parietal) are placed at the three extreme, marginal points of the posterior cortical sheet, and the progression from level 1 to level 2 to level 3 cortices follows the path toward the geometrical center of the cortical sheet, which is the area of the inferior parietal lobule.

Anterior cortex is different from the posterior cortex in terms of its basic neuroanatomy. It consists of only one lobe. The frontal lobe can also be viewed as organized in terms of level 1 to level 2 to level 3 progression. This organization, however, can be best conceptualized as a partial gradient: level 1–level 2–level 3. In this gradient, level 1 is represented by motor cortex (Brodmann area

4); level 2 by premotor cortex (Brodmann area 6 and, in part, 8); and level 3 by prefontal cortex (Brodmann areas 9, 10, and, in part, 8). In our review of cortical gradients, we will be concerned mostly with the dorsolateral prefrontal cortex.

Although such partial gradiental organization characterizes every cortical lobe, in the posterior cortex they are aligned pairwise so as to make the following alignment possible: level 1–level 2–level 3–level 2–level 1. This is the basic architecture of a cognitive gradient. One can easily see that a gradient is constructed of a pair of lobe-specific partial gradients directed toward each other. The concept of a partial gradient as applied to the frontal cortex is not fundamentally different from the concept of the cognitive gradient as applied to the posterior cortex. They both are expressions of the fundamental principle of cognitive-neuroanatomical isomorphism. By using the motor–premotor–prefrontal partial gradiental arrangement as the fundamental organizational feature of the frontal lobe, we will see how gradiental elaborations will then emerge within the lateral hemispheric context.

## *The Basic Frontal Lobe Gradient*

Having defined the general organization of the frontal functional gradient, we are now ready to specify its constituents in some detail.

## The Motor Cortex

The level 1 element of the frontal gradient consists of the motor cortex (Brodmann area 4), which is somatotopically organized in the way which roughly parallels the somatotopical organization of the postcentral, somatosensory cortex. It occupies the anterior wall of the central sulcus and adjacent parts of the precentral gyrus (Carpenter, 1976). Both in terms of its somatotopical organization and in terms of its function, it is comparable with the level 1, primary cortical projection areas of posterior gradients. Motor cortex is the point of origin of the pyramidal system and constitutes therefore the primary cortical motor output station.

## The Premotor Cortex

The level 2 element of the frontal gradient consists of premotor cortex (Brodmann area 6 and, according to some authors, also parts of Brodmann area 8). Unlike the motor cortex, lesions of premotor cortex do not lead to loss of movement, to permanent paralysis or paresis. However, disintegration of sequential organization of complex skilled movements or ad hoc motor sequences takes place (Foerster, 1936; Luria, 1980). It is not the strength of the movements, or the ability to perform isolated, single movements that suffers, but rather the dynamics of the motor act, its kinetic organization. This may take two forms which are often combined.

Transition from one motor element to another within the motor sequence may be impaired, and it often takes the form of motor perseveration. To be precise, motor perseveration may take two forms: a deficit of transition from one motor act to another; and a deficit of termination of a motor act, which leads to the excessive repetition or maintenance of the same discrete motor act (the phasic version) or posture (the tonic version) (Goldberg, 1987; Goldberg & Bilder, 1986; Goldberg & Costa, 1986; Goldberg & Tucker, 1979; Luria, 1965, 1980). Denny–Brown (1958) considered the latter type of perseveration central to frontal lobe pathology. He considered it a manifestation of the "magnetic reaction," the central mechanism of frontal pathology in Denny–Brown's opinion, due to the release from the normally exerted frontal inhibitory function. This was the basis for the term "magnetic apraxia," introduced by Denny–Brown to describe the devastating effects of perseveratory interminability of action upon motor behavior.

Even when the execution of motor sequences is available in principle and the transition from one motor element to another can take place, the plasticity of such transitions may suffer. The continuous movement then becomes broken down into discrete, disjointed components.

These two types of deficient sequential motor organization, that of motor transition and that of the plasticity of motor transition, correspond to the dysfunction of "principal" and "background" components of movements in Bernstein's terminology (1947, 1967). The deficit of the "background" movement components has been termed by some authors "melokinetic apraxia" (Fulton, 1937; Hecaen & Albert, 1978; Nielsen, 1946). The deficit of the "principal" components of movements leads to the picture similar to what some authors terms "limb-kinetic" apraxia (Heilman & Gonzales Rothi, 1985; Liepmann, 1920).

On the basis of these various clinical observations, various authors concluded that the function of premotor cortex consists of sequential organization of discrete movements into organized and smooth sequential patterns.

## The Prefrontal (Dorsolateral) Cortex

The prefrontal cortex has been usually associated with the highest levels of neural control. Although it is possible to talk about general, unifying characteristics of the "prefrontal syndrome," and to view all of the prefrontal cortex as a functionally distinct entity, major differences exist between different aspects of the prefrontal cortex as well as between the corresponding variants of the "prefrontal syndrome" (Damasio, 1979; Goldberg, 1985; Luria, 1980; Pribram, this volume). In this discussion, we will concentrate on the function of the dorsolateral aspect of the prefrontal cortex. It lies on the continuation on our frontal gradient and constitutes its level 3 component.

Damage to the dorsolateral aspect of the prefrontal cortex is usually associated with a plethora of clinical manifestations, among which the following are most prominent: *perseveration,* which is pervasive both horizontally (affecting virtually every behavioral domain) and vertically (disrupting virtually every level of neurocognitive control) (Goldberg, 1987; Goldberg & Bilder, 1986; Goldberg & Tucker, 1979; Luria, 1980); *aspontaneity,* which may take two forms: inertia of initiation and inertia of termination (Bilder & Goldberg, 1987; Goldberg, 1986; Luria, 1980); *field-dependent behavior,* which may take the form of "utilization behavior" (Goldberg & Costa, 1986; Lhermitte, 1986; Lhermitte, Pillon, & Serdaru, 1986; Luria, 1980); regression to *imitative behaviors* (echolalia and echopraxia) and *stereotypic behavior* (Luria, 1980).

In attempting to conceptualize this plethora of deficits and trying to find a common denominator behind them, one notes the supramodal, ubiquitous nature of these deficits. Perseverations, aspontaneity, and so on, can be observed following other focal lesions, but then they are limited to a particular sensory modality, type of situation or level of processing. They can be characterized in terms of their material or modality specificity. Following dorsolateral prefrontal damage, on the other hand, these deficits are universal in terms of their impact (Goldberg & Bilder, 1986, 1987). Because of this superordinate nature of the elements of the "prefrontal syndrome," they are often referred to as "executive" deficits.

Attempts to find the normal mechanism, the function whose breakdown leads to the prefrontal, "executive" syndromes have led to a variety of theories and speculations (Goldberg & Bilder, 1986; Goldstein, 1975; Luria, 1980; Stuss & Benson, 1984; Teuber, 1964). In the present context the following fact should be emphasized: both phylogentically, and in terms of its ontogenetic differentiation, the dorsolateral prefrontal cortex is an extension of and elaboration upon the premotor cortex (Kononova, 1940, 1948; Polyakov, 1966). This means that it may be of heuristic value to conceptualize also the functions of the dorsolateral prefrontal cortex as an extension of and elaboration upon those of the premotor cortex. Just as the premotor cortex has been invested with the function of sequential organization of motor patterns, so can the function of the prefrontal cortex be seen in sequential organization of behavior at large. The continuity between motor controls and cognitive controls at large has been particularly emphasized in the work of Nicholas Bernstein (1947, 1967). The concept of various cognitive controls as internalized overt behaviors also figured prominently in the work of several cognitive and developmental psychologists (Bruner, 1966; Bruner & Goodnow, 1956; Vygotsky, 1962).

Current attempts to capture the nature of prefrontal function use descriptors like "programming of behavior," "formulation of plans," "sequential organization of behavior," "maintenance of behavior selectivity." Although each of these descriptors emphasizes a somewhat different aspect of cognitive control, they all tap into an intuitively parsimonious construct, which for the lack of a better term, we call the "executive function." It is not the purpose of this review to decide whether there is a single, monolithic "executive function" or whether we are dealing with a group of related cognitive controls. What needs to be emphasized, however, is that this function or class of functions are much closer in terms of their cognitive constituents to motor than to perceptual functions. Just as a complex motor act requires a smooth alignment of motor elements into a coordinated sequence, so does a strictly cognitive act require the selection and organization into a coordinated pattern of pre-existing cognitive routines. One can therefore say that the prefrontal cortex is critically involved in the ad hoc coordination of cognitive elements into patterns dictated by the current behavioral context.

I think that this affinity between the premotor and prefrontal functions is fundamental, and it certainly fits into the notion of motor–premotor–prefrontal cortical gradient. The following important elaboration of the prefrontal function upon the premotor function, however, has to be noted. When we describe the role of the premotor cortex with respect to elementary cognitive acts, we emphasize its role as the "sequential organizer." When we discuss the role of prefrontal cortex with respect to cognitive routines, we have to introduce an additional dimension. The prefrontal controls are both linear, sequential and vertical, hierarchic. The hierarchic nature of complex controls has been emphasized both in neural and cognitive models (Bernstein, 1947, 1967; Miller, Galanter, & Pribram, 1960). Although the distinction between motor and cognitive processes is not strictly dichotomous in terms of the presence or absence of the hierarchic aspect of controls involved, it is clear that the more complex is the desired sequential output, the greater degree of hierarchic controls and the complexity of *nestedness* of subroutines is required for its realization. It is the prefrontal cortex that can be thought of as being critical for the hierarchic organization of complex cognitive controls (Goldberg & Bilder, 1987).

We can therefore describe the frontal gradient in terms of the following continuum: motor control (furnished by level 1 motor cortex)–sequential organization of complex motor patterns (furnished by level 2 premotor cortex)–hierarchic/sequential organization of any type of behavior (furnished by level 3 prefrontal cortex in its dorsolateral division). As with respect to the posterior gradients, clear agreement also exists between neuroanatomical and functional continuities in the anterior brain. The motor-prefrontal gradient is not hemisphere-specific. It reflects the fundamental principle of organization of the anterior cortex as a whole.

Having defined the basic organizing principle of the anterior brain, we will now concentrate on its hemispheric elaborations. As before, we will focus on the properties of the left hemisphere.

## Neurolinguistic Digression II: Broca's Aphasias

Before proceeding with the discussion of the hemisphere-specific gradient, a general discussion of the so-called Broca's aphasia is required.

The neuroanatomical definition of Broca's area is somewhat ambiguous. It encompasses a premotor component (the inferior part of Brodmann area 6) and an associative one (the area of frontal operculum, which corresponds to Brodmann area 44) (Benson, 1985; Goodglass & Geschwind, 1976; Luria, 1980). Cognitive descriptions of the Broca's aphasia also encompass two distinct components: disintegration of kinetic, sequential organization of articulatory output; and agrammatism. These two symptoms are usually regarded as components of the same syndrome with the same neuroanatomical substrate. One wonders, however, whether at a neuroanatomically finer level of analysis a double dissociation may be obtained between the two cognitive aspects of Broca's aphasia on the one hand, and the two neuroanatomical components of the Broca's area on the other hand. If this is correct, then the usual co-occurrence of these two aspects of Broca's aphasia is a consequence of the physical adjacency of corresponding cortical territories rather than of a unitary, shared cognitive mechanism.

It is the first, akinetic, aspect of Broca's aphasia that is emphasized in Luria's taxonomy of aphasias. He uses the term "efferent (kinetic) motor aphasia" (Luria, 1970, 1980). Disorder of articulation is viewed by Luria as the central feature of this syndrome. Luria maintains that the deficit is not so much related to the production of separate articulemes, as it is to the capacity for smooth transitions between them. He views the mechanisms of Broca's aphasia as related to the kinetic, sequential aspects of oral praxis. Denny–Brown (1963) concurs with this interpretation of Broca's aphasia. He points to the association of Broca's aphasia with buccolinguofacial apraxia, that is, an inability to engage in nonverbal motor sequencing involving oral apparatus (Jackson, 1931/1932). The view of Broca's aphasia as "speech apraxia" is shared also by other authors (Johns & Darley, 1970; Trost & Canter, 1974). It is proposed here that the akinetic aspect of Broca's aphasia is caused by damage to the inferior part of the premotor area (Brodmann area 6) in the left hemisphere. I will refer to this type of linguistic deficit with Luria's term "efferent motor aphasia."

Agrammatism associated with lesions in the Broca's areas has been emphasized by many authors (Goodglass & Geschwind, 1976; Hecaen & Albert, 1978; Luria, 1970, 1980). Earlier in this chapter I proposed that this phenomenon is an expression of the disruption of predicative basis of language, which is in turn based on internal representation of actions. I will not repeat the argument here but refer the reader to an earlier section of this chapter, "Neurolinguistic Digression 1."

It is proposed here that the disruption of the predicative aspect of language (which presumably underlies Broca's agrammatism) is caused by the damage to the frontal operculum (Brodmann area 44) which is usually classified as associative rather than premotor cortex (Carpenter, 1976). I will refer to this type of linguistic deficit as agrammatical aphasia. This term is chosen merely as a concession to tradition. In the scheme of things developed here it is, in fact, a misnomer, since I believe that the deficit underlying the Broca's agrammatism is essentially semantic.

It has to be stressed that the distinction between two "Broca's aphasias" proposed here clearly represents a minority opinion. Both Benson (1985) and Hecaen and Albert (1978) hint, however, at the existence of "variants" of Broca's aphasia.

We are now prepared to proceed with the discussion of the remaining gradient of the anterior portion of the left hemisphere.

## Left Inferior Motor-prefrontal Cognitive Gradient

This continuum is neuroanatomically defined by its two extreme points: the inferior portion of the motor strip (Brodmann area 4) and the dorsolateral prefrontal area, respectively. The inferior part of the motor strip is, together with its premotor counterpart, the area of motor control of oral apparatus. The functions of the dorsolateral prefrontal cortex have been extensively described earlier, with the emphasis of the global, executive nature of prefrontal control.

In defining the middle elements of this continuum, we first turn to the inferior part of the premotor cortex in the left hemisphere (Brodmann area 6). This is the territory whose damage leads to efferent motor aphasia (we follow here the terminological distinction between two hypothesized variants of Broca's aphasia introduced earlier). Both on clinical and on neuroanatomical grounds, the normal function of this area can be inferred as that of sequential organization of articulatory patterns, a special case of the general function of sequential motor organization mediated by premotor cortex at large.

As we move farther toward the middle of this gradient, we encounter its central component. This is the associative (Brodmann area 44) aspect of the Broca's area. According to the hypothesis advanced earlier (see "Neurolinguistic digression I"), this is the area whose damage produces agrammatical aphasia.

In order to be able to speculate about normal functions of this area, one has to recall the earlier discussion of neuropsychological mechanisms of agrammatism. It was proposed earlier (see "Neurolinguistic digression I") that the agrammatism of Broca's aphasia is a consequence of the disruption of the predicative structure of language, which is based in its turn upon the linguistic representation of actions. It was further proposed that, in line with the notion of the distributed nature of the cerebral representation of the lexicon, the cerebral substrate of the linguistic representation of actions is neuroanatomically intertwined with the cerebral substrate of actions themselves.

It is premotor cortex (Brodmann area 6) which can be reasonably assumed to be central to the cortical representation of actions. It is proposed here that the associative area of the frontal operculum, which is neuroanatomically located close to the bulk of area 6, and to the motor/premotor representation of linguistic codes, is critically in charge of the motor-linguistic interface. This interface takes the form of the cerebral representation of that lexical domain which denotes actions, and hence of the predicative aspects of language.

As we proceed along the axis defined by the two extreme points anteriorly, away from the motor extreme and toward the dorsolateral prefrontal extreme, we encounter the territory whose damage leads to the syndrome of "frontal dynamic aphasia." This is the area immediately anterior of the frontal opperculum, and it roughly corresponds to Brodmann area 45. First described by Kleist (1934) under the name of *Antriebsmangel der Sprache* (defect of speech initiative), this syndrome was extensively studies by Luria (1965, 1980). Although this syndrome is often classified as "aphasia," it can be argued that linguistic structures per se are intact, and that the deficit is that of linguistic behavior rather than of language per se. The patient's discourse is characterized by aspontaneity and lack of initiation. It is difficult for the patient to initiate a conversation. Repetition is considerably more intact than those forms of linguistic activity that require spontaneous speech. To the extent that a speech sample can be obtained from the patient, it is likely to be replete with perseveration. This perseveration, however, can be better described as thematic rather than linguistic. In a dialogic situation, the patient with "dynamic aphasia" is likely to be echolalic. There will be no flaws, however, in the phonological, articulatory, lexical, or grammatical aspects of his or her verbal output.

The deficit implicit in this syndrome can be best described as an executive deficit selectively affecting language behavior but nothing else. Indeed, all the executive failures which characterize the dorsolateral prefrontal syndrome are present also in "dynamic aphasia." The difference is that in the former these symptoms are pervasive and affect every behavior, whereas in the latter they are limited to verbal behavior.

We can therefore conclude that the area in question, which is located on the junction between premotor and prefrontal cortices in the left hemisphere, normally serves the function of executive-linguistic interface. It provides executive control over linguistic behavior.

## *Summary of Anterior Cortical Cognitive Gradients*

We will designate level 1 motor cortex as M1; level 2 premotor cortex as PM2; and level 3 dorsolateral prefrontal cortex as PF3. The M1-PM2-PF3 organization is viewed as a fundamental, symmetrical description of the frontal lobe. Hemispheric elaborations are introduced upon it in a secondary fashion.

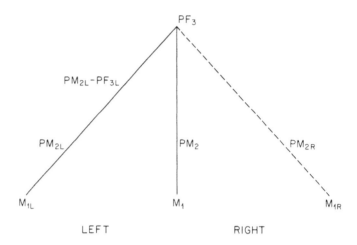

**FIGURE 3** Gradiental structure of anterior cortex. M1—"primary" motor cortex (Brodmann area 4); PM2—"secondary" premotor cortex (Brodmann area 6 and in part 8); PM2L—the left inferior part of premotor cortex; PF3—dorsolateral prefrontal cortex (Brodmann areas 9, 10, and in part 8); PM2L-PF3L—the left frontal operculum and pars triangularis (Brodmann areas 44, 45). These abbreviations refer to corresponding areas in the left hemisphere when amended by L, and the right hemisphere when amended by R. Damage to PM2 leads to melokinetic and limb-kinetic apraxias; PF3—executive syndrome; PM2L—speech apraxia; PM2L-PF3L—syntactical agrammatism (when more posterior) and dynamic aphasia (when more anterior). (Reproduced from the *Journal of Clinical and Experimental Neuropsychology*).

Schematic representation of the gradiental structure of the anterior brain is provided in cortex is provided in Figure 3.

Like in the case of posterior cortex, a structure of cognitive continua characterizes the left anterior cortex. These are: motor-prefrontal (motor-executive) partial gradient, and inferior motor-prefrontal (linguo-executive) partial gradient. It is presumed that a complementary pattern of elaborations can be uncovered for the right anterior brain.

## *Summary of Cortical Cognitive Gradients*

We have completed our review of cortical cognitive gradients. These gradients form a diamond-like structure, with a triangular arrangement in every

Composite schematic representation
of cortical gradiental structure

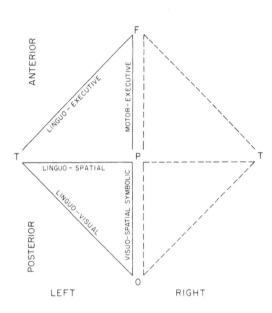

**FIGURE 4** Composite schematic representation of cortical gradiental structure. O, T, P, and F denote occipital, temporal, parietal, and frontal poles, respectively. Visuospatial symbolic, linguovisual, linguospatial, and linguoexecutive gradients are left-hemispheric elaborations on occipitoparietal, occipitotemporal, temporoparietal, and inferior motor-prefrontal gradients, respectively. The motor-executive (motor-prefrontal) gradient is presumed to be symmetrical. (Reproduced from the *Journal of Clinical and Experimental Neuropsychology).*

cortical quadrant (Figure 4). We will briefly review the components of this structure.

| | |
|---|---|
| *Left posterior quadrant:* | Occipitoparietal (visuospatial symbolic) gradient |
| | Temporoparietal (linguospatial) gradient |
| | Occipitotemporal (linguovisual) gradient |
| *Left anterior quadrant:* | Motor-prefrontal (motor-executive) gradient |
| | Inferior motor-prefrontal (linguoexecutive) gradient |

This gradiental structure of the left hemisphere is a result of hemispheric elaboration upon a more fundamental, symmetrical organization, applicable to both hemispheres. It can be characterized as follows:

Occipitoparietal (visuospatial) gradient
Temporoparietal (auditory-spatial) gradient

Occipitotemporal (visuo-auditory) gradient
Motor-prefrontal (motor-executive) gradient

It is presumed that an elaboration of this fundamental underlying structure in the right hemisphere leads to a double-triangular gradiental structure similar in its architecture to the one described for the left hemisphere.

It is proposed that the cognitive gradient constitutes a fundamental unit of neocortical functional organization. In combination, cognitive gradients define the pattern of the horizontal neocortical functional organization. This horizontal principle, together with the vertical (hierarchic) principle, define two aspects of basic (symmetrical) cortical organization. A cognitive gradient is the fundamental unit of the horizontal organization in the same way as a hierarchic level is the fundamental unit of the vertical organization.

Hemispheric specialization is viewed in this scheme of things as a secondary elaboration upon the (fundamentally symmetrical) horizontal and vertical principles of organization.

The horizontal functional organization of neorcortex of which the cognitive gradient is a unit, is a reflection of cognitive-neuroanatomical isomorphism. By cognitive-neuroanatomical isomorphism I mean the fact that the neuroanatomical metrics of distances between cortical regions and cognitive metrics of distances between cortical regions are in close agreement. Two cortical areas are similar in terms of their cognitive functions if, and only if, they are neuroanatomically close. The fact that various neuropsychological syndromes can be arranged in the gradiental fashion in the given sense constitutes, in my opinion, a powerful evidence in favor of cognitive-neuroanatomical isomorphism.

## THEORETICAL IMPLICATIONS OF THE GRADIENTAL MODEL

### Mosaic vs. Continuous Principles of Functional Cortical Organization

In the course of our review of neuropsychological syndromes and corresponding, functionally distinct neocortical regions we introduced the degree of specificity, which may be perceived as a throwback toward the Gall-style mosaic localization. In fact, I am about to draw exactly opposite conclusions.

Two opposite views on the nature of brain-behavioral relationships are logically possible:

1. Brain-behavioral mapping is essentially mosaic.
2. Brain-behavioral mapping is essentially continuous.

The first, mosaic, principle presupposes that the relationship between the neuroanatomical cortical and functional cortical metrics is random. In other words, it denies the existence of close agreement between cognitive and neuroanatomical geometries . According to the mosaic principle, two cortical regions can be neuroanatomically adjacent but functionally distant and vice versa. Random pattern of relationship between two geometries presupposes abrupt, discrete borders between functionally distinct cortical regions.

The second, continuous, principle of cortical localization of functions presupposes an orderly relationship between neuroanatomical and functional cortical metrics. In its strongest form, it presupposes neuroanatomical-functional isomorphism. Because the continuous principle dictates that if two cortical areas are neuroanatomically adjacent, they are also functionally proximal, it does not necessitate abrupt, discrete borders between functionally identifiable cortical regions. Instead, gradual transititions are emphasized.

By demonstrating the existence of cognitive cortical gradients, we have provided a strong argument in favor of the continuous principle of functional cortical organization and against the mosaic principle.

The mosaic-continuous dichotomy is closely related to two other dichotomies which reflect alternative views of cerebral organization. These are the modular-interactive dichotomy and the prededicated-emergent dichotomy. I will discuss them systematically.

## Modular vs. Interactive Principles of Functional Cortical Organization

By the modular principle of organization, I mean a system consisting of encapsulated units connected among themselves only through input-output relationships. Once the input has been received by a module from other modules, the processing taking place in the given module is not influenced by external events or influences until after the output stage.

By the interactive principle of organization, I mean a system in which every unit has multiple connections with other units. The informational exchange between units is not limited to input-output relations but occurs continuously.

The modular principle emphasizes the spatial discreteness of functional units and the temporal discreteness of "bursts" of informational exchange between units.

The interactive principle emphasizes spatial continuity between functional units and temporally continuous, uninterrupted information flow between units. In this type of system, it may be more appropriate to talk about somewhat arbitrarily specified "locations" in the network than about "units" in an absolute sense. Furthermore, it may be more appropriate to describe information processing in continuous terms of flow than in discrete terms of stages. The opposite is true for the modular system.

Neuroscientific concepts dealing with the brain-behavioral relationships have always been swinging like a pendulum between these two extreme visions of the brain. Early mosaic localizations of Gall and Kleist clearly represented the early precursors of the modular point of view. Lashlean notions of equipotentiality represented the opposite extreme. Hughlings Jackson introduced the notion of the hierarchic organization of the brain which can be restated as the principle of "controlled distributedness of functions." This design incorporates both modular and interactive features. Nikolai Bernstein and Alexandr Luria were among the most important proponents of this eclectic point of view in more recent times.

Diagram drawers of contemporary behavioral neurology and proponents of the interpretation of most neuropsychological disorders as "disconnection syndromes" pushed the pendulum back to the modular extreme, and Karl Pribram pulled it again toward the interactive extreme by introducing the holographic model of the brain.

The modular view of brain-behavior relations has recently become prominent again owing to the formulations of Fodor (1983, 1985), who is in fact responsible for introducing the term "module" into cognitive psychology (the term has been traditionally used by neurophysiologists and those concerned with more cellular, automatic information-processing units which can be thought of as the informational basic primitives of the brain and can be linked to rather distinct neural entities, such as neurons characterized by receptive fields with particular properties, or neuronal columns [Barlow & Hill, 1963; Hartline & Ratcliff, 1946; Hubel & Wiesel, 1962, 1963; Mountcastle, 1961; Purpura, 1970]).

Brain-behavioral conceptual deliberations of the global kind described heretofore are usually concerned mostly with the neocortex, and it is the cortical territory where the modular-interactive battles are usually fought.

The two dichotomies, mosaic vs. continuous, and modular vs. interactive, appear to be related. In considering the four possibilities obtained by treating the two dichotomies as orthogonal dimensions, one concludes that logically all four combinations are possible. Intuitively, however, some are more plausible than others. A mosaic-interactive design of cortical organization strikes one as a rather impractical one, since it implies intensive interactions between neuroanatomically distant regions. A modular-continuous design sounds like a rather redundant arrangement, since it presupposes an order (cognitive-neuroanatomical isomorphism) where it is not really required. This reasoning is based on the assumption that in a system composed of insulated processing units (modules) connected with cables, the geometry of the modular distances is not critically important. It would be more important in a continuous interaction system. Mosaic-modular and continuous-interactive designs reflect the more plausible relationships between the two dichotomies in question. This means that by providing support for the continuous nature of cortical functional organization, we are at the same time indirectly supporting the hypothesis of the interactive rather than modular cortical functional organization. Since the concept of continuous organization as it developed in our discussion is most compelling with respect to the middle, associative segments of the previously discussed cognitive gradients, it can be proposed that also the interactive principle is most applicable to these middle segments of the cognitive gradients. This can be restated in the following fashion: Associative, intermodal cortical regions are the ones which most strongly adhere to the interactive principle of organization as opposed to the modular one. Secondary, higher-order modality specific cortices are also likely to adhere predominantly to the interactive principle. The notion of the modular principle of functional organization at the cortical level is more tenable with respect to primary cortical projection areas.

In order to consider the relationship between modular and interactive principles of functional cerebral organization in a truly comprehensive way, one has to go beyond the scope of the neocortex and at the very least consider also thalamocortical interactions.

Such interactions are beyond the scope of this chapter, but they have been discussed elsewhere with special reference to the issues of modularity vs. interactiveness (Goldberg, in press B).

## *Prededicated vs. Emergent Principles of Functional Cortical Organization*

Finally, I will consider the impact that our conclusions regarding the primacy of the continuous principle of functional cortical organization has on the distinction between prededicated and emergent principle of functional cortical organization.

By the prededicated principle of functional cerebral organization I mean the situation when the functions of cerebral structures or regions are genetically prespecified.

By the emergent principle of functional cerebral organization I mean the situation when a priori constraints upon the functional designations of cerebral structures or regions are rather limited, and they *assume* their function through self-organizing processes in neural networks as a result of their interaction with the environment. It is presumed that such self-organizing processes within neuronal networks follow certain rules, among which the *economy principle* is central.

Assuming that we want to understand the relative roles of the prededicated and emergent aspects in the functional organization of the neoroctex, can the knowledge of the continuous nature of the functional neocortical organization provide any guidance?

The two dichotomies, mosaic vs. continuous, and prededicated vs. emergent are not orthogonal. They are related in the following sense: The assumption of the functional neural network organization which is mosaic and emergent at the same time would constitute a virtual impossibility. This is due to the fact that the mosaic principle of organization implies a random relationship between functional and neuroanatomical regional proximities. To the extent that we believe in the adaptive wisdom of the design of the brain, it is clear that a self-organizing neural network cannot develop in this fashion, since it would be impractical and cumbersome. A self-organizing neural network can be expected to follow the principle of spatial economy, which means adherence to the principle of functional-neuroanatomical isomorphism.

We can therefore conclude that if the functional characteristics of a neural network have *emerged* as a result of systemic self-organizing processes, the network is extremely unlikely to be organized in a mosaic fashion. It is almost certainly organized in a continuous fashion. Conversely, if a network is organized in a mosaic fashion, one can conclude with near-certainty that its functional properties have been prededicated in a rather specific and strong way.

This means that had my conclusion been that the neocortical functional organization is fundamentally mosaic, I would be concluding in the same breath that it is strongly prededicated.

As it stands, I have concluded that the functional organization of the neocortex is fundamentally continuous. I do not think that this conclusion favors a particular choice within the prededicated vs. emergent dichotomy in a logical sense. Logically, it is compatible with either possibility. Intuitively, however, it favors the likelihood of a substantial role of the *emergent* principle in the neocortical functional organization. While fully realizing that our intuitions are often idiosyncratic and arbitrary, I would like, nevertheless, to pursue the possibility further.

If we believe that the pattern of the functional cortical organization captured by the gradiental scheme is a result of self-organizing processes in the neural network at least to some, substantial degree, we have to immediately limit the scope of applicability of the specific pattern of brain-behavioral relations thus described. We have to conclude that in this form it reflects *only* the invariant aspects of cortical localization in an adult, mature brain of an individual who has been a product of statistically prevalent cultural and experiential circumstances. This pattern of localization *does not* reflect neocortical functional organization in children. Furthermore, one has to conclude that there is no such thing as a single pattern of child functional neocortical organization. What we are dealing with, instead, is a *process of change* which is asymptotically directed toward the resultant, adult pattern of cortical functional organization, which can be viewed as reflecting certain statistical environmental invariants. We have to draw, in other words, the distinction between the *a priori* and *resultant* aspects of functional organization.

Furthermore, even with respect to the resultant pattern of localization, we have to ask the following questions: Does localization really exist in the sense that there are distinct cortical areas intrinsically invested with certain distinct functions? Or is our discrete nomenclature of cortical areas (which are presumed to be invested with distinct functions) nothing more than an inevitable outcome of attemping to describe essentially continuous distributions in finite terms, by imposing a finite taxomony? If the latter is the case, then our so-called neocortical functional units are nothing more than discrete "flags" to approximate gradients which are essentially continuous and without distinct borders. The advantage of such a model is that it enables us to interpolate the functional decription of any arbitrarily delineated locus along a continuous cognitive gradient. We are not bound any longer by a finite list of "syndromes" and corresponding normal areas with distinct "functions" against which we have to match our real life clinical cases in a template fashion. So, paradoxically, it is precisely the refutation of the mosaic principle of organization that enables us to specify "functions" of any arbitrarily outlined cortical area through interpolation. The gradiental principle of neocortical functional organization makes such interpolation possible precisely because it refutes the mosaic principle and assumes continuity based on functional-neuroanatomical isomorphism.

Finally, having put to question the existence of functionally distinct cortical areas, I am compelled to put to question the existence of distinct cognitive functions themselves, regardless of the nature of their cerebral representation. Indeed as I have concluded that neocortical functional "loci" may be nothing more than attempts to describe an intrinsically continuous neuronal spread in observable, finite terms, so we can apply the same reasoning to an essentially psychological rather than biological level of description. Assuming the existence of continuous gradients of interactions among a limited number of cognitive primitives, continuous distributions of combinations of "shades" of these cognitive primitives emerges in a neural network in a genuinely gradiental fashion. Our elaborate taxonomies of distinct cognitive functions may be nothing more than attempts to describe in finite terms essentially continuous patterns of "mixing" of these (relatively few) cognitive primitives. The gradiental approach allows one to make distinct predictions regarding the geometry of these functional distributions. Imagine, for instance, a congenitally blind person with a good language facility, who learned about physical objects predominantly with reliance on tactile inputs. In such a person anomic aphasia would be caused by a stroke along the temporoparietal rather than temporo-occipital gradient, somewhere in the region of the supramarginal gyrus rather than in the posterior part of the middle temporal gyrus.

The conclusion of the fictitiousness of the absolute borders between cognitive functions should come as no surprise to cognitive psychologists who are becoming increasingly prepared to emphasize the relativity of borders between memory and attention, memory and encoding, attention and executive controls, and so on. What many cognitive psychologists may be reluctant to accept, is that our concepts of the brain and cognition are not mutually independent. As there is a strong affinity between the "faculty" view of psychology and the "modular" view of the brain, so an equally strong affinity exists between the gradiental view of the brain and the fictitiousness of the concept of a finite number of cognitive functions. It is an epistemological ploy to which we inevitably have to resort in our inquiry, but it does not reflect the ontology of cognitive processes.

It has to be noted that these final paragraphs constitute nothing more than the exploration of logical consequences stemming from the proposition of the fundamentally emergent nature of functional organization of the neocortex. Nothing in this discussion can be regarded as a definitive proof of this principle. Strong evidence favoring the continuous nature of brain-behavioral mapping in neocortex was provided, and this is *consistent* with the emergent nature of functional neocortical organization, nothing more and nothing less. One does not *necessitate* the other.

There is almost certainly room both for the prededicated and the emergent principles in the functional organization of neocortex. The former is likely to be most applicable to the primary cortical projection areas, and the latter to the tertiary, associative cortices. In this respect the transition from the emphasis on functional prededication to the emphasis on the emergent functional organization probably constitutes a basic evolutionary trend in the phylogeny of the central nervous system which parallels the quantitative increase of the neural network complexity and provides for more adaptive and flexible principles of organization. It is a transition from the description of functional properties of the brain in terms of long explicit lists of functions and their locations, toward an open-ended self-organization attainable within quantitatively highly complex (but minimally prededicated) neural networks and governed by compact general rules applicable to an open class of specific situations. The principle of functional-neuroanatomical isomorphism and its gradiental expression is an example of such a general rule.

The transition from the prededicated to the emergent principles of organization can be traced within the neocortex when one compares primary with secondary, and secondary with associative tertiary cortical areas. This transition is probably even more striking when one compares subcortical (e.g., thalamic) principles of functional organization with neocortical ones. The examination of the differences between and the interplay of the discrete, modular, prededicated principle of cerebral organization and the continuous, interactive, emergent principle of organization is probably most elucidating when the thalamocortical relationships are considered. It is there that the dialectical interplay between these two radically opposite principles of cerebral organization becomes most apparent.

It has been proposed by some authors that only modularly organized functions can be successfully investigated, whereas the continuous interactive processes are in effect closed to systematic inquiry. Even if this were correct, nature is under no obligation to accommodate the intellectual ambitions of cognitive psychologists, neuropsychologists, and the like. I do believe, however, that the gradiental approach to functional cerebral organization offers a way of systematic and rational examination even of those processes which cannot be presumed to be modular either from a neuroanatomical or functional point of view.

## ACKNOWLEDGMENTS

The work on this chapter was made possible by a fellowship at the Institute for Advanced Studies, Hebrew University of Jerusalem. An abbreviated version of this chapter appears in the *Journal of Clinical and Experimental Neuropsychology*.

## REFERENCES

Ajuriaguerra, J. de, Hécaen, H., & Angelergues, R. (1960). Les apraxies varietes cliniques et lateralisation lesionelle. *Revue Neurologique, 102,* 566–594.

Albert, M. L., Reches, A., & Silverberg, R. (1975). Associative visual agnosia without alexia. *Neurology, 25,* 322–326.

Barlow, H. B., & Hill, R. M. (1963). Selective sensitivity to direction of motion in ganglion cells of the rabbit's retina. *Science, 39,* 412–414.

Bauer, R. M., & Rubens, A. B. (1985). Agnosia. In K. M. Heilman & E. Valenstein (Eds.), *Clinical neuropsychology* (2nd ed., pp. 187–242.

Beauvois, M.-F. (1982). Optic aphasia: A process of interaction between vision and language. *Philosophical Transactions of the Royal Society, London, B298,* 35–47.

Beauvois, M.-F., Saillant, B., Meininger, V., & Lhermitte, F. (1978). Bilateral tactile aphasia: A tacto-verbal dysfunction. *Brain, 101,* 381–401.

Bender, M. B., & Feldman, M. (1972). The so-called "visual agnosia." *Brain, 95,* 173–186.

Benson, D. F. (1985). Aphasia. In K. M. Heilman & E. Valenstein (Eds.), *Clinical neuropsychology,* New York, Oxford University Press, pp. 17–47.

Benson, D. F., & Geschwind, N. (1969). The alexias. In P. J. Vinken & G. W. Bruyn (Eds.), *Handbook of clinical neurology: Disorders of speech, perception and symbolic behavior.* New York: Elsevier, pp. 112–140.

Benson, D. F., Segarra, J., & Albert, M. L. (1974). Visual agnosia-prosopagnosia: A clinicopathological correlation. *Archives of Neurology, 30,* 307–310.

Benton, A. (1985). Body schema disturbances: Finger agnosia and right-left disorientation. In K. M. Heilman & E. Valenstein (Eds.), *Clinical neuropsychology.* New York: Oxford University Press, pp. 115–129.

Benton, A. L., Smith, K. C., & Lang, M. (1972). Stimulus characteristics and object naming performance in aphasic adults. *Journal of Communicative Disorders, 5,* 19–24.

Bernstein, N. A. (1947). *The construction of movements*. Moscow: Medgiz, (in Russian).

Bernstein, N. A. (1967). *The coordination and regulation of movements*. Oxford, England: Pergamon Press.

Bilder, R. M., & Goldberg, E. (1987). Motor perseveration in schizophrenia. *Archives of Clinical Neuropsychology, 2*, 195–214.

Bisiach, E. (1966). Perceptual factors in the pathogenesis of anomia. *Cortex, 2*, 90–95.

Brown, W. S., Lehman, D., & Marsh, J. T. (1980). Linguistic meaning-related differences in evoked potential topography: English, Swiss–German and Imagined. *Brain and Language, 11*, 340–353.

Brune, J. S. (1966). On cognitive growth, I, II. In J. S. Bruner, R. R. Oliver, & P. M. Greenfield (Eds.), *Studies in cognitive growth: A collaboration at the Center for Cognitive Studies*. New York: Wiley, pp. 1–67.

Bruner, J., & Goodnow, A. (1956). *A study of thinking*. New York: Wiley.

Caramazza, A., Berndt, R. S., & Brownell, H. H. (1982). The semantic deficit hypothesis of the naming deficit: Perceptual parsing and object classification by aphasic patients. *Brain and Language, 15*, 161–189.

Carpenter, M. B. (1976). *Human neuroanatomy*. Baltimore: Williams & Wilkins.

Coughlan, A. K., & Warrington, E. (1978). Word comprehension and word retrieval in patients with localized cerebral lesions. *Brain, 101*, 163–185.

Damasio, A. (1979). The frontal lobes. In K. M. Heilman & E. Valenstein (Eds.), *Clinical neuropsychology*. New York: Oxford University Press, pp. 360–412.

Damasio, A. R., McKee, J., & Damasio, H. (1979). Determinants of performance in color anomia. *Brain and Language, 7*, 74–85.

Dejerine, J. (1914). *Semiologie des Affections du Systeme Nerveux*. Paris: Mason.

Denny–Brown, D. (1958). The nature of apraxia. *Journal of Nervous and Mental Disorders, 126, 1*, 9–33.

Denny–Brown, D. (1963). The physiological bases of perception and speech. In H. Halpern (Ed.), *Problems of dynamic neurology*. Jerusalem: Jerusalem Post Press, pp. 1–33.

De Renzi, E., Pieczulo, A., & Vignolo, L. A. (1968). Ideational apraxia: A quantitative study. *Neuropsychologia, 6*, 41–52.

De Renzi, E., & Spinnler, H. (1966). Visual recognition in patients with unilateral cerebral disease. *Journal of Nervous and Mental Disorders, 142*, 513–525.

Faglioni, P., Spinnler, H., & Vignolo, L. A. (1969). Contrasting behavior of right and left hemisphere-damaged patients on a discriminative and a semantic task of auditory recognition. *Cortex, 5*, 366–389.

Fodor, J. A. (1983). *The modularity of mind*. Cambridge, MA: MIT Press.

Fodor, J. A. (1985). Precis of the modularity of mind. *Behavioral and Brain Sciences, 8*, 1–42.

Foerster, O. (1936). Symptomatologie des Erkankungen des Gehirns. Motorische Felder und Bahnen. Sensible corticale Felder. In O. Bumke & O. Foerster (Eds.), *Handbuch der Neurologie* (Vol. 6). Berlin: Springer.

Foix, C. (1916). Contribution à l'etude de l'apraxie ideomotrice. *Revue Neurologique, 1*, 285–298.

Foix, C. (1922). Sur une variete de troubles bilateraux de la sensibilité par lesion unilaterale du cerveau. *Revue Neurologique, 29*, 322–331.

Freud, S. (1891). *Zur Auffassung der Aphasien.* Leipzig, Germany: Deuticke.

Freund, C. S. (1889). Über optische Aphasie und Seelenblindheit. *Archiven für Psychiatrie und Nervenkrankheit, 20*, 276–297, 371–416.

Friedman, R. B., & Albert, M. L. (1985). Alexia. In K. M. Heilman & E. Valenstein (Eds.), *Clinical Neuropsychology.* New York: Oxford University Press, pp. 49–73.

Fulton, J. F. (1937). Forced grasping and groping in relation to the syndrome of the premotor area. *Archives of Neurology and Psychiatry, 31*, 27–42.

Gardner, H. (1973). The contribution of operativity of naming capacity in aphasic patients. *Neuropsychologia, 11*, 213–220.

Gerstmann, J. (1940). Syndrome of finger agnosia, disorientation for right and left, agraphia and acalculia. *Archives of Neurology and Psychiatry, 44*, 398–408.

Geschwind, N. (1965). Disonnexion syndromes in animals and man. *Brain, 237–294*, 585–644.

Geschwind. (1967). The varieties of naming errors. *Cortex, 3*, 97–112.

Geschwind, N., & Kaplan, E. (1962). A human cerebral deconnection syndrome. *Neurology, 12*, 675–685.

Goldberg, E. (1985). Amnesia, tardive dysmentia, and frontal lobe disorder in Schizophrenia. *Schizophrenia Bulletin, 11*, 255–263.

Goldberg, E. (1987). Varieties of motor perseveration: Comparison of two taxonomies. *Journal of Clinical and Experimental Neuropsychology*, 710–726.

Goldberg, E. (in press-a). Associative agnosia and the functions of the left hemisphere. *Journal of Clinical and Experimental Neuropsychology.*

Goldberg, E. (in press-b). The gradiental approach to neocortical functional organization. *Journal of Clinical and Experimental Neuropsychology.*

Goldberg, E., & Bilder, R. M. (1986). Neuropsychological perspectives: Retrograde amnesia and executive deficits. In L. Poon (Ed.), *The handbook of clinical memory assessment in older adults.* Washington, DC: American Psychiatric Association Press, pp. 55–68.

Goldberg, E., & Bilder, R. (1987). Frontal lobes and hierarchic organization of neurocognitive control. In E. Perecman (Ed.), *Frontal lobe revisited.* New York: JRBN Press, pp. 159–187.

Goldberg, E., & Costa, L. D. (1981). Hemisphere differences in the acquisition and use of descriptive systems. *Brain and Language, 14*, 144–173.

Goldberg, E., & Costa, L. D. (1986). Qualitative indices in neuropsychological assessment: An extension of Luria's approach to executive deficit following prefrontal lesions. In I. Grant, & K. M. Adams (Eds.), *Neuropsychological assessment of neuropsychological disorders.* New York: Oxford University Press, pp. 48–64.

Goldberg, E., & Tucker, D. (1979). Motor perseveration and long-term memory for visual forms. *Journal of Clinical Neuropsychology, 1*, 273–288.

Goldstein, K. (1916). Über korticale Sensibilitatsstorungen, *Neurol ogische ZbltCitung 19*, 825–827.

Goldstein, K. (1975). Functional disturbances in brain damage. In S. Arieti (Ed.), *American handbook of psychiatry*. New York: Basic Books.

Goodglass, H. (1980). Disorders of naming following brain injury. *American Scientist, 68,* 647–655.

Goodglass, H., Barton, M. J., & Kaplan, E. F. (1968). Sensory modality and object-naming in aphasia. *Journal of Speech and Hearing Research, 11,* 488–496.

Goodglass, H., & Geschwind, N. (1976). Language Disorders (Aphasia). In E. C. Carterette & M. Friedman (Eds.), *Handbook of perception*. New York: Academic Press.

Goodglass, H., Heyde, M. R., & Blumstein, S. (1969). Frequency, picturability, and the availability of nouns in aphasia. *Cortex, 5,* 104–119.

Goodglass, H., Klein, B., Carey, P., & Jones, K. (1966). Specific semantic word categories in aphasia. *Cortex, 2,* 74–89.

Grober, E., Perecman, E., Kellar, L., & Brown, J. (1980). Lexical knowledge in anterior and posterior aphasics. *Brain and Language, 10,* 318–330.

Hartline, H. K., & Ratcliff, F. (1946). Inhibitory interaction of receptory units of the eye of Limulus. *Journal of General Physiology, 121,* 400–417.

Head, H. (1926). *Aphasia and kindred disorders of speech* (2 vols.) London: Cambridge University Press.

Hecaen, H. (1967). Approche semiotique des troubles du geste. *Language, 5,* 67–83.

Hecaen, H. & Albert, M. L. (1978). *Human Neuropsychology*. New York: Wiley.

Hecaen, H., & Angelerques, R. (1963). La Cecité psychique. Paris: Masson.

Hecaen, H., Angelerques, R., & Houillier, S. (1961). Les varietés cliniques des acalcul-ies au cours des lesions retrorolandiques: Approche statistique du probleme. *Revue Neurologique, 105,* 85–103.

Hecaen, H., Goldblum, M. C., Masure, M. C., et al. (1974). Une nouvelle observation d'agnosie d'object. Deficit de l'association, ou de la categorisation, specifique de la modalité visuelle? *Neuropsychologia, 12,* 447–464.

Heilman, K. M., & Gonzales Rothi, L. O. (1985). Apraxia. *Clinical neuropsychology.* New York: Oxford University Press, pp. 131–149.

Henschen, S. E. (1925). Clinical and anatomical contributions on brain pathology. *Archives of Neurology and Psychiatry, 13,* 226–249.

Hermann, G., & Poetzl, O. (1926). *Über die Agraphie und ihre Localdiagnostischen Beziehungen*. Berlin: Krager.

Hoff, H., Gloning, J., & Gloning, K. (1954). Über Alexie .*Wiener Zeitschrift für Nervenheilkunde. 10,* 149–162.

Hoff, H., & Pötzl, O. (1935). Über ein neues parieto-occipitaler syndrom (Seelen-lahmung des Schauens Storung des korperschemas Wegfall de zentrlen Schens). *Journal für Psychiatrie und Neurologie, 52,* 173–218.

Hubel, D. H., & Wiesel, T. N. (1962). Receptive fields, binocular interaction and functional architecture in the cat's visual cortex. *Journal of Physiology, 160,* 106–154.

Hubel, D. H., & Wiesel, T. N. (1963). Shape and arrangement of columns in the cat's striate cortex. *Journal of Physiology, 165,* 559–568.

Jackson, J. H. (1931/1932). *Selected writings of Hughlings Jackson.* London: Hodder & Stoughton. 1931 (vol. 1), 1932 (vol. 2).

Jakobson, R. (1964). Toward a ainguistic typology of aphasic impairments. In A.U.S. de Reuck & M. O'Connor (Eds.), *Disorders of language.* London: Churchill, pp. 21–42.

Jakobson, R., & Halle, M. (1956). *Fundamentals of language.* The Hauge: Mouton.

Johns, D. F., & Darley, F. L. (1970). Phonetic variability in aphasia of speech. *JSHR, 13,* 556–583.

Kleist, K. *Gehirnpathologie.* (1934). Leipzig: Barth.

Kononova, E. P. (1940). Development of the frontal region in the postnatal period. *Trudi Instituta Mozga, 5,* (in Russian).

Kononova, E. P. (1948). Development of the human frontal lobes during the intrauterine period. *Trudi Instituta Mozga, 6* (in Russian).

Levin, H. S., & Spiers, P. A. (1985). The acalculias. In K. M. Heilman & E. Valenstein (Eds.), *Clinical neuropsychology.* New York: Oxford University Press, 112–114.

Lhermitte, F. (1986). Human autonomy and the frontal lobes, II: Patient behavior in complex and social situations. The "environmental dependency syndrome." *Annals of Neurology, 19,* 335–343.

Lhermitte, J., & de Ajuriaguerra, (1938). Asymbolie tactile et hallucinations du touches. *Etude anatomoclinique. Revue Neurologique,* 492–495.

Lhermitte, F., & Beauvois, M. F. (1973). A visual-speech disconnection syndrome: Report of a case with optic aphasia, agnostic alexia and colour agnosia. *Brain, 96,* 695–714.

Lhermitte, F., Chedru, F., & Chain, F. (1973). A propos d'un cas d'agnosie visuelle. *Revue Neurologique, 128,* 301–322.

Lhermitte, F., Pillon, B., & Serdaru, M. (1986). Human autonomy and the frontal lobes, I. Imitation and utilization behavior: A neuropsychological study of 75 patients. *Annals of Neurology, 19,* 326–334.

Liepmann, H. Apraxia, (1920). *Ergbn. des ges. Med. 1,* 516–543.

Liepmann, H. (1900). Das Kranskheitsbild der Apraxie. *Monatsschr. Psychiat. u. Neurol., 8.*

Liepmann, H. Drei (1908). Aufsatze aus dem Apraxiegebiet (Vol. 1). Berlin: Karger.

Lissauer, H. (1890). Einfall von Sedonblindheit nebst einen Beitrag zur Theorie der-selben. *Arch für Psychiat., 21,* 222–270.

Luria, A. R. (1965). Two kinds of motor perseverations in massive injury of the frontal lobes. *Brain, 88,* 180–192.

Luria, A. R. (1966). *The human brain and psychological processes.* New York: Harper & Row.

Luria, A. R. (1970). *Traumatic aphasia.* The Hague: Mouton.

Luria, A. R. (1974). *The working brain.* London: Penguin Press.

Luria, A. R. (1980). *Higher cortical functions in man* (2nd ed.). New York: Basic Books.

Luria, A. R., & Tsvetkova, L. S. (1968). The mechanisms of dynamic aphasia. *Foundations of Language, 4,*

Miceli, G., Mazzuchi, A., Mann, L., & Goodglass, H. (1983). Contrasting cases of Italian agrammatic aphasia without comprehension disorder. *Brain and Language, 19,* 65–97.

Miceli, G., Silver, M. C., Villa, G., & Caramazza, A. (1984). On the basis for the agrammatic's difficulty in producing main verbs. *Cortex, 20,* 207–220.

Miller, G. A., Galanter, E., & Pribram, K. H. (1960). *Plans and the structure of behavior.* New York: Holt.

Miller, G. A., & Johnson–Laird, P. N. (1976). *Language and perception.* Cambridge, MA: Belknap Press.

Mishkin, M. (1972). Cortical visual areas and their interaction. (1972). In A. G. Karczmar & J. C. Eccles (Eds.), *The brain and human behavior.* Berlin: Springer, pp. 187–208.

Morelaas, J. (1928). *Contribution à l'étude de l'apraxie.* These. Paris: A. Legrand (Ed.).

Mountcastle, V. B. (1961). Some functional properties of the somatic afferent system. In W. A. Rosenblith (Ed.), *Sensory communication.* Cambridge, MA: MIT Press, pp. 403–436.

Nielsen, J. M. (1937). Unilateral cerebral dominance as related to mind blindness: Minimal lesion capable of causing visual agnosia for objects. *Archives of Neurology and Psychiatry, 38,* 198–135.

Nielsen, J. M. (1946). *Agnosia, apraxia, aphasia: Their value in cerebral localization* (2nd ed.) p. New York: Hocber.

Nielsen, J., & Raney, R. (1938). Symptoms following surgical removal of major (left) angular gyrus. *Bulletin of the Los Angeles Neurological Societies, 3,* 42–46.

North, E. (1971). *Effects of stimulus redundancy on naming disorders in aphasia.* Doctoral dissertation, Boston University.

Polyakov, G. J. (1966). The structural organization of the cortical formation of the frontal lobes and their functional significance. In A. R. Luria & E. D. Homskaya (Eds.), *Frontal lobes and regulation of psychological processes.* Moscow University Press, pp. 38–60.

Pribram, K. H. (in press). The frontal cortex—A Luria/Pribram rapprochement. In E. Goldberg (Ed.), *Tribute to Alexandr Romanovich Luria.* Hillsdale, NJ: Lawrence Earlbaum Associates.

Purpura, D. P. (1970). Operations and processes in thalamic and synaptically related neural subsystems. In F. O. Schmitt (Ed.), *The neurosciences, second study program,* (Chapt. 42, pp. 458–470). New York: Rockefeller University Press.

Rubens, A. B., & Benson, D. F. (1971). Associative visual agnosia. *Archives of Neurology. 24,* 305–316.

Saffran, M. E., Schwartz, M. E., & Marin, O.S.M. (1980). The word order problem in agrammatism. *Brain and Language, 10,* 263–280.

Sittig, O. Über Apraxie eine Klinische Studie. (1931). *Arch. aus der Neur., Psychiat., Psych.* Berlin: Grenz, Karger, S. Verlag. 1–248.

Spinnler, H., & Vignolo, L. A. (1966). Impaired recognition of meaningful sounds in aphasia. *Cortex, 2,* 337–348.

Spreen, O., Benton, A. L., & Van Allen, M. W. (1966). Dissociation of visual and tactile naming in amnesic aphasia. *Neurology, 16,* 807–814.

Stuss, D. T., & Benson, D. F. (1984). Neuropsychological studies of the frontal lobes. *Psychological Bulletin, 95,* 3–28.

Teuber, H.–L. (1964). The riddle of frontal lobe function in man. In J. M. Warren & K. Akert (Eds.), *The frontal granular cortex and behavior.* New York: McGraw–Hill, pp. 410–444.

Trost, J. E., & Canter, G. J. (1974). Apraxia of speech in patients with Broca's aphasia: A study of phoneme production accuracy and error patterns. *Brain and Language, 1,* 63–79.

Vignolo, L. A. (1982). Auditory agnosia. *Philosophical Transactions of the Royal Society,* London, *B298,* 49–57.

Vygotsky, L. S. (1962). *Thought and language,* Cambridge, MA: MIT Press.

Warrington, E. K. (1975). The selective impairment of semantic memory. *Quarterly Journal of Experimental Psychology, 27,* 635–657.

Warrington, E. K. (1982). Neuropsychological studies of object recognition. *Philosophical Transactions of the Royal Society, London,* B298, 16–33.

Weigel–Grump, C., & Koenigsknecht, R. A. (1973). Tapping the lexical store of the adult aphasic: Analysis of the improvement mode in word retrieval skills. *Cortex, 9,* 410–417.

Wernicke, C. (1894). *Grundriss der Psychiatrie.* Psychophysiologische Einleitung.

Whitehouse, P., A. Caramazza, & Zurif E. B. (1978). Naming in aphasia: Interacting effects of form and functions. *Brain and Language, 6,* 63–74.

Yamadori, A., & Albert, M. L. (1973). Word category aphasia. *Cortex, 9,* 83–89.

Zangwill, O. L. (1960). La probleme de l'apraxie ideatorie. *Revue Neurologique, 102,* 595–603.

Zurif, E., A. Caramazza, Myerson, R., & Galvin, J. (1974). Semantic feature representation for normal and aphasic language. *Brain and Language, 1,* 167–187.

# Author Index

# Subject Index